Cell Biology Monographs
Continuation of Protoplasmatologia

Vol. 4

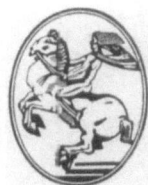

Springer-Verlag
Wien New York

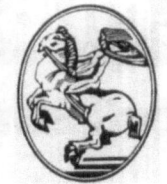

Mitochondria:
Structure, Biogenesis
and Transducing Functions

H. Tedeschi

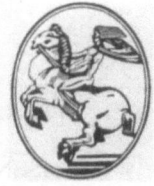

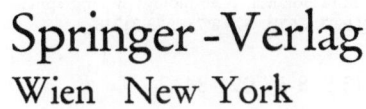

Springer-Verlag
Wien New York

Prof. HENRY TEDESCHI

Department of Biological Sciences
State University of New York at Albany
Albany, N.Y., U.S.A.

With 18 Figures

Library of Congress Cataloging in Publication Data. Tedeschi, Henry. Mitochondria. (Cell biology monographs;
v. 4.) Bibliography: p. 1. Mitochondria. I. Title. II. Series. QH603.M5T4. 574.8′734. 75-31718.

ISBN-13:978-3-7091-8414-1   e-ISBN-13:978-3-7091-8412-7
DOI: 10.1007/978-3-7091-8412-7

To Terry and the children,
Alexander, Devorah, and David,
who make life worthwhile

Preface

In the past few years, the body of experimental work on the structure, function and assembly processes of mitochondria has expanded rapidly. No one person can believe himself or herself completely in control of the burgeoning literature without possessing serious omissions or blind spots.

In the present monograph I have attempted a critical evaluation of the literature. I believe that the common thread of single authorship outweighs the shortcomings of one person presenting many disparate viewpoints. It is my hope that the end product represents a comprehensive and coordinated review of the subject matter to the present date.

Although the bulk of this monograph was completed by October 1974, I have made some attempts to update several of the sections at later times.

Albany, N.Y., November 1975   H. TEDESCHI

Contents

A. Structure of Mitochondria

1. General Organization

a) Conventional Thin Section Electron Microscopy

Transmission electron microscopy of thin sections has provided most of the basic information responsible for our present general concept of mitochondrial organization. Observations on material from a variety of sources have confirmed that the ground plan of mitochondria is generally the same from one type of cell to another (*e.g.*, see VOGELL 1963, STEINERT 1969). The view first proposed by PALADE (1953) and SJÖSTRAND (1953) seems correct, at least in general outline. In thin sections, mitochondria appear to be enclosed by two membranes. An outer membrane delineates the mitochondrial-cytoplasmic interface. The inner membrane enclosing the mitochondrial matrix forms infoldings (the cristae) projecting into the mitochondrial lumen. The cristae can be lamellar or tubular. The size of the space between the two membranes differs depending on the technique used. With freeze-substitution of fresh specimens, for example, the membranes appear closely apposed (MALHOTRA 1966). A close apposition of inner and outer membranes is also shown in freeze-cleavage under at least some conditions (*e.g.*, HACKENBROCK 1968, 1972) although the two membranes appear to separate in the condensed state. Generally, however (with negative staining or conventional fixation), a significant space is apparent between the two membranes. Several kinds of junctions between mitochondrial membranes have been reported (*e.g.*, NEWCOMB *et al.* 1968, HALL and CRANE 1970, TANI *et al.* 1971, BARTÓK *et al.* 1973, MORTON *et al.* 1973, SAITO *et al.* 1974). These structures can take the form of a dense midline in the intracristal space or, alternatively, of ladder-like connections spanning the space between membranes. Apparently, the appearance of these connections depends on physiological conditions (*e.g.*, hydration after a period of dehydration, BARTÓK *et al.* 1973). Although they may be virtually absent normally, in most mitochondria they appear after brief delays in fixation (SAITO *et al.* 1974). These results suggest that, in at least some cases, the junctions are not normally present but they do reflect a molecular organization of mitochondrial components. At least in special functional states this molecular organization becomes apparent at these special junctions.

The presence of connections between cristae or between the inner and outer membranes is perhaps related to the observations that in rat heart mitochondria, a pretreatment with trypsin is needed to separate the outer and inner membranes of isolated mitochondria (SCHOLTE 1973).

Although transmission electron microscopy has provided the general outline of mitochondrial structure, it has provided surprisingly little detail. The visible details of the membranes seem to depend drastically on the preparatory procedures (e.g., see LENARD and SINGER 1968, SJÖSTRAND and BARAJAS 1968, HARMON et al. 1974) and it is difficult to decide what is preparatory artifact. There is little agreement even about the thickness of the mitochondrial membranes. For example, after glutaraldehyde fixation the inner membrane is about 100 Å (HARMON et al. 1974). However, OsO_4 postfixation reduces the thickness to about 80 Å. Direct fixation with OsO_4 results in a thickness of about 75 Å; fixation in permanganate produces a thickness of 75–100 Å. A procedure using protein cross-linking with glutaraldehyde and special embedding procedures (SJÖSTRAND and BARAJAS 1968) produces a thickness of about 180 Å. In contrast, X-ray diffraction studies of centrifugally sedimented wet mitochondrial membranes suggest a thickness of 115–120 Å (THOMPSON et al. 1968). Since bilayers prepared from mitochondrial lipids are much thinner (maximally about 56 Å, GULIK-KRZYWICKI et al. 1967) these results suggest a considerable structural complexity. Lipids extracted from mitochondria can show a lamellar arrangement of 114 to 122 Å in thickness (GULIK-KRZYWICKI et al. 1967). This structure can be explained by a more complex model than a single lipid bilayer.

At high resolution, the mitochondrial membranes appear double as befits unit membranes. Accordingly, they could be interpreted to consist primarily of bimolecular lipid layers. However, the greater thickness already mentioned, the persistance of the double appearance after the extraction of virtually all the lipid (FLEISCHER et al. 1967), and the high proportion of protein in the membrane (e.g., see ROUSER et al. 1968) make this simple explanation unlikely. In thin sections no protein molecules are generally detectable [except perhaps for F_1; e.g., see TELFORD and RACKER (1973) and discussion below in section A 1 b] and it would seem reasonable to assume that most of the mitochondrial membrane proteins are embedded in the membranes. In fact, globular subunits are suggested by some electron microscope techniques (e.g., SJÖSTRAND and BARAJAS 1970). The serious protein denaturation accompanying conventional fixation (LENARD and SINGER 1968) and other artifacts (e.g., SJÖSTRAND and BARAJAS 1968) preclude a simple evaluation of this idea. In addition, the granulation is not detected with X-ray diffraction techniques on fresh specimens (THOMPSON et al. 1968) and it does not become apparent from electron microscopy after lipid extraction (FLEISCHER et al. 1967). As we shall see, however, electron microscope observations following freeze cleavage techniques are entirely in agreement with the concept that globular proteins are contained within a lipid framework. Nevertheless as much as 60 per cent of the proteins of the mitochondrial inner membrane can be stripped with 7 per cent acetic acid in agreement with the notion that about half the proteins are present in the water interface and not embedded in the lipid framework (FLEISCHER et al. 1972).

In recent years, the more common use of serial sections has allowed the recognition of a more complex mitochondrial arrangement. For example, in budding yeast, serial sections indicate the probable presence of a single giant branched mitochondrion (HOFFMAN and AVERS 1973). Each mitochondrion appears to be 30–60 µm in length and 0.2–0.6 µm in diameter. Other studies using serial sections with several yeast strains failed to confirm a single large mitochondrion, suggesting that this is not a general occurrence (GRIMES et al. 1974). During the growth phase of Euglena, mitochondria are very large and branched (OSAFUNE 1973). Observations with the light microscope also suggest that at least during growth periods, mitochondria of mammalian fibroblasts in culture may be unusually long (SCHNEDL 1974). The observations with human fibroblasts suggest interconnections between straight sections. The straight portions of the mitochondria appear as long as 100 µm.

Rat hepatocyte mitochondria appear as two distinct populations, either rod or V-shaped, in a two to one proportion (BERGER 1973). In addition, there is a size gradient depending on their position in the cell (LOUD 1968, BERGER 1973). Serial sections also reveal occasionally large and highly branched mitochondria (BRANDT et al. 1974).

In addition to the continued and more sophisticated use of thin section techniques in the past few years, new approaches have provided information on the organization of mitochondria. Two of these approaches, negative staining (Section b) and freeze-cleavage (Section c) will be examined in some detail.

b) Negative Staining Techniques

Studies of freshly isolated mitochondria using negative staining with ammonium molybdate provide some information on mitochondrial organization. The stain penetrates the space between the two mitochondrial membranes and the mitochondrial infoldings, suggesting that the space is substantial, at least in isolated preparations (MUSCATELLO et al. 1972). The negative staining methods (see HORNE 1965) used on large organelles such as mitochondria have not been sufficiently evaluated. Deformation of the specimen would take place particularly during drying and from local osmotic differences (see REIMER 1967).

In techniques where mitochondrial or submitochondrial preparations are surface spread (e.g., PARSONS 1963), the cristae have a tubular appearance. The inner membrane is studded with particles having a spherical head and a rod-like attachment to the membrane (the so-called lollipop arrangement). These structures are thought to correspond to F_1 (see Section C 2); whether they correspond to structures present in vivo has been debated. The particles may have been extruded from the membrane by the preparatory procedures. However, they do appear in some studies using conventional fixation and staining (e.g., GOMPEL 1964, ASHURST 1965, RUPEC 1969, HANZELY and SCHJEIDE 1971, TELFORD and RACKER 1973, ZAAK 1974) arguing that they may well be present in vivo. Their apparent absence in most preparations could be the result of their lability or lack of contrast (see TELFORD and RACKER 1973). Conversely, the notion that they may be normally embedded

1*

in the membrane fabric is supported by their visualization in thin sections only after phospholipase treatment (KRAUSE 1967). However, these particles have been observed in profile in freeze-fractured preparations (e.g., TEWARI e. al. 1971, 1972).

Surface spread mitochondria from *Tetrahymena* negatively stained with phosphotungstate or ammonium molybdate have tubular, detached cristae (KREBS et al. 1972). The walls of the tubules treated in this way have a mosaic appearance suggesting the presence of subunits inside the cristae. A similar arrangement is shown by procedures in which the membranes are spread out on the surface of a sucrose solution, after which they are fixed with glutaraldehyde, postfixed with osmium tetroxide and subsequently stained with uranyl acetate and lead citrate. These or similar procedures could offer alternatives to techniques more commonly in use.

c) Freeze-Cleavage

Freeze-cleavage (e.g., see BRANTON and DEAMER 1972, BULLIVANT 1973) is a technique particularly suited for the examination of membrane structure. In freeze-cleavage, tissues are frozen rapidly and then fractured by means of a prechilled blade. The fractured face is etched (i.e., sublimed) and then shadowed and replicated with platinum and carbon. The degree of etching can be varied depending on the structures to be exposed.

The procedure is illustrated in Fig. 1. The technique has proved valuable as an alternative to conventional electron microscopy, since it requires no fixation or staining. In addition, it has provided a view of membrane structure not previously available. The resolution of the technique has been estimated to be about 20 Å, presumably because of the limitations of the shadowing procedure. The technique of fracturing membranes on a glass surface has introduced the possibility of combining freeze-fracture to biochemical analytical techniques (PARK and PFEIFHOFER 1974).

The possible artifacts encountered by this technique are not entirely clear because the effects of the various procedures are not easy to evaluate. Gross disruptions or crystal formation can be detected by evaluation of the morphology seen with freeze-etching (BANK and MAZUR 1973, BANK 1974). Similarly, freeze-cleavage makes it possible to examine preparations which have been fixed with a conventional fixative and compare the morphology to that of unfixed preparations (e.g., MCINTYRE et al. 1973). The two approaches are not entirely satisfactory since the judgements are necessarily arbitrary. In addition, these approaches are most likely to detect only gross alterations; they are not likely to be helpful when the changes are subtle.

The effect of the cooling rate can be evaluated in a variety of ways after a freezing-warming cycle (see MAZUR 1970 for a review). The viability of the cells can be examined as an indicator of preservation (MOOR 1964, RAPATZ et al. 1966, SHERMAN and KIM 1964, SAKAI 1971, MAZUR and SCHMIDT 1968, BANK and MAZUR 1972, MAZUR et al. 1969, SHIMADA and ASAHINA 1972). Similarly, other criteria can be used as well. The lysis of cells such as red blood cells (MORRIS and FARRANT 1972) can be used as a criterion of breakdown. The activation of normally cryptic enzymes (e.g., because of a semi-permeable barrier) can be used as an index of disruption, as was done in the case of ATPase, for example (TAKEHARA and ROWE 1971). Similarly, selected enzymes (FISHBEIN and STOWELL 1969) can be examined for their inactivation as a function of cooling parameters. Alternatively, cells subjected to a freezing-thawing cycle can also be observed by conventional electron micro-

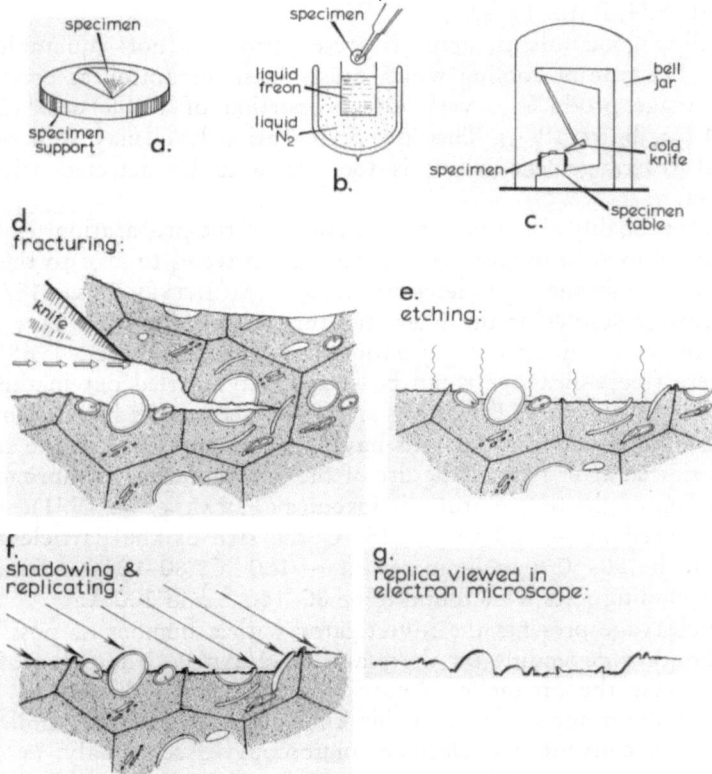

Fig. 1. Freeze etching. (*a*) placement of specimen on copper disc (*b*) rapid freezing of specimen (*c*) placement in precooled vacuum chamber (*d*) fracturing with cooled microtome knife (*e*) etching freshly fractured surface (*f*) shadowing and replication with platinum and carbon. After dissolving the specimen, viewing of the specimen with the electron microscope. (From BRANTON and DEAMER 1972, used by permission.)

scopic techniques (*e.g.*, SHERMAN 1972). The significance of the results of these studies in relation to freeze-cleavage is not clear. Presumably, damage detected by any one of these approaches has an ultrastructural correlate. A detectable damage in the assays should produce some morphological alteration. However, the thawing procedure can also produce damage, for example, by allowing a span of time for the action of disruptive hydrolytic enzymes (SOUZU 1973).

Using any one of these parameters it has become clear that the rate of cooling is an extremely significant factor. Using the viability of the cells as a criterion, the rate of cooling generally exhibits an optimum. Above or below the optimal rate the viability is decreased. As might be expected, the viability optimum varies depending on the nature of the cells used, the medium in which they are suspended, or the presence of protective agents (such as glycerol, PVP and dimethylsulfoxide) (*e.g.,* see MAZUR *et al.* 1969). The rate of cooling during the preparation of a specimen for freeze-cleavage is generally much greater than this optimum (*e.g.,* BANK and MAZUR 1973, GLOVER and GARVITCH 1974, BANK 1974).

Generally, good ultrastructural preservation is not equatable to cell survival. The rate of cooling which causes least disruption as observed with freeze-cleavage produces a very low proportion of viable cells (BANK and MAZUR 1973, BANK 1974). This low preservation level may well represent a structural rearrangement which is too subtle to be detected with present approaches.

Artifacts probably also occur at other stages of the preparation. In lymphoid cells, glycerol used to prevent crystal formation seems to lead to the aggregation of the membrane particles into clusters (MCINTYRE *et al.* 1973). Most freeze-cleavage studies of the finer structure of mitochondria have made use of glycerol to avoid crystal formation (*e.g.,* HACKENBROCK 1968). In the cases where freeze-cleavage could be successfully carried out in the presence and absence of glycerol (TEWARI *et al.* 1971), the results have been reported to be the same although the details have not been presented. The size of the particles viewed after freeze-fracture of the mitochondrial membrane seems to be a function of the temperature of fracture (TEWARI *et al.* 1971). In *Phycomyces* prepared at — 100 to — 115 °C the size of the particles has been reported to be 50–60 Å in diameter, at — 150 °C, 80–100 Å. In other cells the corresponding sizes were found to be 80–100 Å and 200 Å.

Freeze-cleavage presents the investigator with a number of possible views of mitochondria depending on the plane of cleavage. The plane of fracture may transverse the organelle. Apart from occasional differences in detail, the view of the mitochondrion in this kind of section is very similar to that obtained with conventional electron microscopy. Accordingly, external and internal membranes are visible in the usual pattern (MOOR and MÜHLETHALER 1963, BRANTON and MOOR 1964, BULLIVANT and AMES 1966, BAUER and TAMAKA 1968, HACKENBROCK 1968, KEYHANI *et al.* 1969, WRIGGLESWORTH *et al.* 1970, KEYHANI and KRIZ 1969, RUSKA and RUSKA 1969, VAIL and RILEY 1971, HACKENBROCK 1972, MELNICK and PACKER 1971, PACKER 1972, TEWARI *et al.* 1971, 1972).

The contracted state and the expanded state have been observed in response to metabolic condition (HACKENBROCK 1968, TEWARI *et al.* 1972, VAIL *et al.* 1972) or the osmotic pressure of the medium (WRIGGLESWORTH *et al.* 1970) as previously reported with conventional electron microscopy. In two studies fibers were reported in the matrix of mitochondria in the contracted state (HACKENBROCK 1968, WRIGGLESWORTH *et al.* 1970). However, in another study (TEWARI *et al.* 1972) they have been reported to be present in the matrix in the expanded state. In addition, fibers continuous with the external surface of the outer membrane have also been observed (see also Section A 2 b).

In the freeze-cleavage studies of various cells the plane of cleavage frequently exposes membranes. The evidence is consistent with the view that the preferential location of the plane of fracture is between two leaflets of the membranes at hydrophobic sites. This preferential fracture is probably the result of a weakening of hydrophobic bonds caused by the restrictions on the surrounding water imposed by the lowering of the temperature (FRANK and EVANS 1965, KAUZMANN 1959). This view is supported by studies carried

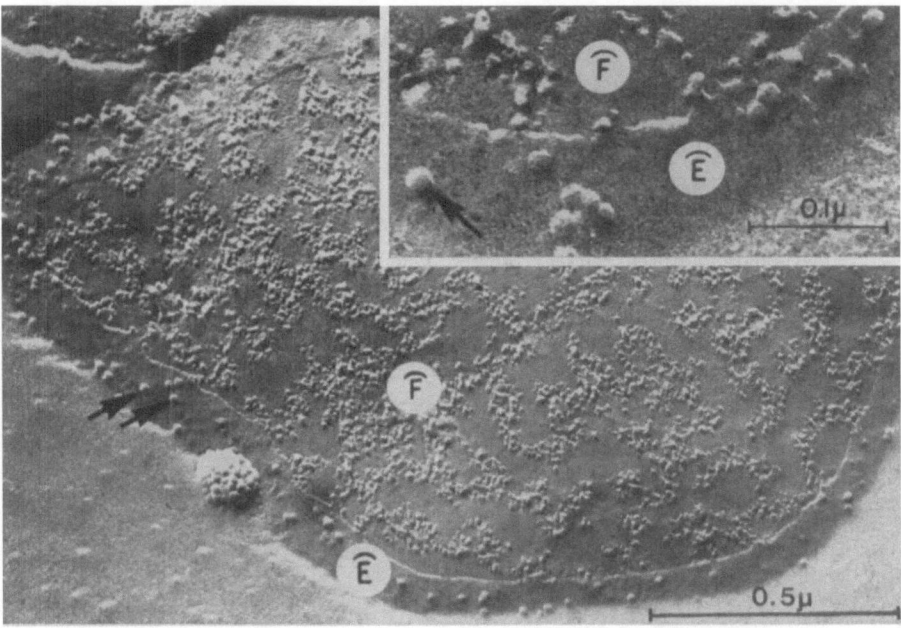

Fig. 2. Membrane faces of an etched, ferritin-conjugated blood cell ghost. Ferritin molecules (arrows) are associated with the etched faces (E) but are not visible on the fractured faces (F). (From PINTO DA SILVA and BRANTON 1970, used by permission.)

out with model systems and biological membranes. Data obtained after the fracture of stearate layers labelled with C^{14} are consistent with the view that the cleavage occurs predominantly in the plane of the hydrocarbon chains (DEAMER and BRANTON 1967). The presence of a ridge at the base of exposed membrane faces is consistent with the view that the fracture exposes the inner surface of a bileaflet membrane (BRANTON 1966, 1967, BRANTON and PARK 1967, MEYER and WINKELMANN 1967).

Several other experiments support this interpretation. When ferritin is conjugated to red blood cell ghosts (PINTO DA SILVA and BRANTON 1970), the ferritin molecules are visible on the surface which has been etched past the fracture point. They are not visible in the fractured face, which therefore represents a layer below the point marked by the ferritin. This is shown in Fig. 2. The ridge between these two surfaces supports this interpretation. A similar interpretation can be reached in studies in which the outer surface of the red blood cell was labelled with actin (Tillack and Marchesi 1970) and sea urchin egg nuclei were marked with ribosomes (Wartiovaara and Branton 1970).

The exposure of the inner surface of the membranes shows globular particles thought to represent protein molecules. This interpretation is supported by freeze-fracture studies carried out with liposomes (Vail et al. 1974). The liposomal fractured faces appear perfectly smooth unless the liposomes were formed in the presence of hydrophobic proteins. The interpretation of the

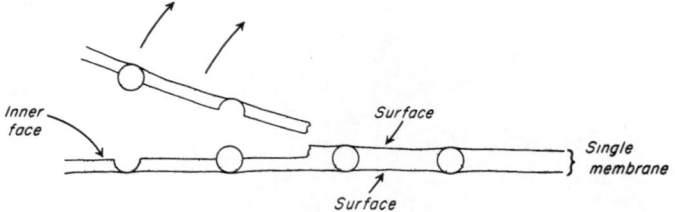

Fig. 3. Interpretation of the fracture process showing how the inner faces are exposed. (From Branton and Deamer 1972, used by permission.)

Table 1. *Characterization of Freeze-Fracture Faces of Mitochondria and Derived Inner and Outer Membrane Preparations* (from Melnick and Packer 1971)

	Density (particle/μm²)		Observed profiles (%)		
	Concave	Convex	Cross sections	Patchwork	Fracture faces
Mitochondria			21	15	64
Inner membrane	990	2290	7	4	89
Outer membrane	2120	578	3	2	95

fracture process just discussed and the exposure of the globular proteins is diagrammed in Fig. 3.

The fractures have revealed particles in mitochondrial membranes which sometimes appear in an hexagonal array (Ruska and Ruska 1969, Wriggles-worth et al. 1970, Hackenbrock 1972). The fractured faces and the globular particles can be assigned to inner or outer membranes. The hexagonal arrays apparently correspond to the outer membrane (Hackenbrock 1972, Packer 1972). The assignment can be made, for example, by actually isolating inner and outer membranes and then examining the preparations with the freeze-fracture technique (Melnick and Packer 1971). Alternatively, examination of the fracture faces permits making assignments when more than one plane of cleavage is visible (*e.g.,* see Hackenbrock 1972). The procedure can best be illustrated with an electron micrograph (Fig. 4). Since the membranes have a concave appearance they are viewed from the inside. The ladder effect of the fracture permits interpretation of the image. The part indicated by a single arrow corresponds to the outer membrane, that indicated by a double arrow to the inner membrane.

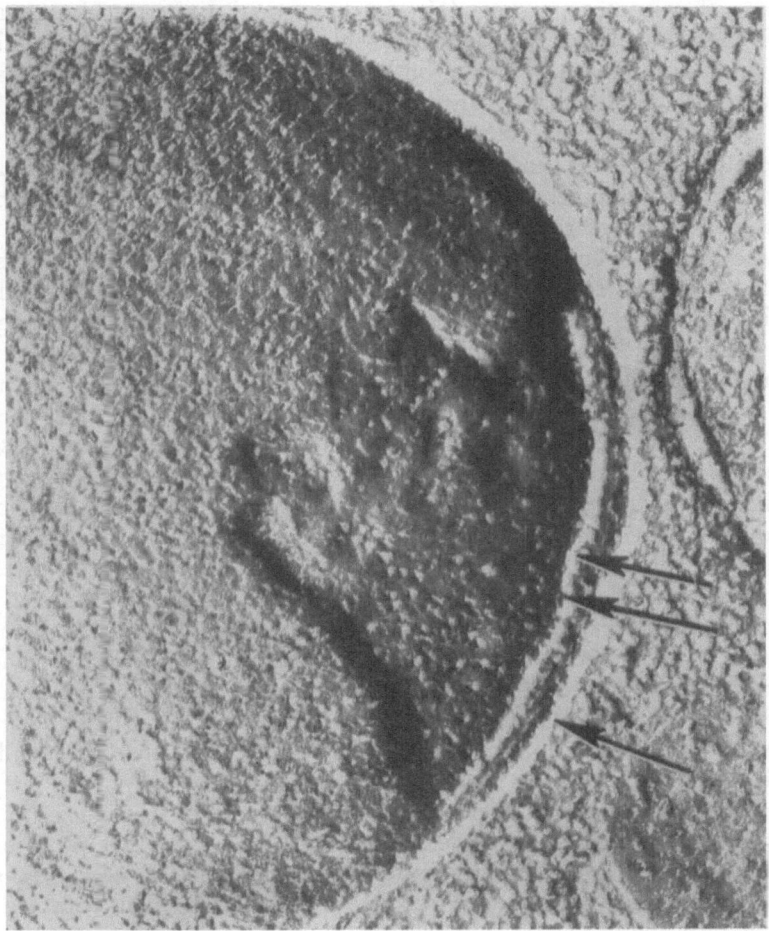

Fig. 4. Concave fracture faces of the outer (single arrow) and inner (double arrow) mitochondrial membranes. (From HACKENBROCK 1972 b, used by permission of the author and the New York Academy of Sciences.)

Studies carried out with freeze-fracture have permitted estimating the size and distribution of the particles enclosed by the mitochondrial membranes (HACKENBROCK 1972, 1973, PACKER 1972, 1973). In isolated membrane preparations (MELNICK and PACKER 1971) the particles remain attached predominantly to one of the two faces of either the outer or inner membrane (Table 1) (see also PACKER 1973). This suggests an asymmetry in the mitochondrial membranes also found in other membranes (BRANTON and DEAMER 1972). The particles appear to be more abundant in the inner membrane (MELNICK and PACKER 1971, TEWARI et al. 1971) and still more frequent in the cristae (TEWARI et al. 1971).

The particles appear clustered in the membrane (WRIGGLESWORTH et al. 1970, HACKENBROCK 1972, PACKER 1972). As already mentioned, in the outer membrane they appear arranged in an hexagonal pattern (HACKENBROCK 1972, PACKER 1972) and clusters are visible at least under some conditions. A redistribution of the particles in both inner and outer membranes has been reported to occur with changes in metabolic conditions (HACKENBROCK 1972, 1973). They appear more clustered in the energized state. Evaluation of these results is difficult since they have not been presented in detail, and in addition, their significance is not clear. Both inner and outer membranes are involved in these rearrangements, whereas presumably only the inner membrane should be concerned with the metabolic changes. Results presented by PACKER (1973) for the distribution of particles during metabolically induced oscillatory mitochondrial structural changes show no changes in the distribution in the inner membrane.

A comparison of the size of the particles in the inner and outer membrane reveals a difference between these two populations (HACKENBROCK 1972, 1973). The particles appear smaller in the outer membrane (major distribution peak approximately 80 Å) than in the inner membrane (major peak approximately 100 Å under non-energized conditions). The size distribution seems to vary depending on whether the mitochondria are in a non-energized (presence of antimycin) or energized (in the presence of succinate) state. The size of the particles of the outer membrane seems to increase upon energization. Similarly, the particles of the inner mitochondrial membrane shift from a major peak at 100 Å to distribution peaks in the range of approximately 110 to 125 Å. These results are difficult to evaluate in view of the possible artifacts in both size and distribution of the particles as already discussed. The energization procedure may indirectly alter the conditions in which the freezing and cleavage have been carried out.

The significance of the particles observed with freeze-cleavage is far from clear in terms of specific biochemical roles. In *petite* yeast lacking a number of components (*e.g.,* cytochrome oxidase, cytochromes b and c_1) freeze-cleavage reveals an appearance which is very similar to that obtained with wild-type mitochondria (PACKER *et al.* 1973).

2. Special Organization and Inclusions

Although the general structure of mitochondria is surprisingly similar in a variety of systems, a number of general variations in shape, size and internal organization have been noted in different cells. In particular, a number of variations have been noted in the general morphology of the cristae and a number of inclusions.

a) Prismatic or Atypical Cristae

The conventional lamellar or tubular arrangement of cristae is present in most mitochondria. In some tissues, although the conventional cristae are the most frequent, other arrangements are apparent in inclusions which are thought to correspond to mitochondria. In these inclusions, prismatic structures which are likely to correspond to cristae are present in regular hexagonal arrays. A sample of the literature on this type of structure is summarized in Table 2.

At this time, it is difficult to decide whether this arrangement corresponds to a preparatory artifact or to an organization present *in vivo*. The extreme regularity of these structures and, in at least some cases, their position in relation to matrix filaments suggest that they reflect a molecular regularity in the system, regardless of whether the structures are present in this form in the intact cell. The fact that similar results have been obtained with a variety of fixatives (*e.g.*, BLINZINGER *et al*. 1965) lends supports to this interpretation.

Table 2. *Atypical and Prismatic Cristae*

Tissue or cells	Configurations	Sample references
Cricothyroid muscle of bat	angular cristae, creases and prismatic cristae	a
Astrocytes of hamster	prismatic tubules in hexagonal arrangement	b, c, d
Lizard glia	hexagonal array, cross section does not appear triangular	e
Glia in pineal system of hamster		f
Vinegar eelworm	triangular cross section, doughnut-shaped 800 Å outer diameter encircled by opaque particles	g

a) REVEL *et al*. 1963. b) BLINZINGER *et al*. 1965. c) MORALES and DUNCAN 1971. d) DUNCAN and MORALES 1973. e) GRAY 1960. f) SHERIDAN and REITER 1970. g) ZUCKERMAN *et al*. 1973.

At this time it is difficult to decide whether all the structures discussed correspond truly to mitochondria. Granting a correspondence to mitochondria, the relationship between the prismatic structure on the one hand, and normal cristae or other mitochondrial inclusions which exhibit crystal-like regularity on the other, is still difficult to evaluate. Little can also be said about their possible functional significance. Future work may throw some light on these aspects.

b) Filaments and Tubules

There are many reports of filaments in mitochondria. Some of the filaments have been shown to be DNase sensitive. Presumably, they correspond to DNA and will be discussed later. Other filaments probably distinct from these also have been reported. Generally, they appear in crystalline-like complexes or inclusions (see Table 3). At times the inclusions are enclosed in a membrane visible with the electron microscope. Most commonly they are not. The filaments may be held together in a rhomboidal or thread-like structure with a regular spacing. The filaments may appear straight or have a helical or beaded appearance. Other filaments form tubules or microcylinders in the range of 270 to 350 Å in diameter (*e.g.*, LIN 1965,

KUROSOMI *et al.* 1966) although smaller tubules have also been reported (outer diameter 130 Å, inner 60 Å, KJAERHEIM 1967). In at least some cases the tubules have been shown to contain a central filament (LIN 1965, KUROSOMI *et al.* 1966). In some of these microtubules it has been possible to demonstrate six filaments per tubule (LIN 1965).

The nature of these inclusions and their possible interrelationship, if any, are still unknown. Their possible association with lipid disorders (ROUILLER and JÉZÉQUEL 1963, SVOBODA and MANNING 1964) suggest an involvement in lipid metabolism. The involvement of lipid in forming helical structures has been proposed (LUCY and GLAUERT 1964). Some of the tubular arrangements are very reminiscent of enzyme crystals such as uricase or catalase (*e.g.*, see VALENTINE and HORNE 1962, HRUBAN and SWIFT 1964).

Filaments have also been claimed to appear in mitochondria dried at the critical point (PIHL and BAHR 1970). The preservation is extremely poor and it is difficult to decide on the meaning of the results. Filaments are also visible in some plant mitochondria (CAILLOUX and GENEVÈS 1966) maintained in a humid atmosphere.

Microfilaments about 5 nm in diameter have been observed in yeast (MAY 1974 b) where they form bundles. Microtubules and inclusions resembling protein crystals have been also found in yeast (MAY 1974 a), Microfilaments have been seen in sub-mitochondrial membrane preparations (*e.g.*, STILES *et al.* 1968, KRAUSE 1968) and in studies carried out with freeze-fracture (Section A 1 c). The repeated observation of microfilaments suggests that the question of the presence of contractile proteins in mitochondria needs reexamination. OHNISHI and OHNISHI (1962 a, b) and NEIFAKH and KAZAKOVA (1963) reported finding an actomyosin-like protein in rat liver mitochondria. Unfortunately, these findings could not be confirmed (LEHNINGER *et al.* 1962, VIGNAIS *et al.* 1963, CONOVER and BÁRÁNY 1966, DARGEL 1967, BEMIS *et al.* 1968).

Various other cases of filamentous inclusions have been tabulated by SUZUKI and MOSTOFI (1967, their Table 1).

c) Amorphous Inclusions

Dense amorphous inclusions apparently not enclosed by membranes have been reported in various materials. Some examples have been collected in Table 4. Other specialized structures seem to occur which are not common to other tissues or organisms. For example, a hexagonal crystalline-like inclusion has been observed in the frog oocyte (WARD 1962) and in the mitochondria of *Hydra* (DAVIS 1967).

d) Intramitochondrial Granules

Apart from ribosomes, generally two types of granules have been observed. A small dense granule has been found in some tissues, for example, in liver cells. These granules are not intrinsically dense (ANDRÉ and MARINOZZI 1965), but depend on the deposition of fixatives such as Os for their density. The granules are removed by microincineration (THOMAS and GREENAWALT 1968), and when fixed with aldehydes they are solubilized by organic solvents

Table 3. *Mitochondrial Filaments and Tubules*

Thickness	Source	Arrangement	Sample references
80–100 Å	normal human liver	rhomboidal crystal-like structure (2000–3000 Å), strands 200 Å apart	a
65–75 Å	thyroid follicular cells, treated	105–115 Å peak to peak distance in crystal	b
60 Å	human liver	helical? in crystal body	c
30 Å	rat liver	helical, 120 Å pitch	d
30 Å	rat astrocytes	helices, 120 Å pitch, 140 Å diameter (possibly DNA)	o
40–80 Å	human reticulocyte cells	40–80 Å filaments	r
55 Å	thick limb of Henle, glycerol treated rats	sometimes 87 Å apart in bundles 280 Å in periodicity	e
55 Å	same as above treated with organic solvents	striated inclusion 350 Å periodicity	f
	low protein diet	helical or beaded in "crystal" arrangement	g
large tubules	yeast	50–60 Å filaments	s
Tubules 100 Å	adrenal cortex of rat	tubules: outer diameter, 130 Å and inner, 60 Å fiber; periodicity, 100 Å	h
		tubules 100 Å in diameter, wall 25 Å thick, tubules in groups of 15–40	i
Tubules 100 Å thick, wall 25 Å	hibernating snake renal tubules	bundles of tubules and dense globular substance (340 Å) with dense core: tubules in groups of 15–40	m
Tubules 270–330 Å	rat pinealocyte	270–330 Å, 6 filaments making up microtubule; central filament present	n
Tubules 240–260 Å	*Euglena*, growth phase		q
	silk worm thoracic gland	filaments in bundle	p
Tubules	yeast		t

a) WILLS 1965. b) FUJITA and MACHINO 1964. c) MUGNAINI 1964 a. d) BEHNKE 1965. e) SUZUKI and MOSTOFI 1967. f) WILLIAMS 1967. g) SVOBODA and HIGGINSON 1964. h) KJAERHEIM 1967. i) SAITO and FLEISCHER 1971. m) KUROSOMI *et al.* 1966. n) LIN 1965. o) MUGNAINI 1964 b. p) BEAULATION 1966. q) OSAFUNE 1973. r) ISHIHARA *et al.* 1973. s) MAY 1974 b. t) MAY 1974 a.

Table 4. *Amorphous Inclusions*

Material	References
Snake renal tubules	a
Testes	b, c, d
Adrenal cortex	e, f
Corpus luteum	g
Pathological human conditions	h, i, m
Hyperplastic mouse epididimis	n
Estrous uterine epithelium	n, o
Aged *Tetrahymena*	p
Liver and kidney in dietary deficiences	q

a) KUROSOMI *et al.* 1966. b) CERVOS-NAVARRO *et al.* 1964. c) CHRISTENSEN and FAWCETT 1961. d) YAMADA 1965. e) SHERIDAN and BELT 1964. f) WEBER *et al.* 1962. g) SATO and KUROSOMI 1965. h) LUFT *et al.* 1962. i) ROUIELLER and JÉZÉQUEL 1963. m) TANDLER and SHIPKEY 1964. n) FREI and SHELDON 1961. o) NILSSON 1958. p) ELLIOTT and BAK 1964. q) HARTROFT 1964.

(ASHWORTH *et al.* 1966). Another type of granule is intrinsically electron dense and may contain Ca^{2+} and Mg^{2+} (GREENAWALT *et al.* 1964, PEACHEY 1964, PORTER 1964, ZUDUNAISKY *et al.* 1968). Observations with the electron microscrope suggest that the transported divalent cations are deposited on preexisting granules (PEACHY 1964, PORTER 1964). The release of Ca^{2+} (or Mg^{2+}) from isolated mitochondria in response to the addition of 2,4 dinitrophenol does not correlate well with changes in the number of granules (PASQUALI-RONCHETTI *et al.* 1969), in agreement with this view. The granules that are soluble in organic solvents may be capable of binding divalent cations and hence, the two kinds of granules may represent two distinct physiological states rather than two distinct granules.

When the divalent cations are taken up by isolated mitochondria in the presence of phosphate, electron-dense areas appear as large granular deposits (*e.g.*, GREENAWALT and CARAFOLI 1966, VASINGTON and GREENAWALT 1968). The deposition is initially at the internal membrane of the cristae (GREENA-WALT *et al.* 1964, GREENAWALT and CARAFOLI 1966, VASINGTON and GREENA-WALT 1968) either in isolated mitochondria (GREENAWALT *et al.* 1964, GREENAWALT and CARAFOLI 1966) or water-extracted mitochondria (VASINGTON and GREENAWALT 1968). The number of eventual areas of deposition (*e.g.*, GREENAWALT and CARAFOLI 1966) clearly exceed that of the original granules. These results are not in agreement with the concept that deposition can only occur in pre-existing granules.

e) DNA Containing Fibers

Fibrous structures have been found within clear areas on the mitochondrial matrix. Under standard conditions of OsO_4 fixation, they appear as bars approximately 400 Å in diameter (NASS and NASS 1963 b). With uranyl acetate fixation fibrils can be seen which range in thickness between 15 and 40 Å. Generally these fibrils resemble the strands in *E. coli* attributed to DNA (NASS and NASS 1963 a).

The strands probably correspond to DNA since they are DNase sensitive but are unaffected by other hydrolytic treatments (NASS and NASS 1963 b). H³-thymidine incorporation, as seen with electron microscopy autoradiography, occurs in the clear areas suggesting that the incorporation does occur at the sites of these fibers (NASS and NASS 1963 b, MEEK and MOSES 1963).

The fibers appear in the mitochondria of several species and therefore probably are a general feature of mitochondria (NASS *et al.* 1965, SCHUSTER 1965). Mitochondrial DNA is discussed from the point of view of mitochondrial assembly in Section B 1.

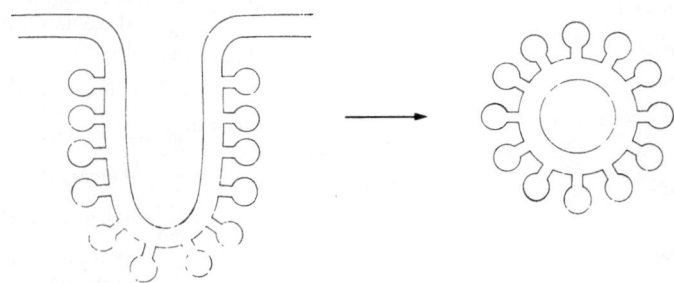

Fig. 5. Diagrammatic representation of the formation of inside-out submitochondrial particles (shown on the right) from the inner membrane of mitochondria (represented on the left). The lollipops represent the oligomycin sensitive ATPase molecules and are shown to illustrate the polarity of the particles.

3. Topography of the Mitochondrial Transducing Systems

There is general agreement about the distribution of functions in the various mitochondrial compartments (for reviews see ERNSTER and KUYLENSTIERNA 1970 and FESSENDEN-RADEN and RACKER 1971). The inner mitochondrial membrane functions in oxidative phosphorylation, permeability and active transport. In addition to the respiratory chain components, it is also the site of succinate dehydrogenase and β-hydroxybutyrate dehydrogenase. Except for the succinate and β-hydroxybutyrate dehydrogenases, the enzymes of the tricarboxylic acid cycle as well as those of fatty acid oxidation are probably in the matrix. The details are shown in Table 5.

The location of the various components of the respiratory chain in the inner mitochondrial membrane is still under study [see HARMON *et al.* (1974) for a review]. These experiments and others which will be discussed later (Section C 4) are facilitated by the availability of sub-mitochondrial particles which have reversed their sidedness (*i.e.*, their membranes are inside out) in relation to intact mitochondria. They have probably been formed by a pinching off process, illustrated in Fig. 5. It should be noted, however, that most submitochondrial particles are probably a mixture (CRANE *et al.* 1956

Table 5. *Localization of Enzymes in Mitochondrial Compartments*
(from ERNSTER and KUYLENSTIERNA 1970, used by permission)

Outer membrane	Intermembrane space	Inner membrane	Matrix
"Rotenone-insensitive" NADH-cytochrome c reductase (NADH-cytochrome b_5 reductase; cytochrome b_5)	Adenylate kinase Nucleoside diphosphokinase Nucleoside monophosphokinase	Respiratory chain (cytochromes b, c_1, c, a, a_3, succinate dehydrogenase; succinate-cytochrome c reductase; succinate oxidase; "rotenone-sensitive"	Malate dehydrogenase Isocitrate dehydrogenase (NADP-spec.) Isocitrate dehydrogenase (NAD-spec.)
Monoamine oxidase		NADH-cytochrome c reductase; NADH-oxidase; choline-cytochrome c reductase cytochrome c oxidase respiratory chain-linked phosphorylation)	Glutamate dehydrogenase
Kynurenine hydroxylase	Xylitol dehydrogenase (NADH-spec.)?		α-Ketoglutarate dehydrogenase (lipoyl dehydrogenase)
ATP-dependent fatty acyl-CoA synthetase			Citrate synthetase
Glycerolphosphate-acyl transferase		β-Hydroxybutyrate dehydrogenase	Aconitase
lysophosphatidate acyl transferase		Ferrochelatase	Fumarase
Lysolecithin-acyl transferase		δ-Aminolevulinic acid synthetase?	Pyruvate carboxylase
Cholinephosphotransferase		Carnitine palmityltransferase	Phosphopyruvate carboxylase
Phosphatidate phosphatase		Fatty acid oxidation system?	Aspartate aminotransferase
Phospholipase A_{11}		Fatty acid elongation system	Ornithine-carbamoyl transferase
Nucleoside diphosphokinase		Xylitol dehydrogenase (NADP-spec.)?	Fatty acyl-CoA synthetase (s)
Fatty-acid elongation system			Fatty acid oxidation systems? (β-hydroxybutyryl-CoA dehydrogenase)
Xylitol dehydrogenase (NAD-spec.)?			Xylitol dehydrogenase (NADP-spec.)?

and ASTLE and COOPER 1974). The sidedness of the particles can be evaluated by a number of criteria. The globular units which probably correspond to F_1 are located on the inner surface of the inner mitochondrial membrane and hence on the external surface of inverted particles. For these reasons their presence can be used as a morphological marker with negative staining of the preparations (*e.g.*, MALVIYA *et al.* 1968). Intact mitochondria and particles of equivalent sidedness can make use of endogenous cytochrome c, whereas inverted particles cannot (CRANE *et al.* 1956 and CHANCE and FUGMAN 1961).

Table 6. *Localization of Component in the Inner Mitochondrial Membrane*

Component	Localization	Evidence	References
Cytochrome c	outer surface	utilization of cytochrome c by deficient mitochondria	CRANE *et al.* 1956
		antibodies to cytochrome c	DI JESO *et al.* 1969
			SCHNEIDER and RACKER 1969
		diazobenzene sulfonic acid labelling	SCHNEIDER *et al.* 1972
		cytochemical staining with 3′,3-diaminobenzidine	ANDERSON *et al.* 1975
F_1	inner surface	antibodies to F_1, diazobenzene sulfonic acid labelling, and F_1 as a morphological marker	FESSENDEN-RADEN und RACKER 1966, CHRISTENSEN *et al.* 1969, TINBERG *et al.* 1974
		cytochemical determination of ATPase activity	OGAWA and MAYAHARA 1969
NADH dehydrogenase	inner surface	dependence of metabolism on NADH permeability	PURVIS *et al.* 1961, BIRT and BARTLEY 1960
		ferricyanide reduction	VON JAGOW and KLINGENBERG 1970
		diazobenzene sulfonic acid inhibition	TINBERG *et al.* 1974
	possibly across	diazobenzene sulfonic acid inhibition	TINBERG *et al.* 1974
Succinate dehydrogenase	inner surface	dependence of metabolism on succinate permeability	QUAGLIARIELLO and PALMIERI 1968
		antimycin sensitive ferricyanide reduction	KLINGENBERG and BUCHOLZ 1970
		diazobenzene sulfonic acid inhibition	TINBERG *et al.* 1974
Glycerol phosphate dehydrogenase	outer surface	ferricyanide reduction	KLINGENBERG and BUCHOLZ 1970
Cytochrome c_1	uncertain:		
	outer surface	antibody (possibly impure)	SCHNEIDER and RACKER 1971
	inner surface	ferricyanide reduction	see HARMONE *et al.* 1974
	inside membrane	ferricyanide reduction	KLINGENBERG 1972
Cytochrome b	inside membrane	ferricyanide lack of reactivity	GRINIUS *et al.* 1972 see also WIKSTRÖM 1973

Table 6 (*continued*)

Component	Localization	Evidence	References
Cytochrome c oxidase (cytochrome a-a$_3$)	across membrane	antibody	MOCHAN et al. 1970
		diazobenzene sulfonic acid labelling	SCHNEIDER et al. 1972
		polylysine crosslinking	SCHNEIDER et al. 1972
Cytochrome a	outer surface	inhibition of cytochrome oxidase by diazobenzene sulfonic acid	SCHNEIDER et al. 1972
Cytochrome a$_3$	inner surface	N$_3$— inhibition	PALMIERI and KLINGENBERG 1967 (see HARMON et al. 1974)

Various techniques have been devised to test the location of respiratory chain components in relation to the semipermeable membrane. These techniques involve the interaction of specific mitochondrial components with reagents to which the mitochondrial membrane is impermeable during short exposures. These chemicals should then interact predominantly with one kind of particle. For example, antibodies to cytochrome c interact only with the cytoplasmic side of the mitochondria and have little effect on the inverted particles (DI JESO et al. 1969, SCHNEIDER and RACKER 1971). Diazobenzenesulfonic acid reacts with mitochondrial cytochrome c but only slightly with cytochrome c of inverted particles (SCHNEIDER et al. 1972). Hence cytochrome c is probably normally located at the external surface of the mitochondrial inner membrane. Similarly, ferricyanide or ferrocyanide, acting as electron acceptor or donor, respectively, are capable of interacting with some of the mitochondrial components. Since they do not diffuse significantly through the mitochondrial membrane they can also be used to localize mitochondrial components. This reasoning and experimental approach have been used to localize various components in relation to the inner membrane. The results and the various techniques are displayed in Table 6.

More recent results with cytochrome oxidase suggest that all polypeptides are accessible externally except for the two larger polypeptides which may be buried in the cytochrome oxidase complex (EYTAN and SCHATZ 1975).

B. The Assembly of Mitochondria

Mitochondria are involved in their own assembly. Although a good deal is now known about this topic, many of the details are still unclear and in the process of being elucidated.

Conceivably, mitochondria could have a semi-autonomous or autonomous role in their own assembly by providing genetic information coding for their components and the machinery necessary for the transcription and translation of their macromolecules. Although there is no question that the mitochondrial contribution to their own organization is of fundamental significance, most presently available evidence suggests that the genetic and translational role is quantitatively rather small. Mitochondria-like structures can be synthesized by yeast lacking functional mitochondrial DNA or protein synthesizing capabilities (see LINNANE and HASLAM 1970, PERLMAN and MAHLER 1970). Although the inner membrane of these organelles is poorly developed, all tricarboxylic acid-cycle enzymes, and parts of the respiratory chain (e.g., succinic dehydrogenase and NADH dehydrogenase) are present along with DNA polymerase and the G and T factors of protein synthesis (SCRAGG 1971). Few polypeptides are coded in the mitochondrial DNA and synthesized in mitochondria. The assembly appears to be the result of a subtle interplay between the nuclear genes translated in the cytoplasm and the mitochondrial genes translated in the mitochondria. Mitochondria contain DNA, which is distinct from nuclear DNA, and the machinery capable of transcribing and translating the information contained in mitochondrial DNA into protein molecules (ASHWELL and WORK 1970, SCHATZ 1970, RABINOWITZ and SWIFT 1970, BORST and KROON 1969, MASON et al. 1972, TZAGOLOFF et al. 1973).

The section which follows (Section 1) will examine mitochondrial DNA and its genetic role. The discussion will then be followed by consideration of the transcription of this DNA (Section 2) and a presentation of the protein synthetic process in mitochondria (Section 3). The synthesis of lipids (Section 4), the assembly of mitochondria (Section 5), the interactions between the mitochondrial and the cytoplasmic synthetic systems (Section 6) and the nucleus (Section 7) are presented in separate sections.

1. Mitochondrial DNA and Its Genetic Role

The evidence that mitochondrial DNA has a genetic role is indirect, but nevertheless compelling. Mutations affecting the respiratory capacity of mitochondria have been known for many years. In a number of cases the transmission of these mutant genes is extrachromosomal [e.g., the petite mutants of yeast (EPHRUSSI et al. 1949 a, b, EPHRUSSI 1950, 1953, 1956) and the poky mutants of Neurospora (MITCHELL and MITCHELL 1952, MITCHELL et al. 1953)]. Similarly, a number of extrachromosomal mutants for resistance to antibiotics has been isolated. The genetics of mitochondria and chloroplasts has been reviewed recently by GILLHAM (1974).

There is considerable evidence that the extrachromosomal genetic markers involved in mitochondrial function are contained in the mitochondria themselves, since they can be transmitted by microinjections of mitochondria in Neurospora (DIACUMAKOS et al. 1965) or Paramecium (BEALE et al. 1972). At least in some cases of petite mutants (ϱ^-), the mitochondrial DNA is altered (MOUNOLOU et al. 1966, MELHOTRA and MAHLER 1968, CARNEVALI et al. 1969). In some of the ethidium bromide induced petites, the mitochondrial DNA is probably absent (MICHAELIS et al. 1971, NAGLEY and LINNANE 1972). A number of nonchromosomal mutants resistant to antibiotics has been isolated (see MAHLE 1973). The loss of mitochondrial DNA from the cells leads to the loss of respiratory functions and of antibiotic sensitivity or resistance (GINGOLD et al. 1969, COEN et al. 1970, BOLOTIN et al. 1971, NAGLEY and LINNANE 1972). Mutations for antibiotic resistance or respiratory deficiency are reflected in the DNA properties (MAHLER et al. 1971 a). For example, loss of all genetic markers generally produces either a grossly aberrant DNA, or the DNA is entirely missing. Loss of one marker alone (e.g., ϱ^-) among several present could lead to a DNA which is closer to wild type DNA in at least some of its properties (e.g., buoyant density). Similar correlations can be made from data obtained using hybridization techniques (GORDON and RABINOWITZ 1973).

The exposure to ethidium bromide (BOLOTIN et al. 1971, DEUTSCH and SLOMINSKI 1971, DEUTSCH et al. 1974) for varying periods of time leads to a differential loss of markers. Long exposures lead to the loss of all markers used. Shorter exposures produce petite cells with all or some of the antibiotic resistance markers missing.

The frequently of the loss of both the ϱ^- and drug resistance is higher than expected on the assumption that the two events are independent (e.g., DEUTSCH et al. 1974), suggesting that the markers are in the same structure, i.e., that they are linked. In hybrid cells derived from a human line and embryonic rat or mouse cells, mitochondrial DNA of the different species seems to be capable of recombination. The results suggest that the recombined components are held together covalently (DAWID et al. 1974). Evidence has been presented in Paramecium (ADOUTTE 1974) and yeast (CALLEN 1974 a, b) suggesting that extrachromosomally transmitted drug resistant markers can also recombine.

All these results support the notion that some relationship is likely to exist between at least some mutations affecting mitochondrial organization and mitochondrial DNA. The known genetic markers would seem to be arranged in the same DNA. In addition to the evidence supporting the concept that mitochondrial DNA performs a genetic function, other evidence points to a semi-conservative mechanism of mitochondrial DNA replication which is also in harmony with a genetic role. This evidence will be discussed below after a discussion of the properties of mitochondrial DNA.

The properties of mitochondrial DNA from various sources are summarized in Tables 7 and 8. Generally, in animals, the molecule is circular with a circumference of about 5 to 6 μm. In protists and plants it is much longer (15 to 30 μm) and generally, but not always, circular. The DNA circles are present with superhelical turns or super-twists (HELINSKI and CLEWELL 1971). The mitochondrial DNA of protists, such as Neurospora (LUCK and REICH 1964) and yeast (TEWARI et al. 1965, MOUSTACCHI and WILLIAMSON 1966, CORNEO et al. 1966) has a distinct base composition and can be separated from that of nuclear DNA by its lower density. The separation from nuclear DNA can be carried out by gradient centrifugation or elution from hydroxy-apatite (BERNARDI et al. 1972) or polylysine (BLAMIRE et al. 1972) columns. In metazoans the differences in base composition are not as marked. In these

Table 7. *Size and Structure of Animal mtDNAs*
(from BORST and FLAVELL 1972, used by permission)

Species	Structure	Size (μm)
Chordata		
Mammals	Circular	4.7–5.6
Birds	Circular	5.1–5.4
Amphibia	Circular	4.9–5.8
Fish	Circular	5.4
Echinodermata		
Echinoidea	Circular	4.6–4.9
Arthropoda		
House fly	Circular	5.2
Annelida		
Urechis caupo	Circular	5.9
Nematoda		
Ascaris lumbricoides	Circular	4.8
Platyhelminthes		
Hymenolepis diminuta	Circular	4.8

Table 8. *Size and Structure of mtDNAs from Protists and Plants*
(from BORST and FLAVELL 1972, used by permission)

Species	Structure	Size (μm)	References
Protozoa			
Tetrahymena pyriformis	Linear	15	a
Fungi			
Ascomycetes			
Saccharomyces	Circular	25	b
Neurospora crassa:			
strain 1118	Circular	20	c
strain 5256	Circular	19	d
strain 5297	Circular	0.5–19	d
strain Em 5256	Linear	26	e
Higher plants			
Pisum sativum	Circular	30	f

a) SUYAMA and MIURA (1968), SCHUTGENS (1971), FLAVELL and FOLLETT (1970), CHARRET (1970), ARNBERG *et al.* (1972). b) HOLLENBERG *et al.* (1970), BLAMIRE *et al.* (1972). c) CLAYTON and BRAMBL (1972). d) AGSTERIBBE *et al.* (1972). d) SCHÄFER *et al.* (1971). f) KOLODNER and TEWARI (1972).

cases, the presence of the DNA in the form of circular coils and twisted supercoils can be used to advantage. Dyes capable of extensive intercalation (for example, ethidium bromide) effect the buoyant density of circular DNA differently from that of linear DNA (HUDSON et al. 1969, BAUER and VINO-GRAD 1971). Consequently, the circular mitochondrial DNA can be separated readily from other kinds of DNA by centrifugation in CsCl-ethidium bromide gradients. The properties of mitochondrial DNA have been reviewed extensively (BORST and FLAVELL 1972, BORST 1972).

After denaturation, the mitochondrial DNA of all animals studied can be separated into two strands which differ in density (DAWID and WOLSTENHOLME 1967, BORST and RUTTENBERG 1969, BORST and AAIJ 1969, LEFFLER et al. 1970, MORA et al. 1970, NASS and BUCK 1970, SKINNER and KERR 1971, CORNEO et al. 1968 a, b, CLAYTON et al. 1970, MAIO 1971). The density difference between complementary strands ranges from 5 mg per cm³ in the sea urchin (DAWID and WOLSTENHOLME 1967) to 44 mg per cm³ in the chick (BORST and RUTTENBERG 1969). At least in HeLa cells, the difference has been shown to be the result of the difference in the thymine content of the two strands (ATTARDI et al. 1970). The two strands are generally described as the heavy or H strand and the light or L strand.

Studies carried out with ribonuclease H, extracted from chick embryos, suggest that the closed circular DNA contains ribonucleotides, about 10 per DNA duplex (GROSSMAN et al. 1973).

Some of the early studies on the replication of the mitochondrial DNA were difficult to interpret in terms of specific mechanisms, although they left no doubt that the mitochondrial DNA was conserved in some way (REICH and LUCK 1966, PARSON and RUSTAD 1968, BORST and KROON 1969). More recent works (GROSS and RABINOWITZ 1969, SENA 1971), however, confirm the notion long suspected that the replication is semi-conservative.

One of the studies (GROSS and RABINOWITZ 1969) uses tritiated 5-bromine-2′-deoxyuridine (BUDR), injected into rats to serve as both a radioactivity and a density tracer. BUDR substitutes for thymine deoxyribonucleoside. The newly synthesized DNA is heavier than the original DNA. The introduction of strand breakage and denaturation [necessary in mitochondrial DNA to avoid a "snapback" into the native configuration (DAWID and WOLSTENHOLME 1967)] allows the separation of the two strands. The difference in the density between the two separated strands is twice that between the labelled and unlabelled native DNA. Hence, the results are entirely consistent with a semi-conservative mechanism of DNA replication.

Electron microscope observations of spread mitochondrial DNA circles have shown two types of structures which may correspond to replicative intermediates. Both would be substantially in agreement with semi-conservative replication. A small number of branched circles (theta circles) have been found in rat liver mitochondrial DNA (KIRSCHNER et al. 1968). These circles contain two branches of equal length, ranging from 0.2 to 4.2 μm. All parts of the molecule appear double stranded. These configurations resemble those described by Cairns for the replicative E. coli chromosomes and accordingly

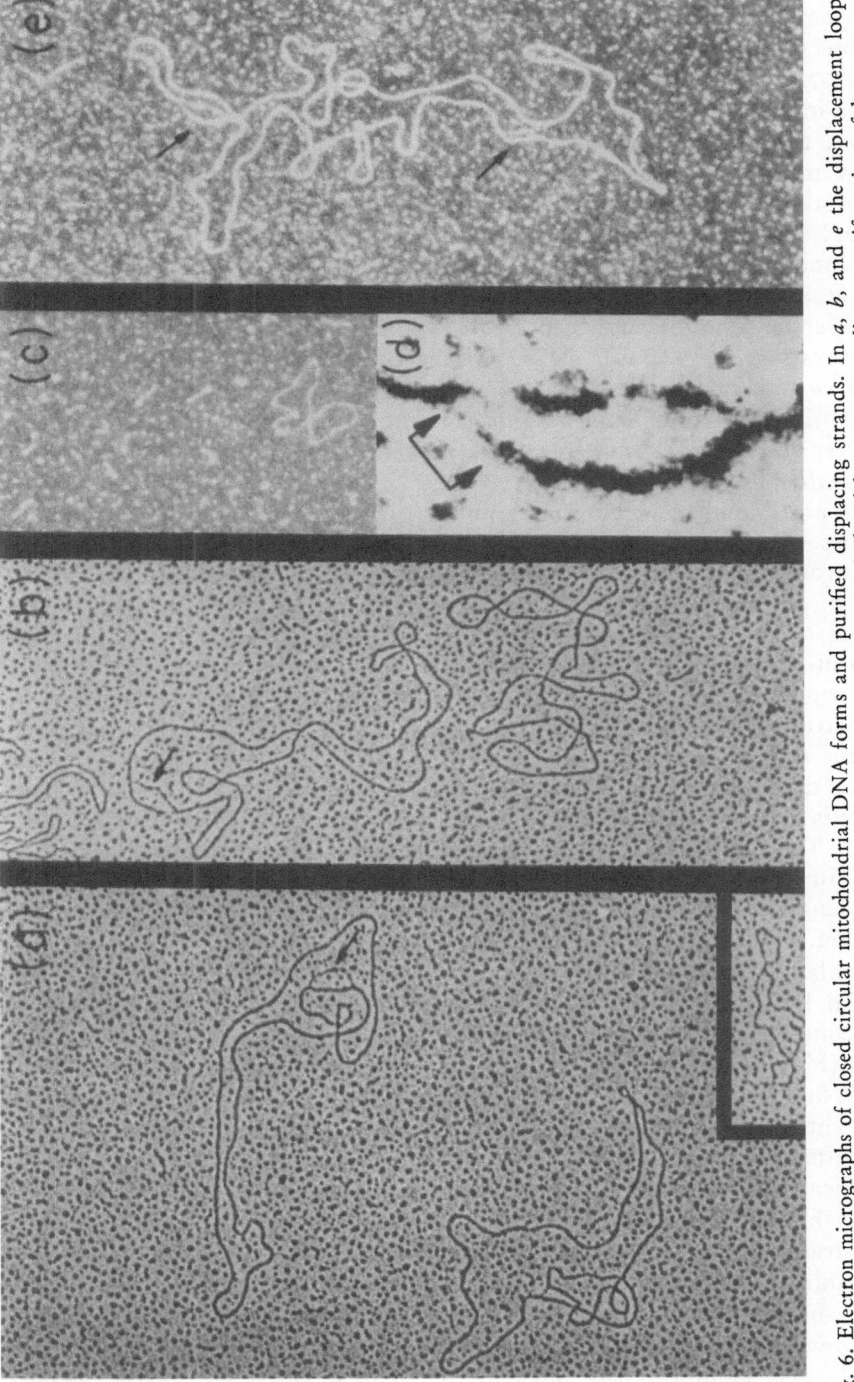

Fig. 6. Electron micrographs of closed circular mitochondrial DNA forms and purified displacing strands. In *a*, *b*, and *e* the displacement loops are shown by arrows. In *a* a single stranded ϕX DNA is present. *c* shows 7 S DNA isolated by sucrose gradient centrifugation of heat treated closed mitochondrial DNA. *d* shows an enlargement of a D-loop. The thin region between the arrows indicates single strandedness. *e* shows mitochondrial DNA from LD cells with two displacement loops. (From KASAMUTSU *et al.* 1971 b, used by permission.)

it would be tempting to consider them intermediates in mitochondrial DNA replication. Replication loops with two double stranded branches have also been observed in *Tetrahymena* in the presence or absence of ethidium bromide (UPHOLT and BORST 1974, ARNBERG *et al.* 1974, CLEGG *et al.* 1974). Ethidium bromide inhibits the synthesis of mitochondrial DNA. After 10 to 15 hours, however, the synthesis resumes partially. The molecules observed with the electron microscope appear linear with the presence of replication loops. Further studies with the linear DNA of *Tetrahymena* agree with the notion that DNA replication starts in the middle, or approximately the middle, of the molecule. It then proceeds in both directions (ARNBERG *et al.* 1974, CLEGG *et al.* 1974).

A different kind of branched circle has been studied in mouse L cells (KASAMATSU *et al.* 1971 a, b, 1973, ROBBERSON *et al.* 1972) and in the DNA formed by isolated mitochondria from chick liver (TER SCHEGGET and BORST 1971 a, b). These forms have also been found in mitochondria isolated from chick liver (ARNBERG *et al.* 1971), chick thyroid gland (PAOLETTI *et al.* 1972) and *Tetrahymena* (ARNBERG *et al.* 1972).

These possible intermediates account for a large proportion of the circular molecules. The structures appear as a closed circular duplex in which a short single strand (the E strand) is attached to the light mitochondrial strand, locally displacing the heavy DNA to form a strand loop (the D loop). The E strand (Fig. 6) is relatively short, from 0.015 to 0.02 μm in length. The configurations observed suggest a replicative cycle represented in Fig. 7. This scheme represents a semi-conservative replication. The D loops are shown in the electron micrographs in Fig. 6 (KASAMATSU *et al.* 1971 b). In this figure the displacement loops are marked by arrows. The E strand is shown in part c of the figure. Part e shows a double length circle (see below). Two arguments can be used to support this interpretation (KASAMATSU *et al.* 1971 b). The E strand only hybridizes to the light strand of the mitochondrial DNA. In addition, in a strain of mouse containing a high proportion of double length circles, some molecules have two D loops, one monomer length apart (Fig. 6 c) (KASAMATSU *et al.* 1971 b).

A similar pattern is revealed by electron microscope studies of other mitochondrial DNAs. In the DNA of *Xenopus laevis*, the D loop occupies 7⁰/o of the contour length, and 76⁰/o of the circles from mature oocytes show this pattern (HALLBERG 1974). In the DNA extracted from NOVIKOFF rat ascites cells (WOLSTENHOLME *et al.* 1973 a, b, KOIKE and WOLSTENHOLME 1974) the daughter segments found represent 2 to 44⁰/o of the total contour length. The results also indicate an additional mode of replication where both strands are replicated sequentially. The prevalence of segments of particular lengths suggests that the replication is halted at discreet points. Replication of both DNA strands has also been detected in the *in vitro* synthesis of DNA by mitochondria from newborn rats (KOIKE and KOBAYASHI 1973).

These findings suggest that in some systems the pattern shown in Fig. 7 is the prevalent mode of replication, whereas in other systems both strands are replicated simultaneously (*e.g.*, in the theta circles or in *Tetrahymena*). Still others exhibit a mixed pattern.

The semi-conservative model for the replication of mitochondrial DNA and more specifically, the model summarized in Fig. 7, are supported by experiments done *in vitro*. The selective inhibition of the replication of the H-strands by sibiromycin underscores the separateness of the replication of the two strands found in some systems (GAUSE and DOLGILEVISH 1975).

Isolated mitochondria are capable of incorporating deoxyribonucleotides and nucleosides into their DNA (BORST and KROON 1969, TER SCHEGGET and BORST 1971 a, b, KAROL and SIMPSON 1968, MITRA and BERNSTEIN 1970, RADSAK *et al*. 1971, KALF and FAUST 1969, TER SCHEGGET *et al*. 1971 a, b). For unknown reasons the incorporation represents only a synthesis of 0.5⁰/₀ of the DNA in these cases.

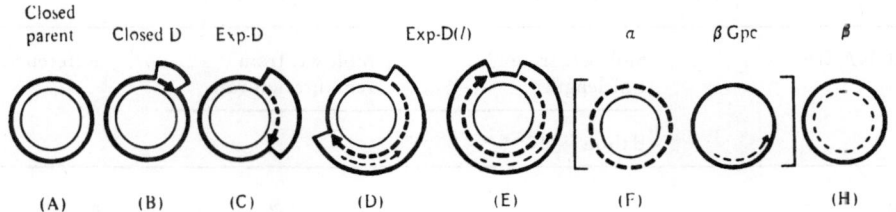

Fig. 7. Replication of mitochondrial DNA arranged in order of increasing degree of replication. Parental strands: solid lines; progeny strands: dashed lines; heavy strands: thick lines; light strands: thin lines. (From ROBBERSON *et al*. 1972, used by permission.)

Using bromo-dUTP as a labelled precursor, the *in vitro* synthesis was found to be conservative (KAROL and SIMPSON 1968). Since the size and characteristics of the hybrid fragments were unknown, the possibility remained that the incorporation could correspond to a repair process.

The fragments synthesized by isolated chick liver mitochondria could be separated from the supercoil by denaturation. It consisted of a short DNA fragment hydrogen bonded to the closed circular duplex (TER SCHEGGET and BORST 1971 a, b). The newly synthesized piece is a non-random segment of the heavy DNA strand (ARNBERG *et al*. 1971, TER SCHEGGET *et al*. 1971 b) in agreement with the idea that the strand corresponds to the E strand previously described.

The replicative pattern of DNA and the characteristics of the mutants discussed argue for a genetic role of the mitochondrial DNA. However, those studies do not throw light on the informational content of the DNA, *i.e.*, the number of messages that could be coded by the DNA. Hybridization kinetics help provide information on the upper limit of the number of messages that could be contained by the DNA. More direct evidence on the number of polypeptides likely to be synthesized by mitochondria and the probable number of mRNA molecules (see Section B 3) will be presented later and provide an independent estimate.

The informational content of the mitochondrial DNA can be estimated from their complexity using renaturation kinetics. Generally, the molecular weight calculated from renaturation kinetics is approximately the same as the molecular weight estimated from the length of the DNA. These findings indicate that a) all DNA molecules in the preparation are equivalent and b) there are no repeated sequences. The data has been collected in Table 9 (BORST and FLAVELL 1972). Not all the studies can be interpreted in a simple and straightforward manner. Some complications have emerged from studies carried out with *Neurospora* (WOOD and LUCK 1969) in some experiments with yeast (CHRISTIANSEN *et al.* 1971) and *Euglena* (TALEN *et al.* 1974). Generally, from these considerations the mitochondrial genome can be estimated to be small; in animal cells about 9.6×10^6 daltons or 15,600 nucleotide pairs. Since 2,500 of the nucleotides are probably

Table 9. *Genome Size of mtDNAs Calculated from Renaturation Rates*
(from P. BORST and FLAVELL 1972, used by permission)

mtDNA from	Mol. wt. from EM length	Mol. wt. from renaturation rate	References
	dalton $\times 10^{-6}$		
Rat	9.6	9.9	a
Guinea pig	11	11	a
Tetrahymena	29	30	b
Saccharomyces	49	63	c
		about 50	d
Pea	66	74	e

a) BORST (1971). b) FLAVELL and JONES (1970). c) HOLLENBERG *et al.* (1970) [corrected for low G. C. according to SEIDLER and MANDEL (1971)]. d) CHRISTIANSEN, C., personal communication to BORST and FLAVELL. e) KOLODNER and TEWARI (1972).

used to code for rRNA and 720 additional nucleotides for 4 S RNA (probably tRNA), the upper limit for the coding capacity of mRNA corresponds to approximately 12,000 nucleotides. However, after allowing for spacers (*i.e.*, DNA portions with regulative but no coding properties) and the sections complementary to the DNA coding for rRNA or tRNA, the portions which could contain the code for mRNA probably correspond to only 5,000 to 6,000 nucleotides (ALONI and ATTARDI 1971 a, c, 1972). Assuming a standard polypeptide of molecular weight of 20,000, this number of nucleotides would code for about 10 polypeptides, in good agreement with more direct estimates of the number of polypeptides synthesized in the mitochondria or of the number of possible mRNA molecules estimated by fractionating RNA containing poly-A (see Section B 3).

The good agreement between the possible number of messages estimated from the DNA complexity and the probable number of mitochondrial mRNA and mitochondrially synthesized polypeptides argues against a nuclear contribution of either mRNA or DNA originating from a nuclear DNA template. Other evidence also argues against a nuclear contribution.

In principle, the question of a nuclear origin of the mitochondrial DNA could be settled by hybridization of mitochondrial DNA to nuclear DNA.

Unfortunately, the experimental procedures are complicated by the fact that a single copy of the mitochondrial DNA would be infinitesimally small compared to the rest of the nuclear DNA (0.001% in a vertebrate). Consequently, even a slight contamination of the nuclear DNA with mitochondrial DNA would produce erroneous results. Early hybridization experiments in fact erroneously suggested a base sequence homology between mitochondrial and nuclear DNA (DU BUY and RILEY 1967, WINTERSBERGER and VIEHHAUSER 1968). These results are not in agreement with later studies. The DNA of mitochondria and that of the nucleus can also be compared by examining their ability to hybridize RNA. RNA from yeast mitochondria hybridizes with both mitochondrial and nuclear DNA. However, when purified by first hybridizing to mitochondrial DNA, the RNA is unable to combine with nuclear DNA (FUKUHARA 1970, COHEN et al. 1970). Experiments have also been carried out using highly labelled RNA produced in vitro by E. coli RNA polymerase and mitochondrial DNA as a template. The hybridization of the RNA with nuclear DNA in the presence of increasing amounts of mitochondrial DNA (TABAK 1972, MICHAELIS et al. 1972) suggests that few mitochondrial DNA copies, if any, are present in the nucleus. In view of the experiments using mitochondrial RNA, the experiments suggest that there are probably no copies of mitochondrial DNA in the nucleus.

Other studies are in agreement with this interpretation. In Xenopus crosses (X. mulleri × X. laevis) the inheritance of the mitochondrial DNA (which differs in the two species in base sequence) is maternal (DAWID and BLACKLER 1972). This finding is consistent with the view that the mitochondrial DNA is extrachromosomal in origin.

The alternative possibility that mRNA is of nuclear origin is also not likely. Mitochondrial protein synthesis ceases abruptly when yeast cells are treated with acridine dyes or ethidium, which attach selectively to mitochondrial DNA (e.g., see SCHATZ et al. 1972). Conversely, mitochondrial RNA continues to be formed in the presence of camptothecin, an inhibitor of nuclear RNA synthesis (BOSMANN 1970, PERLMAN et al 1973). Similarly, in temperature mutants of yeast, mitochondrial RNA and protein synthesis remain unaffected in the absence of nuclear transcription (MAHLER and DAWIDOWICZ 1973). The subsequent re-establishment of normal nuclear transcription at the permissive temperature does not sustain mitochondrial protein synthesis in the presence of ethidium (MAHLER and DAWIDOWICZ 1973). However, the ability of isolated mitochondria to translate added mRNA (e.g., DMITRIATIS and GEORGATSOS 1974) leaves open the possibility that a role may be played by the translation of nuclear mRNA by mitochondria in vivo under at least some circumstances.

The organization of mitochondrial DNA in petite, drug resistant or sensitive mutants has been very helpful in defining the genetic properties of mitochondrial DNA. In some cases the kinetics of the effects of ethidium bromide on cells has provided a good deal of information. Petite mutants of yeast are reduced in genetic complexity. In some mutants, the DNA may be reduced or even absent. However, in others, the amount of DNA is normal. Apparently, the DNA is reiterated to compensate for the loss of genetic markers (e.g., FUKUHARA et al. 1969, BERNARDI et al. 1970, HOLLENBERG et al. 1972, FAUMAN and RABINOWITZ 1972, MICHAELIS et al. 1972, GORDON and RABINOWITZ 1973, FAYE et al. 1973, MICHEL et al. 1974). Studies of the mutagenic effect of ethidium bromide reveal that various petite mutants eliminate or retain different parts of the genome (e.g., GINGOLD et al. 1969). After subcloning the yeast and stabilization of the clones, it becomes evident that the treatment has removed genetic information. The removal is inversely related to the amount of reiteration (NAGLEY et al. 1973). The results are consistent with the interpretation that the DNA replication is inhibited initially. This is then followed by a fragmentation of DNA, after which the remaining portion is reiterated (e.g., NAGLEY et al. 1973, BORST 1974).

Using tRNA hybridization (COHEN et al. 1972, COHEN and RABINOWITZ 1972, CASEY et al. 1974, GORDON et al. 1974, RABINOWITZ et al. 1974) it can be shown that in petite mutants some tRNA-genes may be retained (e.g., leucyl-tRNA) while others may be lost (e.g., valyl-tRNA). In mutants where the ability to hybridize a specific tRNA is retained, the level of hybridization is greater than in the wild type.

Similar results have been obtained with other markers, e.g., GC sequences (HOLLENBERG et al. 1972), AT sequences (SANDERS et al. 1973), ribosomal RNA cistrons (NAGLEY et al. 1974 a) and drug resistance markers (LAZOWSKA et al. 1974). Electron microscope observations of single stranded DNA in petite yeast show that in at least some mutants, portions of the DNA appear double stranded after denaturation, indicating that there are some reiterated segments which are inverted and adjacent to each other (LOCKER et al. 1974).

Selective reiteration characteristic of mitochondrial DNA mutagenesis suggests the possibility of purifying and amplifying specific mitochondrial genes by selecting the appropriate mitochondrial mutants as an experimental tool in elucidating the genetic properties of the mitochondrial DNA (see NAGLEY et al. 1974 b).

In summary, the results collected by a variety of approaches are consistent with the interpretation that the DNA of mitochondria contains information for ribosomal and tRNA. The messages in the mitochondrial DNA molecule are limited in number. Neither the DNA nor the mRNA of mitochondria is likely to be of nuclear origin. Replication of the mitochondrial DNA is by a semi-conservative, probably discontinuous, process. The replication in some cases involves a replication of predominantly one strand, followed by replication of the other strand. In other cases, both strands may be replicated simultaneously. Petite mutants frequently have a normal DNA content. However, this DNA has less information and is more reiterated.

2. Transcription of the Mitochondrial DNA

The synthesis of mitochondrial RNA has been reviewed recently (WINTERSBERGER 1972). Isolated mitochondria incorporate labelled RNA precursors into RNA (LUCK and REICH 1964, KALF 1964, WINTERSBERGER 1964, WINTERSBERGER and TUPPY 1965, NEUBERT and HELGE 1965, NEUBERT et al. 1966 a, NEUBERT and MORRIS 1966, SACCONE et al. 1967, 1969, KROON et al.

1967, SOUTH and MAHLER 1968, SUYAMA and EYER 1968, FUKAMACHI et al. 1972). When labelled RNA is synthesized using P^{32}-GTP as a precursor, digestion with diesterase and alkaline phosphatase liberates 250 nm absorbing material and P^{32} in parallel (WINTERSBERGER 1964). This indicates that the P^{32} is in internucleotide linkages.

The incorporation of precursors into RNA is not likely to be the result of a synthesis resulting from a contamination of the preparation. Mitochondria prepared from sterile animals and under sterile conditions exhibit RNA polymerase activity comparable to conventional preparations (KROON et al. 1967). Furthermore, as already mentioned, some of the mitochondrial RNAs correspond to molecules distinct from their cytoplasmic counterparts. Therefore, contamination of RNA synthesizing machinery from the nucleus is not likely. The RNA synthesizing system of intact mitochondria also exhibits characteristics which differ from nuclear RNA synthesis. For example, the incorporation of C^{14}-ATP into the RNA of intact mitochondria is inhibited by atractyloside which does not affect the nuclear incorporation (SACCONE et al. 1967). Presumably, atractyloside inhibits the entry of adenine nucleotides into mitochondria (e.g., HELDT et al. 1965). The RNA synthesized in vitro by rat liver mitochondria also hybridizes predominantly with one of the two mitochondrial DNA strands, in agreement with the notion that it is transcribed in the mitochondrion and that the process corresponds to that occurring in vivo (AAIJ et al. 1970) (see below).

The mitochondrial origin of several RNAs is supported by hybridization studies. Mitochondrial ribosomal RNA hybridizes only with mitochondrial DNA (SUYAMA 1967, WINTERSBERGER 1967, BORST and GRIVELL 1971, BORST 1972). This has become evident for Neurospora (KÜNTZEL 1971, SCHÄFER and KÜNTZEL 1972), yeast (REIJNDERS et al. 1972, AAIJ and BORST 1972, REIJNDERS and BORST 1972), Xenopus and HeLa cells (WU et al. 1972). At least some tRNAs (see later discussion and DAWID 1972 a, WU et al. 1972, NASS and BUCK 1970, COHEN and RABINOWITZ 1972, CASEY et al. 1972) and RNA containing poly-A segments, thought to correspond to mRNA (e.g., OJALA and ATTARDI 1974) hybridize to mitochondrial DNA.

A good deal is now known about the in vivo transcription of the mitochondrial DNA of HeLa cells (ATTARDI et al. 1970, ALONI and ATTARDI 1971 a, b, c, WU et al. 1972). The mitochondrial RNA labelled with uridine for a long period (48 hours) was hybridized to the separated H and L strands of the mitochondria. The long-labelled RNA hybridizes predominantly to the H strand. Data from rat liver (BORST and AAIJ 1969) and amphibian eggs (DAWID 1972 a) are in agreement with these findings. A maximum of 1.5% of the L strand binds to the RNA in contrast to the virtual 100% binding by the H strand. This complete hybridization was confirmed with both ultracentrifugation and electron microscopy (ALONI and ATTARDI 1972). Experiments carried out with a short pulse give significantly different results (ALONI and ATTARDI 1971 d) from those obtained with prolonged labelling. The level of hybridization to the L strand is sufficiently high to suggest that the two strands hybridize approximately to the same extent. These results suggest that the transcription is symmetric. This interpretation

is probably correct since the RNA self hybridizes to form a structure 60%
of which is RNase resistant and hence in a duplex configuration. With electron
microscopy, a large proportion of the RNA appears to be of the size of the
mitochondrial DNA or larger, suggesting a complete transcription of the
genome. A comparison of the results obtained with the long incubation to those obtained with the short pulses suggest that most of the
RNA which is transcribed is degraded or removed from the mitochondria.
Although after long incubation the bulk of the RNA is derived from tran-
scripts of the H strands some information is derived from the L strand as
well. The 4 S RNA of *Xenopus* hybridizes significantly to the L strand
(DAWID 1972 a) and in the rat, tyrosine and serine tRNA hybridize to the
L strand (NASS and BUCK 1970).

The properties of the RNA polymerases extracted from mitochondria have
been recently reviewed (SACCONE *et al.* 1974).

a) mRNA

There is a good deal of evidence for the synthesis of mRNA in mitochondria.
However, the presently available evidence is consistent with the concept that
it codes for very few messages. We have seen from hybridization kinetics
that the informational content of the DNA is small (see Section B 1).

Hybridization experiments using mRNA also support the notion that the
mitochondrial mRNA has a limited coding capacity (DAWID 1970, 1972 a).
In *Xenopus laevis* eggs, the mitochondrial DNA has a molecular weight of
about 11.7×10^6; 20% of the DNA is accounted for by its hybridization to
rRNA and tRNA. Only 16% of the DNA sequences hybridize to other mitochondrial RNAs and may correspond to mRNA. Similar conclusions have
been reached for yeast and other organisms such as fungi and protozoans
(*e.g.*, see KURIYAMA and LUCK 1973 a, BERNARDI *et al.* 1972, PIPERNO *et al.*
1972, ERLICH *et al.* 1972, SANDERS *et al.* 1973). Some of these organisms
have larger mitochondrial DNA molecules. However, the mRNA coding
capacity of the DNA could not be much greater since the rRNA, tRNA and
spacers account for a greater proportion of the genome.

Hybridization of the DNA from two different *Xenopus* species (*laevis*
and *mulleri*) also support the idea that the capacity of the mitochondrial
genome to produce mRNA is restricted to a few messages (see DAWID and
BLACKLER 1972). The two species can be crossed to produce sterile but
nevertheless viable progeny. The mitochondria of the two species have very
similar properties. Surprisingly, however, only 20% of the DNA hybridizes
to form closely matched heteroduplexes. This 20% corresponds to the
proportion of the DNA coding for rRNA and tRNA. 50% of the sequences
correspond to only slightly matched sequences arguing that most of the rest
of the DNA does not carry a genetic message. The alternative explanation
that the evolution is rapid and has altered the mitochondrial genetic messages
drastically is not convincing. Although it is clear that the mRNA could
only code for a few messages, there is a good deal of evidence that it is
synthesized by mitochondria and probably serves as a messenger for the
synthesis of polypeptides. In *Neurospora* an RNA fraction which differs

from rRNA or tRNA can be isolated from either whole mitochondria or poly-somes (SCHÄFER and KÜNTZEL 1972). This RNA hybridizes with 10⁰/o of the genome and it accounts for 5×10^6 daltons or about 7.5×10^4 nucleotide pairs. Similar evidence is available for *Saccharomyces cerevisiae* (REIJNDERS *et al.* 1972). In this latter study no significant evidence was found for the presence of RNA of nuclear origin. The presence of only a small number of genetic messages in mitochondrial DNA is supported by work in animal mito-chondria, in which eight distinct poly-A containing RNAs (presumed to cor-respond to mRNA) have been found in polysomal units (*e.g.*, HIRSCH *et al.* 1974, OJALA and ATTARDI 1974). These units, together with rRNA and tRNA hybridize to 70⁰/o of HeLa cell mitochondrial DNA (OJALA and ATTARDI 1974).

The synthesis of an RNA fraction likely to correspond to mRNA has also been demonstrated in HeLa cells in the presence of an inhibitor of nuclear RNA synthesis, camptothecin (PERLMAN *et al.* 1973, HIRSCH and PENMAN 1974 b). The mitochondrial RNA formed in the presence of this inhibitor was found to be entirely sensitive to ethidium bromide and hence, to correspond to an RNA synthesized by the mitochondrial system. A considerable portion of the heterogeneous RNA fraction contained a poly-(A) sequence about 50 to 70 nucleotides long, characteristic of eukaryotic mRNA. Studies carried out with temperature mutants of *S. cervisiae* lead to similar results. Yeast temperature mutants are unable to synthesize nuclear mRNA at 36°, although they can at a lower tem-perature. At 36°, mitochondrial RNA and protein synthesis is unaffected (MAHLER and DAWIDOWITZ 1973), and there are no alterations in mito-chondrial polysomal structure or polypeptide chain initiation or elongation. Ethidium bromide, on the other hand, blocks these functions in either the temperature sensitive strain at a permissive temperature (22°) or in the wild type at 36°. Interestingly enough, as already indicated, the results of this study indicate that a contribution of the nucleus to mitochondrial RNA is not likely. When the temperature sensitive cells were first exposed to elevated temperatures for 60 minutes in the presence or absence of ethidium bromide and then shifted to 22° in its presence, the nuclear DNA transcription and cytoplasmic protein synthesis resumed without a return of these mitochondrial activities. These experiments suggest a negligible contribution of mRNA from the nucleus.

The finding that poly (A) is associated with a mitochondrial RNA fraction suspected to be mRNA is of considerable interest. The poly-(A) segment in the mitochondrial mRNA is smaller than the poly (A) segment from cyto-plasmic mRNA (PERLMAN *et al.* 1973, HIRSCH and PENMAN 1973). It has been found in two mammalian systems (human and hamster) and in insects (*Drosophila* and mosquito) (HIRSCH *et al.* 1974), suggesting that the poly (A) segment may be characteristic of all mitochondrial mRNA. Results with yeast are somewhat contradictory. mRNA containing poly-(A) has been reported (COOPERS and AVERS 1974). However, this report conflicts with data obtained from another laboratory (GROOT *et al.* 1974). Mitochondrial systems capable of synthesizing poly-A have been studied (*e.g.*, JACOB *et al.*

1972, JACOB and SCHINDLER 1972, HIRSCH and PENMAN 1974 a). The poly-(A) segment is added post-transcriptionally in a process which is cordycepin sensitive. In contrast the nuclear system is not inhibited by this compound (HIRSCH and PENMAN 1974 a). When the poly-(A) RNA is labelled in the presence of camptothecin (which inhibits nuclear RNA synthesis), the poly-(A)-RNA is found to sediment with polysomes. This RNA is likely to correspond to functioning mRNA since the association with the heavier particles is disrupted by puromycin, which should terminate polypeptide synthesis, and the disruption is inhibited by chloramphenicol, which should block mitochondrial protein synthesis (HIRSCH and PENMAN 1974 b).

The lifetime of the poly-A-RNA was estimated to be about 1.5–2 hours in mitochondria in which new synthesis was blocked with actinomycin or cordycepin. The presence of a poly-(A) segment allows the isolation of mitochondrial mRNA with relative ease [e.g., in oligo-(T) cellulose column]. Acrylamide gel electrophoresis of this fraction resolved eight distinct mRNA species (HIRSCH and PENMAN 1973, HIRSCH et al. 1974, OJALA and ATTARDI 1974). This number corresponds, at least approximately, to the number of polypeptides found to be synthesized by the mitochondrial synthetic system.

Other evidence suggests the synthesis of mRNA. Pulse labelling with radioactive amino acids results in the labelling of particles sedimenting at a speed corresponding to ribosomal dimers and, to a lesser extent, larger aggregates (KÜNTZEL and NOLL 1967). In addition, actinomycin inhibits both the incorporation of radioactive amino acids into proteins (KROON 1963 b, KALF 1964, WINTERSBERGER 1965) and RNA synthesis (e.g., WINTERSBERGER 1966).

The concept that mitochondrial mRNA is produced by the transcription of mitochondrial DNA is supported by experiments carried out in vitro. Mitochondria incorporate H^3 ATP in the presence of UTP, CTP, and GTP (see WINTERSBERGER 1966). The accumulation of labelled RNA is blocked by actinomycin. After the introduction of the inhibitor, the radioactivity decays with a half life of about 15 minutes, in agreement with the concept that it corresponds to a labile RNA fraction.

b) The Machinery for Transcription and Translation

Most of the proteins needed for the transcriptional and translational machinery of mitochondria, probably as many as one hundred distinct proteins, are synthesized in the cytoplasm and are probably coded in the nucleus (e.g., GROSS et al. 1968, KÜNTZEL 1969, NEUPERT et al. 1969, LIZARDI and LUCK 1972, PARISI and CELLA 1971, SCRAGG et al. 1971, BARATH and KÜNTZEL 1972 a, b, GROOT 1974). On the other hand, RNA found in the mitochondria is distinct from cytoplasmic RNA and there is evidence that it is transcribed in the mitochondria.

The RNA present in intact mitochondria is RNase resistant (RIFKIN et al. 1967) and remains present despite extensive purification (WINTERSBERGER and TUPPY 1965).

The 4 S RNA of mitochondria appears to be tRNA since it accepts radioactive amino acids in the presence of the appropriate soluble system. This tRNA differs from cytoplasmic tRNA (BARNETT and BROWN 1967, BARNETT et al. 1967, BARNETT and EPLER 1966) and it binds polynucleotides with different specificities (EPLER and BARNETT 1967). In *Xenopus,* twenty five moles of tRNA are found per rRNA (BORST 1972, DAWID 1972 a). The mitochondrial tRNAs have a distinct base composition (DAWID and CHASE 1972) and they are specific for the corresponding mitochondrial aminoacyl synthetases. In *Neurospora,* at least 14 tRNAs distinct from those in the cytoplasm have been identified on the basis of their amino acid acceptance and synthetase specificity (EPLER 1969, EPLER et al. 1970). Similarly, eight have been found in yeast (CASEY et al. 1972) and five in liver (BUCK and NASS 1969). In *Tetrahymena,* at least several different mitochondrial tRNAs were found to code for the same amino acid and to correspond to different synonym codons. In *E. coli* this tRNA multiplicity has been implicated in the regulation of protein synthesis (NIRENBERG et al. 1966); perhaps the multiplicity of mitochondrial tRNAs has a similar functional significance.

The prokaryotic initiator molecule, fmet-tRNA is also characteristic of mitochondrial protein synthesis and it has been found in many species (RABINOWITZ and SWIFT 1970, ASHWELL and WORK 1970, HALBREICH and RABINOWITZ 1971, SMITH and MARCKER 1968, GALPER and DARNELL 1971, MAHLER et al. 1972, KÜNTZEL 1971). This kind of tRNA, together with the necessary transformylase (HALBREICH and RABINOWITZ 1971) is present only in the mitochondria and not in the cytoplasm.

The mitochondria from *Neurospora crassa* contain amino acyl synthetases for at least 15 different amino acids. At least four of these are specific for mitochondrial tRNA, exhibiting little activity with cytoplasmic tRNAs (BARNETT and EPLER 1966). Similar results have been obtained with liver mitochondria (BUCK and NASS 1960).

The recent literature on mitochondrial ribosomes and rRNA has been recently reviewed (BORST and GRIVELL 1971, BORST 1972, KROON et al. 1972). It is generally recognized that the mitochondrial ribosomes of fungi sediment at about 73 S and they dissociate into two 50 S and 38 S subunits (BORST and GRIVELL 1971, KÜNTZEL 1971, GRIVELL et al. 1971, SCHMITT 1970). Both ribosomal subunits are required for the synthesis of polyphenylalanine directed by poly (U) (GRIVELL et al. 1971). Recent studies with *Neurospora* indicate that the 73 S ribosomes are probably not the functioning ribosomes which probably sediment at 80 S. In contrast to the 80 S ribosomes, the 73 S ribosomes are not active in forming polysomes (AGSTERIBBE et al. 1974).

A complete characterization has been carried out for the ribosomes of the mitochondria of the yeast *Candida utilis* (VIGNAIS et al. 1972). These ribosomes are 72 S and dissociate at low Mg^{2+} into 50 S and 36 S subunits. The mitochondrial ribosomes can dimerize artifactually. The subribosomal units can be separated further in the presence of EDTA. 21 S and 16 S subunits are obtained which are apparently derived from the 50 S and 36 S subunits, respectively. Incorporation of C^{14}-leucine occurs in the 72 S particle and the incorporation is chloramphenicol sensitive and cycloheximide resistant. Puromycin releases the radioactivity suggesting an incorporation into a nascent polypeptide chain.

Ribosomes from animal mitochondria sediment at much lower values, in the neighborhood of 55 S (see BORST and GRIVELL 1971) and they dissociate into 40 S and 30 S subunits. The various reports are in approximate agreement with these values (see BORST 1972, AVADHANI and RUTMAN 1974, GRECO et al. 1973, 1974). The electron micrographs of mitochondrial ribosomes or their subunits from rat liver are very similar to those of bacterial ribosomes except that they appear smaller (ANDRÉ and MARINOZZI 1965). These mitochondrial ribosomes have a much lower buoyant density than either E. coli or cytoplasmic ribosomes, in part accounting for the low sedimentation coefficient (DE VRIES and KROON 1974). The lower density of these ribosomes may be the result of the lower RNA content (DE VRIES and KROON 1974, O'BRIEN et al. 1974). The migration of these ribosomes in a polyacrylamide gel suggests that the volume of the particles is smaller than the cytoplasmic particles and larger than the E. coli ribosomes (DE VRIES and KROON 1974). This conclusion is at variance with the electron microscopic observations. The ribosomes of the mitochondria of the locust (Locusta migratoria) have a sedimentation constant of 60 S with two unequal subunits (40 and 25 S). In contrast, the cytoplasmic ribosomes sediment with a constant of 80 S (KLEINOW 1974).

The sedimentation constant of the mitochondrial ribosomes is not invariably lower than that of the cytoplasmic ribosomes. In Tetrahymena, the mitochondrial ribosomes have approximately the same sedimentation coefficient (80 S) as the cytoplasmic ribosomes (CHI and SUYAMA 1970, CURGY et al. 1974). Both subunits of the Tetrahymena mitochondrial ribosomes sediment at the same rate (55 S) although they are distinguishable on a density gradient (CHI and SUYAMA 1970). Morphologically, the Tetrahymena mitochondrial ribosomes (STEVENS et al. 1974, CURGY et al. 1974) are distinct from either the cytoplasmic ribosomes of the same organism or the E. coli ribosomes; for example, they are larger and more elongated than their cytoplasmic counterparts (CURGY et al. 1974).

Mitochondrial ribosomes resemble bacterial ribosomes in many respects although there are a number of significant differences as well (see BORST 1972, p. 350). Mitochondrial rRNA differs from its cytoplasmic counterpart in base composition, nucleotide sequence, size and secondary structure (RIFKIN et al. 1967, KÜNTZEL and NOLL 1967, BORST and GRIVELL 1971, MITRA et al. 1972, EDELMAN et al. 1970, VERMA et al. 1971, DAWID and CHASE 1972). In addition, the mitochondrial rRNA has more species specific differences than cytoplasmic rRNA (BENDICH and McCARTHY 1970, SINCLAIR and BROWN 1971). At least in Neurospora, the mitochondrial and the cytoplasmic ribosomes are immunologically distinct, showing no cross reaction (HALLERMAYER and NEUPERT 1974 b).

Since the base sequence fingerprints of the small and large rRNA portions are not identical, they constitute two distinct species of RNA.

The lengths of the mitochondrial rRNA from several species have been directly estimated with the electron microscope. In Aspergillus nidulans they are 0.91 and 0.47 µm in length compared with 1.10 and 0.52 µm for cyto-plasmic rRNA (VERMA 1970). In HeLa cells they are both approximately 0.26 µm in length (WU *et al.* 1972, ROBBERSON *et al.* 1971). Molecular weights can be calculated from these measurements by assuming 2.45 Å between bases. The calculated molecular weights can then be compared to those obtained in other systems. Generally, animal mitochondrial rRNA is smaller than the corresponding RNA from fungi and protozoans (see Table 10).

Table 10. *Properties of rRNA's from Eukaryotic Cells*
(from MAHLER 1973, used by permission)

›ecies	Mitochondrial			Cell sap	
	Base composition ($\%$ G + C)	Molecular weight (daltons $\times 10^6$)	$S_{20,w}$ (S)	Base composition ($\%$ G + C)	$S_{20,w}$ (S)
spergillus	30.5, 31.5	1.30, 0.70	23.5, 15.5	51	26.5, 17.0
richoderma viride	31.5, 35.5		$\sim$ 22	50.0, 49.0	
eurospora	34.0, 36.5	1.28, 0.72	23, 16	49.5 $\pm$ 0.5	26, 17
east					
(Candida utilis)	33		21, 16	50	25, 17
(Saccharomyces)	25.0, 27.1	1.2, 0.6	21.5[1], 14.5	47.6, 45.2	26, 17
etrahymena pyriformis	27.9, 30.6	0.82, 0.52	21, 14	43.2, 49.2	26, 17
uglena gracilis	29.8		21.4, 15.9	55.7	24.4, 20.1
enopus laevis (eggs)	40, 43	0.53, 0.30	18.5, 13	63, 53	
Ian (HeLa)	45	0.56, 0.36	16, 12		28, 18
. coli[2]	54, 54	1.04, 0.56	24.0, 16.0		

Note: If more than one value is given, the first corresponds to the rRNA of the large, the second to that of the small ribosomal subunit. Sedimentation coefficients usually determined relative to those of *E. coli* taken as 23.0 and 16.0 S, respectively.

[1] Average of several different reports.
[2] And other bacteria, regardless of DNA base composition.

Hybridization studies allow one to estimate the proportion of the genome involved in the coding for rRNA, tRNA, and mRNA. Mitochondrial 4 S RNA and rRNA hybridize to mitochondrial DNA (see BORST and GRIVELL 1971). Some of these 4 S RNAs are tRNAs. Leucine, phenylalanine, tyrosine, and serine-tRNA have been found to hybridize to mitochondrial DNA in the rat (NASS and BUCK 1970) and leucine, valine, methionine, formylmethionine, glycine, and alanine-tRNA in yeast (CASEY *et al.* 1972, COHEN and RABINO-WITZ 1972).

The two rRNA components hybridize on one cistron each in *Xenopus* (DAWID 1972 a) and in HeLa cell DNA (ATTARDI *et al.* 1970, ALONI and

ATTARDI 1971 c). For 4 S RNA, 5 cistrons have been found for *Xenopus*, 11 for HeLa cells. In the case of animal cells, it has been possible to make an assignment as to the strand coding for the RNA (Wu *et al.* 1972, NASS and BUCK 1970). In HeLa cells it has actually been possible to map the DNA strands with the electron microscope. The gene location was recognized either by observing the presence of large RNA segments or by using RNA covalently bound to ferritin (Wu *et al.* 1972). This map is shown in Fig. 8. Starting at 12 o'clock in the H strand shown (Part A of Fig. 8) the 12 S segment corresponds to the light rRNA (about 1010 nucleotides); site H 2 cor-

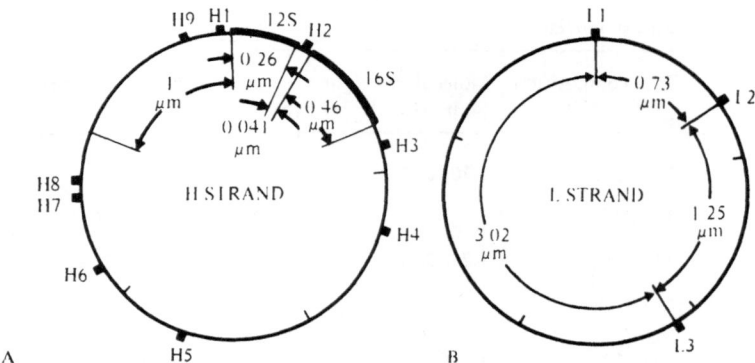

Fig. 8. Circular map of the positions of the complementary sequences for 4 S RNA's on the H and L strands. For the H strands the positions relative to the 12 S and 16 S rRNA shown as H 1 through H 9. The total circumference is 5 μm. (From Wu *et al.* 1972, used by permission.)

responds to 4 S RNA. The 16 S sector corresponds to the heavy rRNA (about 1570 nucleotides). Then, eight 4 S RNA sections follow (H 3-H 9 and H 1). The L strand has three 4 S sequences (Part B of Fig. 8). In rat liver (NASS and BUCK 1970) leucine tRNA and phenylalanine tRNA hybridize to the H strand, tyrosine tRNA and serine tRNA to the L strand. The RNA containing a poly-A sequence and which is thought to correspond to mRNA (HIRSCH *et al.* 1974, OJALA and ATTARDI 1974) has been calculated to account for a large portion of the HeLa cell DNA not already assigned to tRNA or rRNA (ALONI and ATTARDI 1971 a, b, ROBBERSON *et al.* 1971). All three kinds of RNA are thought to account for about 70% of the genome (*e.g.*, see OJALA and ATTARDI 1974). One of the poly-A RNAs found in HeLa cells hybridizes to the L stand, whereas the other seven hybridize to the H strand (OJALA and ATTARDI 1974).

c) Turnover of Mitochondrial RNA

Estimating the turnover of mitochondrial RNA presents a number of practical problems. For example, the inhibitors generally used may also alter the degradation rate (see ATTARDI *et al.* 1970). rRNA has been found to have a half life of about 3 hours, whereas tRNA has been found to be stable (ATTARDI and ATTARDI 1971, PENMAN et al. 1970, DUBIN et al. 1972, ZYLBER et al. 1971). The half life of mitochondrial mRNA has been estimated by following the decay of mitochondrial protein synthesis (i.e., the cycloheximide-resistant protein synthesis) after blocking the synthesis of mitochondrial RNA. The values obtained differ significantly in the various systems. In yeast (with ethidium or acriflavin) the half life is less than 10 minutes (SCHATZ et al. 1972). In HeLa cells (with ethidium or cordycepin) it appears to range from 1 to 3 hours (ZYLBER et al. 1971, LEDERMAN and ATTARDI 1970).

3. Protein Synthesis

The synthesis of mitochondrial proteins has been recently reviewed (e.g., KROON et al. 1972, SCHATZ and MASON 1974). Present evidence suggests that, at most, only a dozen hydrophobic polypeptides are synthesized in the mitochondria (e.g., see SCHATZ and MASON 1974). Three of these are associated with cytochrome oxidase, four with rutamycin (or oligomycin)-sensitive ATPase and one with cytochrome b. Probably some component or components of the adenine nucleotide translocator are also synthesized in the mitochondria (see HASLAM et al. 1974 a) (see Section B 3 b). The nature of the remaining polypeptides is still in question.

As already discussed mitochondrial RNA containing a poly-A sequence is thought to correspond to mRNA. Upon fractionation with acrylamide gel electrophoresis, eight distinct species can be recognized (HIRSCH et al. 1974, OJALA and ATTARDI 1974). This number corresponds at least approximately to the number of polypeptides which are thought to be synthesized in mitochondria.

In this section mitochondrial protein synthesis and its characteristics will be discussed first (Part B 3 a). This will be followed by an evaluation of the role of the mitochondrial protein synthesis in the assembly of the mitochondria (Part B 3 b) and a discussion of the synthesis of specific mitochondrial components (Part B 3 c).

a) Mitochondrial Protein Synthesis and Its Characteristics

There is little question that mitochondria from a variety of sources are capable of carrying out the synthesis of protein in vitro (e.g., see BEATTIE 1971, SCRAGG et al. 1971, NEUPERT and LUDWIG 1971). Some of the components of the mitochondrial system, such as the tRNA or the ribosomes, differ significantly from their cytoplasmic counterparts, as we already discussed. Therefore, the activity detected in isolated mitochondria is not likely to correspond to that of a contaminant. In addition, the mitochondrial system is not inhibited by RNase or cycloheximide which interferes with cytoplasmic protein synthesis. In contrast, it is inhibited by chloramphenicol, lincomycin, and erythromycin—antibiotics which do not affect cytoplasmic synthesis. Some of the differences and the pertinent references are summarized in Table 11. The difference in properties and the different sensitivity to antibiotics of mitochondrial RNA rule out a significant contamination from the cytoplasmic system. The sensitivity of mitochondria and mitochondrial ribo-

Table 11. *Differences of Mitochondrial Protein Synthesis in Relation to the Cytoplasmic Synthetic System*

Difference in properties	References
I. No need for soluble enzyme supplement	a, b
Not inhibited by RNase	c–i
II. Insensitivity to inhibition of cytoplasmic synthesis	j–m
Cycloheximide and emetine insensitivity	o–q
III. Sensitivity to inhibition not affecting cytoplasmic synthesis	
chloramphenicol	e, g, i, n, r
Macrolide antibiotics	j, m

a) KROON 1963 a. b) McLEAN et al. 1958. c) KALF and SIMPSON 1959. d) GREENGART and CAMPBELL 1959. e) KROON 1963. f) WINTERSBERGER 1965. g) MAGER 1960. h) ROODYN et al. 1961. i) KALF 1963. j) CLARK-WALKER and LINNANE 1966. m) LAMB et al. 1968. n) RENDI 1959. o) MAHLER et al. 1971 c. p) PERLMAN and PENMAN 1970. q) HERNANDEZ et al. 1972. r) CHAKVABARTI et al. 1972.

somes from yeast and rat liver to inhibitors of protein synthesis has been evaluated in a recent, thorough study (IBRAHIM et al. 1974).

Bacterial contamination is generally not likely to be a significant artifact. In at least some studies, the incorporation of radioactive amino acids by mitochondrial preparations from sterile animals is comparable to that obtained from conventionally prepared mitochondria (KROON et al. 1967). Nevertheless, unless otherwise demonstrated a contamination from bacterial components is always a disturbing possibility since the *in vitro* incorporation of amino acids into mitochondrial proteins is low (*e.g.*, BEATTIE et al. 1967 a), probably because the newly synthesized polypeptides are rapidly degraded (see WHEELDON et al. 1974).

Generally, the protein synthesizing system of mitochondria has many features in common with that of prokaryotes. In mitochondria, initiation of protein synthesis results in the incorporation of the formylmethionyl moiety in the N terminal position of nascent polypeptides. In at least some organisms the deformylase activity is sufficiently low to permit using the incorporation of the formyl moiety to distinguish mitochondrially synthesized proteins (POLZ and KREIL 1970, MAHLER et al. 1972, 1974, FELDMAN and MAHLER 1974).

The incorporation of formate into polypeptides and formylmethionyl puromycin has been used to determine the upper limit of the mitochondrial contribution to its protein components. Apparently, the overall level of synthesis is about 10% (2% under conditions of derepression) (MAHLER et al. 1972).

Labelled amino acids are incorporated into the interior of the polypeptide chain (KALF and SIMPSON 1959, ROODYN et al. 1961, SUTTIE 1962, KALF 1963, DAS et al. 1964, SINGH et al. 1964, WINTERSBERGER 1965) and the process is puromycin sensitive (SIMPSON 1962, WINTERSBERGER 1965, WHEELDON and LEHNINGER 1966). Some significantly distinctive features of mitochondrial protein synthesis have also emerged. The ribosomes of mitochondria seem to be closely associated with the mitochondrial membranes (*e.g.*, see VIGNAIS *et al.* 1972). This association, together with the finding that certain mitochondrial mutants exhibit antibiotic resistance *in vivo* but not *in vitro*, has prompted LINNANE and collaborators to propose a special ribosomal-membrane arrangement capable of imparting special characteristics to the mitochondrial ribosomes (see LINNANE and HASLAM 1970, C. H. MITCHELL *et al.* 1973, BUNN *et al.* 1970, DIXON *et al.* 1971). These special properties of the ribosomes may well be the result of the hydrophobic nature of the polypeptides produced (see OJALA and ATTARDI 1972, MICHEL and NEUPERT 1973) which may require incorporation into the membrane for continued synthesis. Whether this view is correct is still unresolved. Regardless of the eventual answer in their arrangement in relation to the membrane, the evidence at this time strongly suggests that the ribosomes are present in a conventional polysomal pattern, although some of the experimental results are contradictory. The question of whether polysomes are actually present is of some importance since the conventional synthesis of larger proteins would require relatively long mRNA molecules (and hence, polysomes). Conversely, the synthesis of small polypeptides, later assembled in larger molecules, would only require short mRNA fragments which may not need synthetic units larger than monosomes. *In situ* views in thin sections of the yeast *Candida utilis* shows alignments containing frequently six to eight ribosomes and occasionally up to ten or twelve ribosomes (VIGNAIS *et al.* 1972). Some of the views suggest attachment to a thread which could correspond to mRNA. The particles appear preferentially arranged on the inner mitochondrial membrane. Most of the mitochondrial RNA is present in structures larger than single ribosomes with discrete peaks ranging in size from two to six ribosomes in yeast (*e.g.*, MAHLER *et al.* 1972, MAHLER and DAWIDOWICZ 1973, COOPER and AVERS 1974), and in *Euglena gracilis* (AVADHANI *et al.* 1971, AVADHANI and BUETOW 1972 a, b) and from two to seven ribosomes in HeLa cells (OJALA and ATTARDI 1972). In yeast and in *Euglena* the polysomes are broken down to a single ribosomal peak by treatment with RNase, suggesting that the ribosomes are held together by an mRNA thread. However, the polysomal structures derived from *Neurospora* mitochondria are not dissociated by RNase (see MICHEL and NEUPERT 1973). The results with *Neurospora* suggest that these ribosomes are attached to structures other than RNA. This attachment could be the result of the hydrophobic interactions between nascent polypeptides. Mitochondrially synthesized polypeptides have been found to be very hydrophobic.

The polysomes are active in protein initiation and elongation since they can be labelled *in vivo* by a pulse of labelled leucine or formate (as mentioned, formate is involved in initiation). Since radioactive uracyl labels the polysomes either as a short pulse (suggesting incorporation in mRNA) or after 60 minutes incubation, the formation of the polysomes is likely to have involved mRNA. The results are similar in studies carried out with HeLa cells (OJALA and ATTARDI 1972) or *Euglena gracilis* (AVADHANI and BUETOW 1972 a).

Usually supernatant factors (for example, elongation factors) are similar or interchangeable with those of bacteria (*e.g.*, see KROON *et al.* 1972, KÜNTZEL 1971, RICHTER and LIPMANN 1970, RICHTER 1971).

As already mentioned, the initiation is distinct from that taking place in the cytoplasm. As in bacteria, it requires the involvement of fMet-tRNA$_F$Met by a transformylase. The initiation requires the interaction between ribosomal subunits, initiation factors and the fMet-tRNA (SALA and KÜNTZEL 1970).

The incorporation of lebelled amino acid occurs predominantly in the insoluble membrane protein fraction (ROODYN *et al.* 1961, ROODYN 1962, TRUMAN and KORNER 1962, WINTERSBERGER 1965), mostly in the fraction attributed to the inner mitochondrial membrane (NEUPERT *et al.* 1967, BEATTIE *et al.* 1967 b).

Mitochondria contain a number of glycoproteins (YAMASHINA *et al.* 1965, MARTIN and BOSMANN 1971, ITO *et al.* 1974 b). Most but not all of them seem to be associated with the external mitochondrial membrane and the intramembrane space (ITO *et al.* 1974 a). The function or site of origin of these proteins is not known. The enzyme mannosyltransferase has been found associated with the inner mitochondrial membrane (MORELIS *et al.* 1974), suggesting that at least some of the processing of the glycoproteins could be taking place in the mitochondria.

b) Role of Mitochondrial Protein Synthesis

It is now recognized that mitochondria are assembled by a complex inter-action between two protein synthesizing systems. On the one hand, some of the proteins are synthesized by the cytoplasmic synthetic system, most probably using mRNA coded by nuclear genes. On the other hand, some proteins are synthesized by the mitochondrial system, most probably using mRNA coded by mitochondrial genes. The two systems are intertwined in complex interactions to the extent that interference with either one of the synthetic systems affects the other.

The role of mitochondrial synthesis could be assessed by determining the ability of mitochondria to synthesize proteins *in vitro*. Unfortunately, the *in vitro* capacity to synthesize proteins is much more limited than the estimated *in vivo* synthesis (ASHWELL and WORK 1970). As mentioned, this low rate of synthesis imposes the need to avoid bacterial contamination. The removal of mitochondria from their normal cytoplasmic environment may also remove important regulatory and supportive effects. Despite these objections, the products formed *in vitro* are comparable in number and size distribution to those formed *in vivo* (COOTE and WORK 1971, LEDERMAN and ATTARDI 1973). Nevertheless, the low rate of synthesis makes it one of the least practical methods.

The *petite* mutants of yeast have been found to be incapable of mito-chondrial protein synthesis (SCHATZ and SALTZGABER 1969). Since *petite* mutants appear to possess mitochondria, albeit modified mitochondria (MAHLER *et al.* 1971 a), the role of cytoplasmic synthesis of the mitochondrial proteins could be examined by studying the proteins present in the organelles of *petite*.

Alternatively, antibiotics have been used to inhibit specifically protein synthesis either in mitochondria or in the cytoplasm. Chloramphenicol and erythromycin have been frequently used to inhibit mitochondrial protein synthesis (WINTERSBERGER 1965, LAMB et al. 1968). Cycloheximide, on the other hand, blocks cytoribosomal protein synthesis (So and DAVIE 1968, SISLER and SIEGEL 1967). These inhibitors have been found to act specifically on mitochondrial synthesis in yeast, but may not be specific or effective in other cells (see IBRAHIM et al. 1974).

These approaches have been summarized and examined critically by MAHLER et al. (1971 a, b, 1973) and SCHATZ and MASON (1974). A protein may be considered mitochondrial if the protein is absent in *petite* mutants and if its synthesis in wild type is blocked by inhibitors of mitochondrial protein synthesis but not by inhibitors of cytoplasmic protein synthesis. Hopefully, the protein is also synthesized *in vitro* by isolated mitochondria. The latter criterion only applies where the synthesis does not require some interaction with the cytoplasm. Conversely, a protein can be presumed to be of cytoplasmic origin if it is present in *petites,* if the mutations affecting the protein are transmitted by chromosomal genes and if the synthesis is blocked by inhibitors of cytoplasmic but not mitochondrial protein synthesis.

In vivo pulse labelling in the presence of an appropriate inhibitor followed by removal of the inhibitor has been found useful in pinpointing the site of synthesis of mitochondrial components. Presumably this procedure interferes minimally with the normal mitochondrial-cytoplasmic interactions.

There is little doubt that the mitochondria synthesize some of their own proteins which seem to be coded in mitochondrial DNA. However, quantitatively, this role is minor. By the appropriate use of inhibitors it has been estimated that between 85 to 95% of the total mitochondrial protein is made in the cytoplasm (HENSON et al. 1968, SCHWEYEN and KAUDEWITZ 1970, HAWLEY and GREENAWALT 1970, SCHATZ et al. 1972). This estimate is in good agreement with the 10% calculated as the upper limit of mitochondrial contribution from the incorporation of the formyl moiety (MAHLER et al. 1972, FELDMAN and MAHLER 1974). In fact, the major components of the mitochondrial matrix (ROODYN 1962), the outer membrane (NEUPERT et al. 1967, BEATTIE et al. 1967 b), the inner membrane (HENSON et al. 1968, SCHATZ et al. 1972) and the proteins constituting the transcriptional and translational machinery (SUBIK et al. 1970) are coded for in the nucleus and synthesized in the cytoplasm.

Chloramphenicol or erythromycin treated cells exhibit a deficiency in cytochromes a, a_3, b, and c_1, suggesting at least a partial mitochondrial involvement. On the other hand, the content of cytochrome c, fumarate or malate dehydrogenase, or other easily solubilized enzymes are not decreased by the treatment (CLARK-WALKER and LINNANE 1966, 1967, HUANG et al. 1966, WILKIE et al. 1967, EVANS and LLOYD 1967, KROON and JANSEN 1968, FIRKIN and LINNANE 1968). Yeast *petite* mutants also lack cytochromes a, a_3, b, and c_1 but contain cytochrome c, fumarase, aconitase, and easily solubilized enzymes (see SAGER 1972, p. 259—264 for review).

The *petite* mutants contain F_1 (ATPase) (KOVAČ and WEISSOVÁ 1966,

SCHATZ 1968). However, the system differs from the ATPase system of wild type since it is oligomycin insensitive. This probably indicates that some component of the normal ATPase system has been altered or is lacking.

As suggested by these results, in addition to the synthesis of proteins by mitochondria, mitochondrial proteins are also synthesized by the cytoplasm, suggesting that nuclear genes are also responsible for the coding of mitochondrial proteins. Many chromosomal mutants are known which produce respiratory deficiencies in yeast and *Neurospora* (*e.g.*, see CHEN et al. 1950, EPHRUSSI 1953, RAUT 1953, WAGNER and MITCHELL 1955, PITTMAN 1959, PITTMAN et al. 1960, SHERMAN and SLONIMSKI 1964). The genes coding for the structure of iso-1-cytochrome c (the major cytochrome c of wild-type yeast) are chromosomal (SHERMAN et al. 1965, 1966). Its synthesis has been shown to be governed by at least six distinct genes. Only one of these is the gene coding for the structure of the apoprotein (SHERMAN 1966). This suggests a complex pattern for either regulation or assembly. The synthesis of cytochrome c is cytoplasmic. When rats are injected with C^{14}-lysine, the microsomal cytochrome c was found to be labelled more rapidly than mitochondrial cytochrome c (*e.g.*, GONZÁLEZ-CADAVID and CAMPBELL 1967). Comparable results were obtained with ascites tumor cells (*e.g.*, FREEMAN 1967). These results are in harmony with the idea that cytochrome c is coded by a chromosomal gene and that it is synthesized in the cytoplasm. Apparently, the membrane bound polysomes of the cytoplasm are the ones primarily involved in this synthesis (GONZÁLEZ-CADAVID and DE CORDOVA 1974). These pulse label experiments do not completely exclude the possibility that a highly labelled contaminant is responsible for the radioactivity (*e.g.*, see DAVIDIAN and PENNIALL 1971, SCHATZ and MASON 1974). However, the chromosomal control of the cytochromes and the presence of cytochrome c in *petite* mutants independently confirm the cytoplasmic origin of this component. Other chromosomal mutations have been reported to affect enzymes of the inner membrane (SHERMAN and SLONIMSKI 1964, SUBIK et al. 1970, EBNER and MASON 1972).

Yeast cytochrome c_1 has been recently purified and found to have a molecular weight between 27,000 and 30,000 (ROSS et al. 1974). The synthesis of cytochrome c_1 has been studied in cells labelled with H^3-leucine in the presence or absence of acriflavin (an inhibitor of mitochondrial protein synthesis) (GROOT et al. 1972), or cycloheximide (which blocks cytoplasmic synthesis) (ROSS et al. 1974). Cycloheximide completely blocks the synthesis whereas acriflavin does not. The site of synthesis was accordingly interpreted to be in the cytoplasm. However, the formation of the holocytochrome requires the synthesis of some mitochondrial component (CLARK-WALKER and LINNANE 1967) suggesting that a mitochondrially synthesized component is necessary for the assembly of a functional cytochrome. This polypeptide could perhaps be a component of cytochrome b, since the latter is synthesized in mitochondria (*e.g.*, WEISS et al. 1972).

Mitochondria isolated from chloramphenicol, lincomycin, or erythromycin-treated or anaerobically grown yeast are still capable of incorporating C^{14}-leucine. This suggests that proteins involved in the translational process in mitochondria have originated in the cytoplasm (DAVEY et al. 1969) as in fact shown for the ribosomal proteins of Neurospora crassa (LIZARDI and LUCK 1972).

Cytoplasmic ribosomes have been observed in close apposition to the mitochondrial outer membrane in S. cerevisae (WATSON 1972, KELLEMS et al. 1974 a, b), the yeast Rhodoturula rubra (KEYHANI 1973) and in Dicto-stylium cerevisiae (COTTER et al. 1969). In S. cerevisae, these ribosomes apparently correspond to the 80 S ribosomes which remain attached to the mitochondrial membranes during the isolation of the mitochondria (KELLEMS and BUTOW 1972). The attachment is not an artifact since an isolation medium which blocks the attachment of ribosomes to mitochondria does not change the proportion of ribosomes found attached to the isolated mito-chondria (KELLEMS and BUTOW 1974). The number of ribosomes on the mitochondria varies with the physiological condition (KELLEMS and BUTOW 1974). The cytoplasmic ribosomes attached to the mitochondria synthesize mitochondrial proteins and in vitro a large portion of these are released to the mitochondria (KELLEMS et al. 1974 a, b). The synthesis is likely to be a vectorial process very similar to that observed in the rough endoplasmic reticulum (e.g., REDMAN 1967).

GAITSKHOKI et al. (1974) attempted to distinguish the polysomes engaged in the synthesis of mitochondrial proteins in rat liver homogenates using I^{125} labelled antibodies to mitochondrial antigens. The antibodies were found to bind to cytoplasmic ribosomes present in the post-mitochondrial fraction as well as to polysomes extracted from mitochondria. However, they were not found to bind to polysomes attached to the membranes of the post-mito-chondrial fraction.

c) Synthesis of Specific Proteins by Mitochondria

As already discussed, the role of mitochondrial translations is quantitatively minor. Nevertheless, it is qualitatively significant; the mitochondrial electron transport and phosphorylative system cannot function in the absence of proteins synthesized by the mitochondria (for reviews see TZAGOLOFF et al. 1973 and SCHATZ and MASON 1974). It has been estimated that about 20% of the proteins synthesized in mitochondria correspond to components of cytochrome oxidase (EBNER et al. 1973 b).

As already discussed, there are several ways in which one can estimate the role of mitochondrial or cytoplasmic translation in the assembly of mito-chondria.

The proteins produced by mitochondrial translation can be studied by labelling intact cells such as Neurospora or yeast in the absence of cytoplasmic translation which can be blocked by cycloheximide (SCHATZ and SALTZGABER 1969). The recently developed SDS-polyacrylamide gel electrophoresis permits separating out relatively insoluble proteins and then fractionating them according to their approximate size distribution (SHAPIRO et al. 1967, SHAPIRO and MAIZEL 1969, WEBER and OSBORN 1969). The results of experi-ments with Neurospora, yeast, liver and HeLa cells are similar (COOTE and

WORK 1971, GROOT et al. 1971, SCHATZ et al. 1972, WEISLOGEL and BUTOW 1971, THOMAS and WILLIAMSON 1971, BREGA and BAGLIONI 1971, GALPER and DARNELL 1971, LEDERMAN and ATTARDI 1973, LANSMAN et al. 1974). Roughly 5 to 10 peaks were obtained in the molecular weight range from 10,000 to 95,000.

The study of the size and nature of mitochondrial products is complicated by the possibility of some specific artifacts. The proteins studied could be degraded by proteases (see PRINGLE 1970) or alternatively, proteins may aggregate to form units of much higher molecular weight by virtue of their hydrophobicity. Protease degradation can be avoided at least in part by the use of methylsulfonyl phenyl fluoride (see LANSMAN et al. 1974). Aggregation and protease activity could lead to serious misunderstandings in relation to the basic polypeptide units synthesized in mitochondria. In addition, pulse-chase experiments are presented with the difficulty, that at least in the case of leucine, the intramitochondrial amino acids are favored despite a high level of external amino acid (LANSMAN et al. 1974).

The possibility has been raised that one or several low molecular weight polypeptides act as precursors of mitochondrial proteins. The precursors are assembled into larger molecular weight units (see TZAGOLOFF 1972, MICHEL and NEUPERT 1973). A small number of proteins coded by the mitochondria could function in providing units necessary for the assembly of the functional proteins synthesized in the cytoplasm (e.g., see TZAGOLOFF 1972). This latter idea clearly encounters a stumbling block in the case of cytochrome b which is synthesized in the mitochondria or with cytochrome c oxidase where antibodies to mitochondrially synthesized polypeptides are distinct and inhibit the activity of the complex (POYTON and SCHARTZ 1975 b). However, some evidence supports these two ideas.

Evidence for the synthesis of low molecular weight precursor polypeptide or polypeptides stems from experiments with Neurospora in which the translational products of mitochondrial ribosomes were labelled with H^3-leucine in vivo in the presence of cycloheximide and in isolated mitochondria (MICHEL and NEUPERT 1973). The products were found to be approximately 5,000 to 11,000 in molecular weight with SDS-polyacrylamide gel electrophoresis. A kinetic study was carried out after a short pulse in vivo. The radioactivity appears first in fractions with a molecular weight of 18,000 and 11,000 and a small portion with a molecular weight 20,000 and 40,000. The lower molecular weight components are not unfinished polypeptides since following a much briefer chase, no radioactivity is found in the ribosomes. At later times the proportion of the radioactivity present in the component of higher molecular weight is increased. The results obtained with isolated mitochondria are comparable although the two higher molecular weight components are not formed. These suggest that a low molecular weight product is first produced by mitochondria and is then assembled into larger molecules. Studies carried out with isolated rat liver mitochondria (BURKE and BEATTIE 1974) failed to confirm an early incorporation into a low molecular weight protein.

However, a similar major low molecular weight mitochondrial product (molecular weight of about 7,800) has also been reported in yeast (TZAGOLOFF and AKAI 1972), where it is present in a polymeric form of molecular weight of 45,000. *In vitro* experiments, either with a submitochondrial polypeptide synthesizing system from *Neurospora* (KÜNTZEL and BLOSSEY 1974) or with isolated mitochondria (WHEELDON *et al.* 1974), have found the synthesis of polypeptides of low molecular weight (in the range of 10,000 to 13,000) which may correspond to these presumed precursor proteins.

It is entirely possible that small molecular weight precursors are responsible for forming the larger mitochondrial proteins. However, the final mitochondrial protein products are not likely to originate from a single low molecular weight precursor. The amino acid analysis of three of the units making up the cytochrome oxidase molecule and synthesized in the presence of cycloheximide (SEBALD *et al.* 1973, TZAGOLOFF *et al.* 1974, POYTON and SCHATZ 1975 a) or a low molecular weight component of the ATPase synthesized in the mitochondria (TZAGOLOFF *et al.* 1974) differ significantly in amino acid composition. In addition, antibodies to mitochondrially synthesized polypeptides are specific (*e.g.*, WERNER 1974 a, b, TZAGOLOFF and MEAGHER 1972, POYTON and SCHATZ 1975 b).

As already discussed (B 1), only a limited number of enzymes have been found to require mitochondrial translation: cytochrome oxidase (CLARK-WALKER and LINNANE 1966, KRAM and MAHLER 1967, CHEN and CHARALAMPOUS 1969, WEISS *et al.* 1971, MASON and POYTON 1972), the rutamycin-sensitive ATPase complex (SCHATZ 1968, TZAGOLOFF 1971 b, TZAGOLOFF and MEAGHER 1972), cytochrome b (WEISS and ZIGANKE 1974 a, b), and some component or components of the adenine nucleotide transporter (HASLAM *et al.* 1974 a).

Cytochrome Oxidase

The cytochrome oxidase of yeast consists of at least seven polypeptides (*e.g.*, see TZAGOLOFF *et al.* 1974). These polypeptides range in molecular weight between 8,600 to 35,000 on 7.5% polyacrylamide gels in the presence of sodium dodecyl sulfate (SDS) (RUBIN and TZAGOLOFF 1973 a, b, SHAKESPEARE and MAHLER 1971, MASON *et al.* 1972, MASON *et al.* 1973). The molecular weights obtained with 10% polyacrylamide gel are slightly higher (see RUBIN and TZAGOLOFF 1973 a, MASON *et al.* 1973). The reasons for the difference are still unclear.

The polypeptide composition of cytochrome oxidase is similar for yeast (*e.g.*, MASON *et al.* 1973), *Neurospora crassa*, *Locusta migratoria* (WEISS *et al.* 1971, 1972) and beef heart (RUBIN and TZAGOLOFF 1973 a).

Different isolation procedures (*e.g.*, using isoelectric focusing) also result in the isolation of the seven polypeptides, suggesting that this is the actual number of the subunits (POYTON and SCHATZ 1975 a).

The amino acids of the three mitochondrially synthesized polypeptides were analyzed in *Neurospora* (SEBALD *et al.* 1973). These polypeptides were found to have a higher content of acidic and apolar amino acids than usual. These polypeptides were characterized further in yeast. All have an acidic isoelectric point. Two of the mitochondrially synthesized components of higher molecule weight and two of the cytoplasmically synthesized components were examined for amino acid composition (TZAGOLOFF et al. 1974, POYTON and SCHATZ 1975 a). The mitochondrially synthesized polypeptides were found to have a higher proportion of non-polar amino acids, in agreement with their solubility properties.

The antiserum to one of the mitochondrially synthesized polypeptides (subunit II) inhibited cytochrome oxidase, either in mitochondria, or in submitochondrial particles of the purified complex (POYTON and SCHATZ 1975 b). Similar results were obtained with antisera to some of the cytoplasmically synthesized peptides. The results suggest that both mitochondrial and cytoplasmic products are needed for cytochrome c oxidase function.

The role of yeast mitochondria in the synthesis of cytochrome oxidase has been examined using cycloheximide as an inhibitor of the cytoplasmic protein synthesizing system (RUBIN and TZAGOLOFF 1973 b, MASON et al. 1972, MASON and SCHATZ 1973). The newly synthesized protein was labelled by growing the cells in the presence of H^3-leucine. The cytochrome oxidase components were isolated from the crude extract by immunoprecipitation. The three higher molecular weight components were synthesized in the presence of cycloheximide in a process sensitive to erythromycin (MASON and SCHATZ 1973), acriflavin (MASON and SCHATZ 1973), and chloramphenicol (RUBIN and TZAGOLOFF 1973 b). Essentially the same results have been obtained with Neurospora (SEBALD et al. 1972, 1973, 1974, LANSMAN et al. 1974).

Mitochondria isolated from yeast have been found to synthesize three polypeptides in vitro which correspond in size to those synthesized in vivo in the presence of cycloheximide (POYTON and GROOT 1975). These polypeptides are precipitated by antibodies to the holoenzyme. When complexed to cytoplasmic polypeptides they can also be precipitated by antibodies to these cytoplasmic polypeptides. Accordingly, the polypeptides synthesized in vitro appear to correspond to those synthesized by the mitochondria of intact cells.

Originally in Neurospora (WEISS et al. 1972), only one polypeptide, 20,000 in molecular weight, was identified as a mitochondrial product. However, the study could not exclude the possibility of two other polypeptides of molecular weight 28,000 and 36,000 (SEBALD et al. 1972). More recently, three mitochondrial products have been found to be synthesized in the presence of cycloheximide (LANSMAN et al. 1974, SEBALD et al. 1974). The recovery from cycloheximide inhibition also permits following the fate of newly synthesized mitochondrial components and examining their possible interaction with cytoplasmically synthesized components. In this experimental design the proteins synthesized by mitochondria are pulse-labelled in the presence of cycloheximide. Then the proteins synthesized can be examined for size distribution and enzymatic activity while recovering from cycloheximide. Four proteins originally labelled in the presence of cycloheximide were not found associated with cytochrome oxidase. After a recovery period (2 to 3 hours) three of the four were still present and incorporated into cytochrome oxidase. The size of the three corresponds to that of three of the units synthesized originally. Results obtained with cytochrome oxidase during oxygen adaptation (*e.g.*, CHEN and CHARALAMPOUS 1969) and for rutamycin sensitive ATPase (TZAGOLOFF and MEAGHER 1972) also suggest an assembly requiring both mitochondrial and cytoplasmic products. In the case of the ATPase, the proteins found in the presence of cycloheximide were authentic parts of the ATPase as determined immunologically.

The peak which does not appear after assembly corresponds to a small component (LANSMAN *et al.* 1974, ROWE *et al.* 1974) about 10,000 in molecular weight. Immediately after the pulse labelling procedure, the radioactivity of the low molecular weight peak seems highest, and eventually after recovery it disappears. The component could conceivably correspond to a precursor in the assembly of larger molecules. Alternatively, it could well disappear either as the result of export to the cytoplasm or degradation.

A proposal has also been put forth for higher molecular weight precursors of the mitochondrial proteins on the basis of other experiments using antibodies to cytochrome oxidase. In *Neurospora*, antibodies to purified cytochrome oxidase precipitate seven polypeptides from mitochondrial extracts (WERNER 1974 a, b). The antibody to one of the subunits (subunit 3 of molecular weight 21,000) recognizes two subunits which are not precipitated by the cytochrome oxidase antibody. One of these has a molecular weight of 21,000 (WERNER 1974 a) and another has a molecular weight of 35,000 (WERNER 1974 b). WERNER suggests that the two polypeptides correspond to precursors of subunit 3. In the case of the polypeptide of lower molecular weight the interpretation is bolstered by the finding that it has a half life of 2 minutes. The results also could be interpreted on the basis of a changed reactivity of subunit 3 to the antibody depending on whether it has been integrated into the complex.

In *Neurospora* either in the presence of cycloheximide or chloramphenicol the incorporation of the synthesized polypeptides into cytochrome c oxidase takes place only after the inhibitors are washed off (WEISS *et al.* 1971, SEBALD *et al.* 1972, and SEBALD *et al.* 1974). After incubation with cycloheximide, without removal of the inhibitor, only one component and not three are labelled in cytochrome oxidase (WEISS *et al.* 1971). Again, these results suggest an interaction in the assembly of the finished cytochrome c oxidase.

The accumulation of precursors of the cytochrome c oxidase complex is also suggested in studies carried out with copper depleted *Neurospora* (SCHWAB 1974), which have no detectable cytochrome c oxidase (WEISS and BÜCHER 1970). After introduction of the missing copper cytochrome c oxidase activity begins to appear. Copper-depleted cells were first incubated in C^{14}-leucine. Subsequently they were treated with cycloheximide in H^3-leucine. The polypeptides fractionated from these cells were essentially the same as those obtained from copper-sufficient cells. The H^3-proteins synthesized by the mitochondrial system were essentially the same regardless of the presence or absence of copper. Similar results were obtained after pre-labelling all the proteins in the absence of copper, followed by copper addition. All cytochrome c oxidase subunits were labelled. These results suggest that in the absence of copper the assembly process stops although all polypeptides (except for the heme) are present.

A mutual interplay of mitochondrial and cytoplasmic products in the assembly of cytochrome c oxidase is also indicated in studies of nuclear and extrachromosomal mutants (EBNER et al. 1973). Mitochondrially synthesized subunits seem to be necessary for the assembly of polypeptides coded in the nucleus and analogously, chromosomally coded components are necessary for the assembly of mitochondrially synthesized products. One of the chromosomal mutations resulted in the absence of a mitochondrially produced polypeptide. The mutant phenotype could be supressed by nuclear amber supressors (ONO et al. 1975). These results suggest that chromosomal supressor genes may control a mitochondrially synthesized polypeptide.

The results discussed agree with the notion that the three components of cytochrome oxidase of higher molecular weight are translated in the mitochondria. The four remaining components are presumably synthesized in the cytoplasm. There is some disagreement about the origin of the polypeptide carrying heme a. SCHATZ et al. (1972) and MASON et al. (1973) ascribe it to the cytoplasmic synthetic system, whereas TZAGOLOFF et al. (1974) present evidence for the involvement of a mitochondrially synthesized polypeptide.

Rutamycin or Oligomycin Sensitive ATPase Complex

The rutamycin sensitive ATPase complex of yeast mitochondria can be extracted by the detergent Triton X-100. This lipoprotein complex has been purified in glycerol or sucrose gradients. It has been found to have a molecular weight of approximately 340,000 (TZAGOLOFF and MEAGHER 1971). Polyacrylamide gel electrophoresis in the presence of SDS identifies eight distinct units, although probably two others are present (e.g., see TZAGOLOFF 1974). The complex is composed of a water soluble ATPase (F_1), and a protein involved in the binding of F_1 to the membrane and which confers oligomycin sensitivity to the ATPase (OSCP). Another membrane lipoprotein factor contains at least four polypeptides (TZAGOLOFF and MEAGHER 1972), and is also involved with the binding of the complex to the membrane and possibly oligomycin sensitivity (see section C 1 b and SHANNON et al. 1973). F_1 is made up of five different subunits (SENIOR and BROOKE 1970, TZAGOLOFF and MEAGHER 1971).

F_1 and OSCP are synthesized by the cytoplasmic system as shown by inhibitor studies (TZAGOLOFF 1969, 1970). F_1 is produced by yeast grown in the presence of chloramphenicol whereas its synthesis is inhibited by cycloheximide (TZAGOLOFF 1969). The subunits of F_1 are identical whether isolated from normal or chloramphenicol grown cells (TZAGOLOFF 1969, TZAGOLOFF et al. 1972).

Similarly, OSCP is synthesized in cells derepressed in chloramphenicol, whereas cycloheximide blocks its formation (TZAGOLOFF 1970). The partially purified OSCP from the chloramphenicol cells was found indistinguishable from that obtained from normal mitochondria. Therefore OSCP is probably synthesized in the cytoplasm.

When yeast cells are grown in cycloheximide, in the presence of H^3-leucine, the label is incorporated into components which are precipitated by antibodies to rutamycin sensitive ATPase, and correspond to the four lipoprotein subunits involved in membrane binding (TZAGOLOFF and MEAGHER 1972). Therefore, these four polypeptides are probably synthesized in the mitochondria.

Although F_1 and OSCP are synthesized in the presence of chloramphenicol, they fail to assemble into a rutamycin sensitive ATPase (TZAGOLOFF 1969, 1970, TZAGOLOFF et al. 1972). The results suggest that the assembly requires a mitochondrial product. This inference is supported by additional experiments (TZAGOLOFF et al. 1972). As already discussed, F_1 is synthesized by cells grown in chloramphenicol. The F_1 subunits, fail however to assemble and remain in the post-ribosomal fraction. After removal of the inhibitor the F_1 activity is no longer in this fraction and appears in the mitochondria.

Similarly, mitochondrial particles prepared from glucose repressed yeast bind little rutamycin insensitive ATPase or OSCP. Incubation of the cells in derepression medium increases the capacity to bind, suggesting that a membrane factor has to be formed in order for binding to take place. This membrane factor does not appear when yeast are incubated in the presence of chloramphenicol or cycloheximide. However, it does appear when the yeast are incubated first in chloramphenicol and subsequently in cycloheximide (TZAGOLOFF 1971 b). In contrast, when the order of addition of the inhibitors is reversed the system fails to assemble. These findings suggest that the membrane factors synthesized in mitochondria are necessary for assembly of the system.

Cytochrome b

The possible multiplicity of cytochrome b species has been the subject of discussion in the past few years (e.g., see SLATER 1973, WIKSTRÖM 1973). The cytochrome b of Neurospora discussed in this section has the appropriate absorption characteristics of cytochrome b, and a heme to protein ratio of 1. It is probably present as a dimer.

In Neurospora, cytochrome b has been found to have a molecular weight of about 55,000 after extraction with bile salts (WEISS 1972). Originally, this cytochrome was presumed to be made up of three polypeptides, as seen by SDS-polyacrylamide gel. More recent results suggest a dimer made up of two units which may be identical, approximately 30,000 in molecular weight, in both Neurospora and Locusta migratoria (WEISS and ZIGANKE 1974 a, b, LORENZ et al. 1974). Since, in vivo, the incorporation of H^3-leucine into the cytochrome b is insensitive to cycloheximide but sensitive to chloramphenicol, the site of synthesis is presumed to be mitochondrial.

4. Synthesis of Phospholipids

The lipid composition of the inner and the outer mitochondrial membranes and the acyl chain distribution of the component fatty acids have been examined for a number of cells. The nature of the lipid, at least in relation to the acyl chain, seems to play a significant role not only in the physical properties of the membrane but also in oxidative phosphorylation and in the activity of at least some of the enzymes of the inner mitochondrial membrane (ATPase, cytochrome c oxidase) and of the outer membrane (kynurenine hydroxylase) (JANKI et al. 1974). The nature of the lipid is likely to play a significant role in the transporting ability of mitochondrial carriers (see GAUTHERON et al. 1974). Mitochondria of mammalian tissues (e.g., see LEVY and SAUNER 1967, PARSONS et al. 1967, ROUSER et al. 1968, STOFFEL and SCHIEFER 1968) seem to contain very little neutral lipid (about 6 to 9%, a substantial portion of which is cholesterol). The phospholipids are predominantly phosphotidyl choline, phosphatidyl ethanol amine and diphosphatidyl glycerol (cardiolipin). Together these components account for more than 95% of the phospholipids. Diphosphatidyl glycerol is characteristic of mitochondria and seems to be present predominantly in the inner membrane. It is generally thought that cholesterol is present exclusively or almost exclusively in the outer membrane (PARSONS and YANO 1967). The fatty acid components of the phospholipids have a high degree of unsaturation (FLEISCHER and ROUSER 1965).

The phospholipid composition of the mitochondria of eukaryotic microorganisms such as yeast (JAKOVCIC et al. 1971), Tetrahymena (KENNEDY and THOMPSON 1970 and JONAH and ERWIN 1971) or Neurospora (HALLERMAYER and NEUPERT 1974 a) is similar to that of mammalian tissues. Tetrahymena mitochondria have an unusual phospholipid, 2-aminoethylphosphonolipid. In Neurospora there is a significant concentration of ergosterol (1 : 3 in relation to the phospholipid content) which apparently is present only in the outer membrane. In yeast, the proportion of the different lipids in petite yeast is only slightly different from those present in wild-type, suggesting that the enzymes of lipid metabolism are synthesized in the cytoplasm.

Generally, mammalian mitochondria have a more limited capacity to synthesize phospholipids than yeast mitochondria. They are capable of synthesizing phosphatidic acid, lysophosphatidic acid, phosphatidyl glycerol and diphosphatidyl glycerol (STOFFEL and SHIEFER 1968, McMURRAY and DAWSON 1969, WIRTZ et al. 1972). The other necessary phospholipids are apparently synthesized in the endoplasmic reticulum. A system of soluble enzymes is present which is capable of transferring phospholipids between different membrane systems (e.g., WIRTZ and ZILVERSMIT 1968, 1970, McMURRAY and DAWSON 1969, ABDELKADER and MAZLIAK 1970, JUNGAWALA et al. 1971, MILLER and DAWSON 1972, WIRTZ et al. 1972, EHNOLM and ZILVERSMIT 1973, KAMP et al. 1973, HARVEY et al. 1973, HELMKAMP et al. 1973, KADER 1975). In contrast, the mitochondria of Saccharomyces cerevisae have the capacity to synthesize the major mitochondrial phospholipid components (COBON et al. 1974). The pathways of the mammalian and the yeast system are contrasted in Fig. 9. However, it should be noted that the location of specific enzymatic activities in the mammalian systems should be regarded with caution since the results may differ significantly with the tissue from which the mitochondria were isolated (*e.g.*, see DAVIDSON and STANACEV 1974 and their review of the literature).

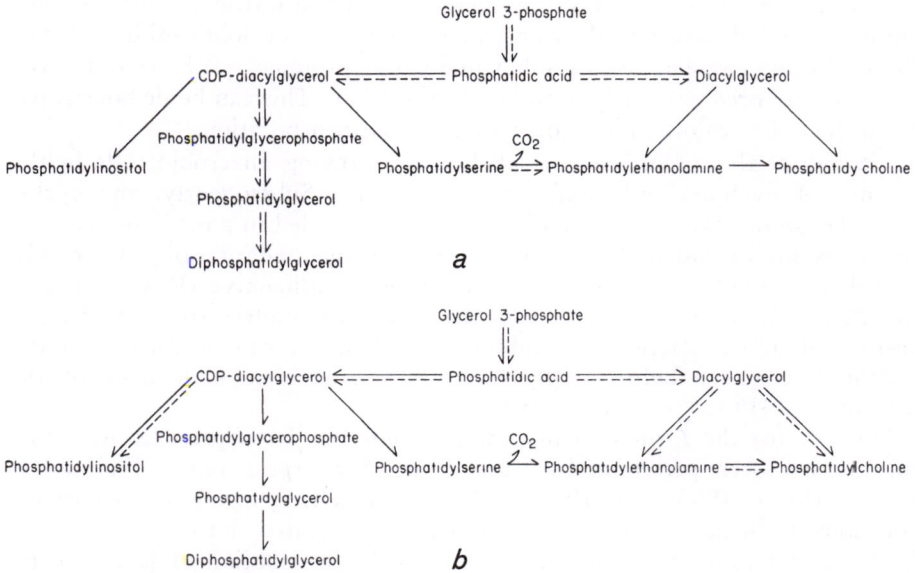

Fig. 9. *a* Major pathways of phospholipid synthesis *de novo* in yeast (‑ ‑‑ ‑‑‑‑‑‑) and mammalian mitochondria (‑‑‑‑‑‑‑‑) excluding base-exchange mechanisms. It is possible that a limited amount of phosphatidylcholine synthesis also occurs in both cases. *b* Major pathways of phospholipid synthesis *de novo* in yeast (——————) and mammalian microsomal fractions (‑‑‑‑‑‑‑‑) excluding base-exchange mechanisms. The microsomal localization of phosphatidylethanolamine synthesis from diacylglycerol in yeast is tentative. (From COBON *et al.* 1974, used by permission.)

5. Mitochondrial Assembly

The mechanisms involved in the assembly of mitochondria are still largely unknown. In cells such as yeast where metabolism can take place either aerobically or anaerobically, the presence of mitochondria can be either repressed (*e.g.*, by the presence of glucose) or induced (*e.g.*, by the introduction of oxygen). These possibilities have been very useful in the study of mitochondrial assembly. The development of mitochondria can be examined by shifting the cells from conditions where mitochondrial functions are not present to an active state (*e.g.*, from an anaerobic to an aerobic system).

In cells grown under anaerobic conditions, subcellular particles are found which contain DNA with a buoyant density characteristic of mitochondrial DNA. These particles also contain an oligomycin sensitive ATPase. This ATPase probably corresponds to F_1 since it is inhibited by the natural inhibitor of F_1 (PULLMAN and MONROY 1963) and the appropriate antibody. The subcellular particles of anaerobically grown yeast were also found to contain succinic and NADH dehydrogenase, flavin and ferrochelatase all of which are also present in normal mitochondria (see SCHATZ 1970). These findings suggest that the genetic system and some of the mitochondrial components are always present as discrete organelles, the promitochondria.

The presence of mitochondrial components under anaerobic conditions and their subsequent assembly into mitochondria after the introduction of aerobic conditions was demonstrated in an experiment using cycloheximide (SCHATZ 1970). In the presence of cycloheximide, the proteins synthesized by the yeast cells are predominantly mitochondrial (90%). This can be demonstrated by the fact that chloramphenicol prevents this incorporation.

Mitochondrial proteins can be labelled by growing anaerobic cells in the presence of cycloheximide and labelled leucine. Subsequently, the cycloheximide can be washed away and the cells resuspended in a medium containing an excess of unlabelled leucine. After oxygen adaptation, the newly formed mitochondria were found to be strongly radioactive (PLATTNER and SCHATZ 1969). These results indicate that the mitochondria are formed from pre-formed units. Particles resembling mitochondria can be seen with the electron microscope before oxygen adaptation, at least with some of the methods used (PLATTNER and SCHATZ 1969).

Evidence for the formation of new mitochondria from pre-existing mitochondria has been presented by LUCK using *Neurospora crassa* choline-less mutants (LUCK 1963 a, b, 1965 a, 1966). In cells growing exponentially exogenous radioactive choline is rapidly incorporated into mitochondria. Upon transfer to a non-radioactive medium, the distribution of label can be followed using radioautography. The labelling was found to be distributed randomly throughout the mitochondrial population. The labelling diminishes as the time of incubation in the non-radioactive medium is lengthened. These results are consistent with the concept that mitochondria are formed from pre-existing mitochondria. The synthesis of new mitochondria would otherwise lead to labelled (the old) and completely unlabelled (the new) mitochondria. Similar experiments can be carried out using choline itself as a density label. The amount of choline incorporated in the mitochondria of choline-less mutants depends on the amount of choline in the medium; the larger the amount of choline incorporated, the lower the density. Shifting growing cultures from low to high choline content produces a mitochondrial population of uniform density (LUCK 1965 b, 1966) and not different kinds of mitochondria.

The demonstration that the mitochondria originate from other mitochondria or from pre-existing structures does not simplify the elucidation of the assembly process. As already discussed many of the mitochondrial proteins are synthesized in the cytoplasm. As discussed above (Section B 4), in mammalian tissues a significant portion of mitochondrial lipids is synthesized in the microsomes. Some of the early evidence suggested that many of the mitochondrial components had the same half life (FLETCHER and SANADI 1966, NEUBERT et al. 1966 b). These data would have agreed with the notion that mitochondria are assembled and disassembled as a unit. Later data suggest that the picture is far more complex. The various mitochondrial components were found to have distinct half-lives (BEATTIE et al. 1966 a, BAILEY et al. 1967, LUSENA and DEPOCAS 1966, TAYLOR et al. 1967, PASCAUD 1964, GURR et al. 1965, VON HUNGEN et al. 1968). In fact, mitochondrial proteins and phospholipids were found to be metabolically independent under a variety of conditions (LUCK 1965 a).

The role of the lipid component of mitochondrial membranes in mitochondrial function and assembly has been evaluated in a number of ways. The isolation of fatty acid auxotrophs (RESNICK and MORTIMER 1966) permitted the demonstration that changes in the fatty acid side chains lead to changes in membrane function (PROUDLOCK et al. 1969, 1971, HASLAM et al. 1973 b). In yeast, when the unsaturated fatty acid content of mitochondria falls below 20%, the yeast can no longer function with non-fermentable substrates. Since the respiratory chain seems normal, the lesion has been presumed to be in the coupling mechanism.

Mitochondria derived from yeast mutants requiring unsaturated fatty acids and grown on a suboptimal concentration of the supplement fail to carry out oxidative phosphorylation (PROUDLOCK et al. 1969, HASLAM et al. 1973 b). This treatment decreases the capacity to transport ions (e.g., valinomycin induced K^+ transport) and increases the permeability to protons. The increase in proton permeability suggests that this change may be responsible for the mode of action of the deficiency (HASLAM et al. 1973 b).

The nature of the fatty acids of the mitochondrial lipids also can be manipulated by changing the conditions of growth and the lipid supplement added to the minimal medium (AINSWORTH et al. 1972, RAISON 1973). Yeast grown anaerobically cannot carry out the unsaturation reactions (BLOOMFIELD and BLOCH 1960). When grown aerobically in the presence of unsaturated fatty acids, the synthesis of unsaturated fatty acids is repressed. Hence, the fatty acid supplement is preferentially incorporated under both sets of conditions. Manipulation of the fatty acid side chains permits testing their role in more detail; for example, it permits demonstrating the temperature dependence of the enzymatic activity on the nature of the lipid side chains. The temperature dependence of enzymatic activity allows the demonstration of temperature transitions in the lipid environment of the enzymes by means of the Arrhenius plots. Cytochrome c oxidase and oligomycin-sensitive ATPase, present in the inner mitochondrial membrane, were found to exhibit temperature transition points characteristic of the lipid supplement used (AINSWORTH et al. 1972, JANKI et al. 1974 a, b, 1975). Similar results were found with the outer mitochondrial membrane marker, kynurenine hydroxylase. The transition temperatures change proportionally to the melting point of the fatty acid supplement.

The assembly of the cytochrome c oxidase, the ATPase and kynurenine hydroxylase during oxygen adaptions was studied (see JANKI et al. 1974 a, b, 1975). The yeast were grown under anaerobic conditions in the presence of a linoleic acid supplement and then shifted to aerobic conditions in a elaidic acid medium. Cytochrome c oxidase was found initially to exhibit two transition temperatures reflecting the supplement used under both anaerobic and aerobic conditions. Gradually, with time, the elaidic acid transition temperature was found to predominate. For ATPase a single transition point was found at all times. However, this transition temperature progressed from the value characteristic of the mitochondria of linoleic acid supplemented yeast to that of elaidic acid supplemented yeast. For kynurenine hydroxylase, the transition temperature is that of linoleic acid for long periods although new enzyme is being synthesized continuously. Using an unsaturated fatty acid auxotroph, it was shown that during oxygen adaptation the formation of ATPase and cytochrome oxidase required a fatty acid supplement whereas kyneurnine hydroxylase did not.

The results have been interpreted tentatively on the basis of three models. In one case the lipids and the enzymes are assembled separately (*e.g.*, for the case of kyneurnine hydroxylase assembly). Eventually the mixing of the lipids in the membrane structure produces a "mixed" transition temperature. For the two other cases, lipid is synthesized and then assembled with precursor proteins before incorporation into the membrane. The newly incorporated lipid tends to remain attached to the complex for the case of cytochrome oxidase. In the case of the ATPase complex, although the lipid and the protein components are assembled in the same manner, the newly formed lipid mixes rapidly with the lipid already present.

6. Interactions in the Assembly of Mitochondrial Components

The assembly of mitochondrial components seems to be the result of a complex interaction between the mitochondrial and cytoplasmic synthesizing systems. The details of this interaction are just beginning to emerge. We have seen how mitochondrial products are needed for the assembly of the proteins produced in the cytoplasm for the case of the rutamycin sensitive ATPase and cytochrome oxidase, and similarly, in some cases cytoplasmic products are needed for the assembly of mitochondrial proteins. Other information from respiratory mutants permits examining other interactions in some detail. Nuclear *petites* have a variety of phenotypes. Some are deficient in specific cytochromes (*e.g.*, aa_3 or b) (SHERMAN and SLONIMSKI 1964, REILLY and SHERMAN 1965). Others have pleiotropic deficiencies (SHERMAN and SLONIMSKI 1964, SUBÍK 1970, GOFFEAU *et al.* 1972, 1973, 1974, EBNER *et al.* 1973 a).

Recently, eighteen respiratory deficient chromosomal mutants have been isolated in yeast. These mutants have retained a normal mitochondrial genome as tested by their ability to complement cytoplasmic mutants. The mutants could be classified into seven complementation groups. Three of these lacked only cytochrome aa_3. More commonly, the effect of a mutation was pleiotropic, where the yeast were deficient in several cytochromes (*e.g.*, aa_3, b, and c_1) and in addition, in some cases, ATPase. SDS polyacrylamide gel electrophoresis showed that these mutants lacked several polypeptides synthesized in mitochondria (EBNER *et al.* 1973 a).

These results suggest three possibilities. The nuclear genes may affect mitochondrial protein synthesis. Alternatively, the nuclear genes are necessary for the assembly of the mitochondrial products, perhaps serving as organizers for the assembly of mitochondria or serving as positive regulators of the mitochondrial genome. In this respect, it is interesting to note that partially purified cytoplasmic proteins have been found to stimulate the synthesis of mitochondrial DNA (D'AGOSTINO *et al.* 1975).

Regardless of mechanism or mechanisms, the interactions appear complex, judging by the number of distinct chromosomal mutations observed to produce pleiotropic effects (*e.g.*, see GOFFEAU *et al.* 1974).

Some of the cytochrome oxidase-less nuclear mutants lack at least one of the cytochrome oxidase components which are synthesized in the mitochondria. These mutants, however, contain components synthesized in the cytoplasm (EBNER *et al.* 1973 b). In contrast, one of the extrachromosomal mutants found lacks all mitochondrially synthesized components and one of the cytoplasmically synthesized components as well (EBNER *et al.* 1973 b). In addition, the cytochrome oxidase components present were loosely bound. These results suggest that proper assembly requires components coded in both the nucleus and in the mitochondria.

A single chromosomal mutation prevents either the assembly or the integration of mitochondrially synthesized components. Complementation analysis of the chromosomal genes studied reveals the involvement of at least five unlinked genes in the coding for cytochrome oxidase (EBNER *et al.* 1973 b). Probably more are involved since cytochrome oxidase is composed of seven polypeptides. The involvement of nuclear genes in the mitochondrially synthesized products suggests that the nuclear genes could be responsible for regulatory components. Alternatively, the mitochondrially synthesized protein could be coded by nuclear mRNA. As we saw there are a number of arguments against this view. In addition, there are probably regulatory genes. For example, in yeast, cytochrome c is controlled by at least six genes (SHERMAN 1964), and several of these are likely to be regulatory in function.

The results of these experiments are also consistent with the view that the mitochondrially coded proteins are needed for the integration of the catalytic subunits which are synthesized in the cytoplasm (EBNER *et al.* 1973 b).

An interaction between mitochondrially and cytoplasmically synthesized polypeptides is also indicated by studies with a yeast temperature mutant (MAHLER *et al.* 1974 a, b). At the restrictive temperature the cytoplasmic synthesis is interrupted at initiation (HARTWELL 1967). After a lag, the mitochondrial synthesis (as estimated from the incorporation of H^3-histidine) is also inhibited. In contrast, the initiation of mitochondrial protein synthesis, indicated by the capacity to synthesize fmet-puromycin, remains normal. An analogous requirement for cytoplasmic polypeptides for the assembly of mitochondrially synthesized components has been previously noted by TZAGOLOFF *et al.* (1972, 1973).

Similarly, in derepression, cytoplasmically synthesized proteins are accumulated in the presence of chloramphenicol. After washing the cells free of the inhibitor the incorporation of mitochondrially synthesized products is not prevented by cycloheximide (BEATTIE *et al.* 1974).

A more general dependence of yeast metabolism on mitochondrial components has been revealed by studies of a nuclear mutant lacking F_1 (EBNER and SCHATZ 1973). This mutant is greatly deficient in cytochromes aa_3, b, and c_1. Despite the presence of a protein synthesizing system in mitochondria, the level of several of the mitochondrial products were drastically decreased. The cytochrome oxidase components synthesized in the cytoplasm were present in a concentration one-tenth of that in the wild type. Since the mutant was unable to grow anaerobically, something other than energy deficiency is responsible for the effect. These finding agree with the concept of inter-dependence of nuclear and mitochondrially coded components.

7. Regulation of Nuclear Genome by Mitochondria

Some of the direct interactions between mitochondrially and cytoplasmically synthesized polypeptides may well determine the final assembly of the mito-chondria. In addition, there is considerable evidence for a mitochondrial control of proteins coded in nuclear DNA. Some of the enzymes coded in the nucleus and synthesized in the cytoplasm appear to be induced when mitochondrial protein synthesis is blocked by appropriate inhibitors. These findings suggest that mitochondria produce a repressor which blocks the expression of nuclear genes.

Treatment of *Tetrahymena* with ethidium bromide induces the biosynthesis of DNA polymerase by the cytoplasm (WESTERGAARD *et al.* 1970, WESTER-GAARD and LINDBERG 1972). In *Neurospora*, both chloramphenicol and ethidium bromide have been found to stimulate the production of elongation factors, methionyl-tRNA transformylase (BARATH and KÜNTZEL 1972 a) and RNA polymerase (KÜNTZEL and BARATH 1972).

Enzymes involved in oxidative metabolism have also been found to be induced by the inhibition of mitochondrial protein synthesis. In *Neurospora* some mutants respire by a pathway which is insensitive to cyanide and antimycin A but is inhibited by salicyl hydroxamic acid (LAMBOWITZ and SLAYMAN 1971, VON JAGOW *et al.* 1973, EDWARDS *et al.* 1973). The alternate oxidase does not involve cytochromes (VON JAGOW and KLINGENBERG 1972, LAMBOWITZ *et al.* 1972 a) and can carry out oxidative phosphorylation (VON JAGOW *et al.* 1973, SLAYMAN *et al.* 1975) apparently at site 1.

The biochemistry of cyanide insensitive respiration in a variety of systems has been recently reviewed (HENRY and NYNS 1975). In wild type *Neuro-spora*, treatment with chloramphenicol also induces the alternate pathway, suggesting that its expression is controlled by a mitochondrial repressor (LAMBOWITZ *et al.* 1972 b, VON JAGOW *et al.* 1972, EDWARDS *et al.* 1974).

The amount of mitochondrial DNA seems to be under the same control mechanism as nuclear DNA (see MAHLER *et al.* 1974 b). The percent of the total DNA accounted for by the mitochondria is constant regardless of ploidy (GRIMES *et al.* 1974). In addition, where *petite* mutant DNA lacks wild-type sequences, the DNA is present in normal amounts (see BORST 1972, MAHLER 1973, NAGLEY and LINNANE 1972, FAYE *et al.* 1973). On the other hand, mitochondrial size and dry mass seem to be independent of mitochondrial DNA content, cell division or nuclear ploidy.

C. Transducing Functions of Mitochondria

1. The Respiratory Assemblies and Oxidative Phosphorylation

a) General Organization

The arrangements of the respiratory chain components of mitochondria which are most generally accepted at this time are summarized in Fig. 10. This scheme includes cytochromes a_3, a, c, c_1, and b and in addition flavoprotein and coenzyme Q. Cytochrome b is thought to be present as two and most probably three spectrographically distinct species (*e.g.*, WIKSTRÖM 1973). Two of these have been designated b_K and b_T (CHANCE *et al.* 1970). The experimental evidence for this scheme together with the properties of the system

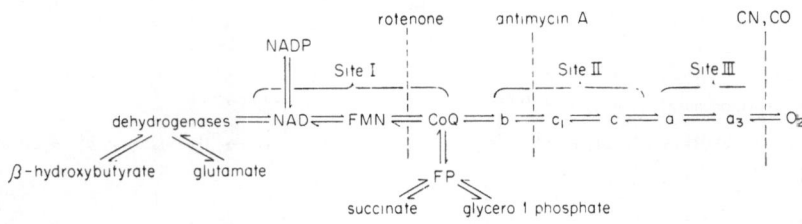

Fig. 10. Scheme for oxidative phosphorylation. The dashed lines indicate the sites of inhibitor blocks. The brackets indicate the approximate region involved in phosphorylation.

have been reviewed repeatedly (*e.g.*, CHANCE and WILLIAMS 1956, LEHNINGER 1965, and KLINGENBERG 1968). This scheme has been derived in part from spectroscopic data together with kinetic studies and data on the effects of a variety of inhibitors. In part it is based on the study of the redox properties of the various components and the dissection of the mitochondria by various disruptive procedures. The approaches making use of disruption and reconstitution have been examined in the thorough review of KAGAWA (1972). The more recent application of EPR techniques has permitted the identification of a number of iron-sulfur proteins which play a role in the respiratory chain (see OHRME-JOHNSON *et al.* 1973, and OHNISHI *et al.* 1970, 1971, 1972 a, b). The arrangement of these iron-sulfur proteins is illustrated in Fig. 11 (OHNISHI 1973). The iron-sulfur proteins have been designated centers 1 to 9. Center 1 is actually constituted of two separate but very similar proteins desginated 1 a and 1 b. Two of the iron-sulfur proteins are associated with succinic dehydrogenase and another (center 9) is the iron-sulfur protein of Rieske (RIESKE *et al.* 1964 a, b).

The sites associated with energy coupling are also indicated in Fig. 10 by the Roman numerals I, II, and III. At each one of these sites 1 ATP is synthesized per electron pair traversing the chain. There are indications that the components of the respiratory chain and the elements involved in the coupling of oxidation to phosphorylation are present in precise stoichiometry, suggesting that they are present in precise functional assemblies. The proportion of the various cytochromes, for example, has been calculated from spectrophotometric data. This is shown in Table 12 (VANNESTE 1966). Similarly, some of the inhibitors of the respiratory chain or the phosphorylative reactions are known to be bound tightly to specific mitochondrial components with a 1 to 1 stoichiometry. Antimycin A binds to one of the cytochrome b species present. Aurovertin (BERTINA *et al.* 1973) and oligomycin (LARDY and LIN 1969) bind to coupling factor F_1, although at different sites. As shown in Table 13, the three inhibitors bind precisely in the same stoichiometry (BERTINA *et al.* 1973) which suggests that 1 F_1 is present per respiratory assembly. The high affinity inhibitor binding sites of the

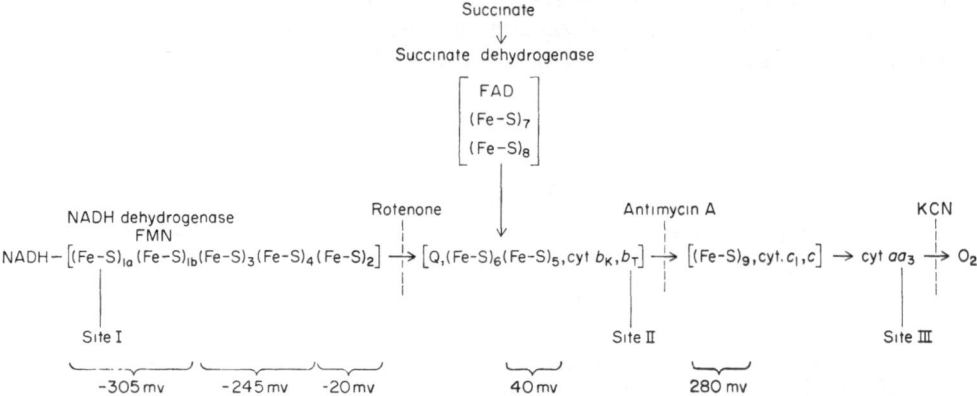

Fig. 11. Respiratory chain components, energy coupling sites and the sites of blocks by respiratory inhibitors. The iron sulfur centers have been numbered for identification. (From OHNISHI 1973, used by permission.)

adenine nucleotide translocator also suggest 1 to 2 sites per respiratory assembly (VIGNAIS *et al.* 1971, 1973 a, b, KLINGENBERG *et al.* 1973).

Evidence reviewed in the next section suggests that cytochrome aa_3, cytochrome b_T and an iron-sulfur protein discussed later, respond to the phosphate potential [*i.e.*, (ATP)/(ADP) (P_i)]. This response suggests the presence of high energy forms of these components involved in the coupling of oxidation to phosphorylation.

SLATER (*e.g.*, 1971, 1974) proposes a mechanism in which two molecules of the b cytochrome are involved in the coupling at site II. This scheme is shown in Fig. 12. The basic catalytic unit, according to this mechanism, would then be a dimer of cytochrome b (bb_i), where b and b_i would represent two distinct cytochromes. The model is based on spectroscopic evidence for the presence of two high energy forms of b which is still under discussion (see below in section C 1 b). The mechanism is compatible with the stoichiometry of 1 ATP synthesized per electron pair traversing site II. There are, in fact, indications that two cytochrome b molecules may be involved in oxidative phosphorylation at site II since the oxidation of cytochrome b (measured as the difference in O.D. between 564 and 575 nm) exhibits second oder kinetics in relation to cytochrome b concentration (HOMMES 1964). In contrast, it exhibits first order kinetics in the presence of the uncoupler, 2,4 di-

Table 12. *Concentration of Cytochromes in Beef Heart Mitochondria*
(from VANNESTE 1966, used by permission)

Cytochrome	Concentration (mμ)	Stoichiometry
aa_3	6.1	4
a_3	3.1	2
a	3.0	2
c	2.7	1.7
c_1	1.5	1.0
b	3.0	2.0

Table 13. *Binding if Inhibitors to Mitochondria* (from BERTINA *et al.* 1973, used by permission)

Source of mitochondria	μgms/gm protein		
	Antimycin	Oligomycin	Aurovertin
Rat heart	0.26	0.27	0.27
Rat liver	0.10	0.12	0.12

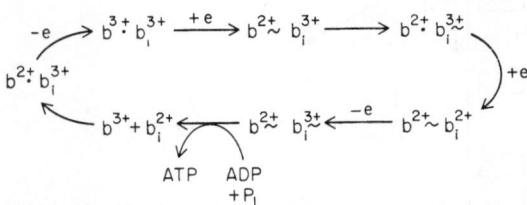

Fig. 12. Coupling of oxidation to phosphorylation involving two molecular species of cytochrome b. (From E. C. SLATER 1971.) The coupling between energy-yielding and energy-utilizing reactions in mitochondria (used by permission).

nitrophenol. A similar mechanism involving two redox carrier molecules could also take place with the first and third coupling sites. There is indeed some evidence for a complex interaction between a and a_3 during oxidation-reduction reactions (LINDSAY and WILSON 1972, LEIGH *et al.* 1974, NICHOLLS and PETERSEN 1974). The possible interaction of cytochromes a and a_3 had been previously proposed in the classical studies of KEILIN and HARTREE (1939).

b) Energetics of the System; Redox Potentials

The energetics of the respiratory chain have been studied by estimating the redox potentials of the respiratory components on mitochondrial or submitochondrial particles.

A number of techniques can be used to measure the potentials of redox components (CLARK 1960). The potentiometric technique has been used most extensively with mitochondria or submitochondrial particles. The redox

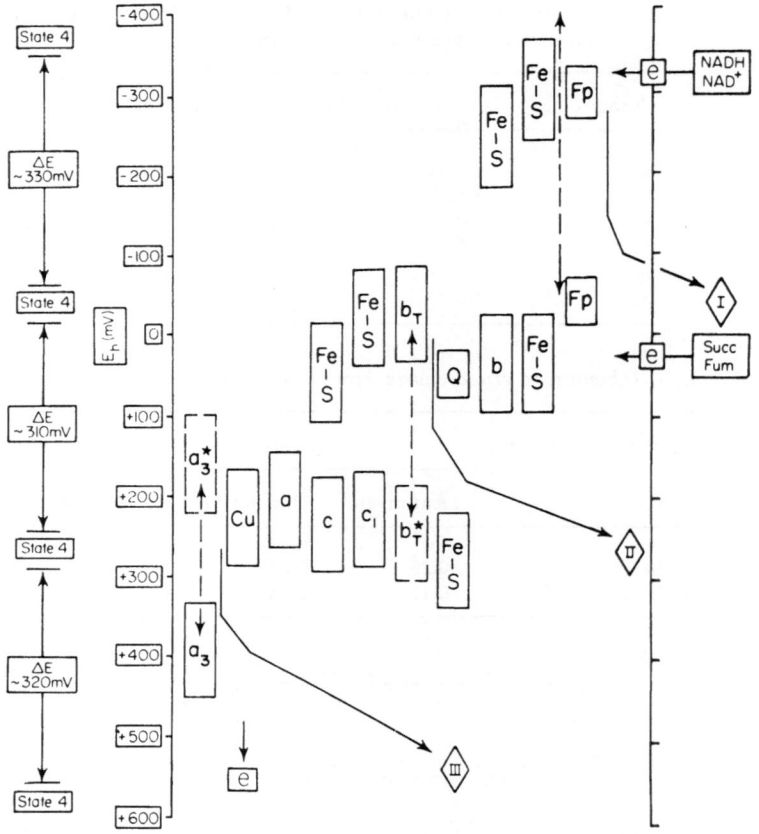

Fig. 13. The redox potentials of the respiratory chain of pigeon heart mitochondria. Each component is represented by a rectangle centered on its half reduction potential at pH 7.2. (From WILSON *et al.* 1973, used by permission.)

state of the various components can be estimated independently from spectro-photometric measurements. In the case of the iron-sulfur proteins the redox state can be estimated by EPR measurements after freezing the sample. The proportion of the reduced and oxidized species of each respiratory carrier can be altered by adding reducing equivalents or electron acceptors. Appropriate artificial electron carriers are necessary to mediate the passage of the electrons from the respiratory chain to the platinum electrode. The methods have been outlined in a number of papers (*e.g.*, WILSON and DUTTON 1970 a, b, DUTTON 1971, WILSON *et al.* 1972 c, 1973). The theory and significance of these measurements has been discussed recently from a general point of view by DUTTON and WILSON (1974, see also the useful discussion in the appendix by DE VAULT).

For hypothetical redox couples of components *A* and *B*, either reduced (subscript *red*) or oxidized (subscript *ox*):

1. $A_{red} + B_{ox} \rightleftharpoons A_{ox} + B_{red}$

Table 14. *Determinations of Midpoint Potentials in Mitochondria*

---

1. Uncoupled mitochondria

Cytochrome oxidase	CASWELL 1968
	WILSON et al. 1972 d
Cytochrome c	DUTTON et al. 1971
Cytochrome b	WILSON and DUTTON 1970 b
	DUTTON et al. 1971
Cu of cytochrome oxidase	TSUDZUKI and WILSON 1971
	ERECIŃSKA et al. 1971
Iron-sulfur proteins	RIESKE et al. 1964 b
	WILSON et al. 1971 a
	OHNISHI et al. 1972
Flavoproteins	ERECIŃSKA et al. 1970
CoQ	URBAN and KLINGENBERG 1969

2. Coupled mitochondria + ATP

Cytochrome b_T	WILSON and DUTTON 1970 a, b
	DUTTON et al. 1971
	LINDSAY et al. 1972
Cytochrome oxidase	WIKSTRÖM and SARIS 1970
	LINDSAY and WILSON 1972
	WILSON et al. 1972 b
Iron-sulfur proteins	OHNISHI et al. 1972 b

---

the difference in redox potential will be:

2. $E = E_m + \dfrac{RT}{nF} \ln \dfrac{(A_{ox})\,(B_{red})}{(A_{red})\,(B_{ox})}$

E_m is the difference in the half reduction potentials, R is the gas constant, T is temperature, and F the Faraday constant. The Gibbs free energy difference ΔG for the redox couples will be:

3. $\Delta G = -\,nF\Delta E$

The E_m values for the various components are shown diagrammatically in Fig. 13 (WILSON et al. 1973, ERECIŃSKA et al. 1974). The studies on which this diagram is based are listed in Table 14. The respiratory chain components fall primarily into three potential groups. One group in the span includes cytochrome oxidase and cytochrome b_T, another in the span including several iron-sulfur proteins, cytochrome b_K and co-enzyme Q and still another involving flavoprotein and iron-sulfur proteins. Cytochrome b_T and a_3 (WILSON and DUTTON 1970 a, b, DUTTON et al. 1971, WILSON et al. 1972 b, c, LINDSAY and WILSON 1972, LINDSAY 1974) and an iron-sulfur protein associated with site I (OHNISHI et al. 1972 b) have been reported to have a midpoint potential which depends on the so-called phosphate potential, *i.e.*, the ratio of (ATP)/(ADP) (P_i) (*e.g.*, WILSON and DUTTON 1970 a, b, LINDSAY *et al.* 1972, DUTTON *et al.* 1972, WILSON *et al.* 1972 b, c). This dependence has been interpreted as indicating a primary involvement in the formation of a high energy intermediate.

The redox couples involved in cytochrome oxidase activity can be expressed as follows (the E_m values are those from WILSON *et al.* 1972 a, and LINDSAY and WILSON 1972):

4. $a^{2+} \rightleftharpoons a^{3+} + e^-$ $E_m = 190\,\mathrm{mv}$

5. $a_3^{2+} \rightleftharpoons a_3^{3+} + e^-$ $E_m = 385\,\mathrm{mv}$

6. $a_{3\sim}^{2+} \rightleftharpoons a_3^{3+} + e^-$ $E_m = 150\,\mathrm{mv}$

The $a_{3\sim}^{2+}$ represent the high energy form of a_3. From these figures it can be calculated that about 5.4 kcal would be available per electron transferred (23 kcal/v $\times$ 0.235 v).

In the case of cytochrome b_T the analysis using analogous equations would indicate that 270 mv would be available, or about 6 kcal per electron (using the values in WILSON *et al.* 1973).

7. $b_T{}^{2+} \rightleftharpoons b_T{}^{3+} + e^-$ $E_m = -30\,\mathrm{mv}$

8. $b_T{}^{2+} \rightleftharpoons b_{T\sim}{}^{3+} + e^-$ $E_m = 245\,\mathrm{mv}$

The changes in E_m produced by energization are consistent with the interpretation that they reflect the presence of a high energy form of the cytochrome. However, other interpretations are possible (see DE VAULT 1971, CASWELL 1971, WIKSTRÖM and BERDEN 1973, LAMBOWITZ and BONNER 1974, LAMBOWITZ *et al.* 1974). One possible interpretation is based on the possibility that the apparent change in E_m reflects reverse electron transport. In the case of cytochrome b, the chemical mediators used to couple the cytochromes to the platinum electrode interact with cytochrome c. Therefore, the equilibration could be taking place through cytochrome c by way of a coupling site. Under these circumstances the apparent change in ΔE_m could simply be the result of reverse electron transport. This view is supported by the block on the redox potential change brought about by antimycin (which blocks the transfer from cytochrome b to c) (DUTTON *et al.* 1972). In addition, it is supported by the failure to demonstrate a change in the apparent midpoint potential of cytochrome b in plant mitochondria (*e.g.*, DUTTON and STOREY 1971, LAMBOWITZ and BONNER 1974). Although the possibility that the coupling differs in the two kinds of mitochondria cannot be eliminated, this is rather unlikely since precisely the same cytochrome b species seem to be present in both systems. On the other hand, the dependence of the midpoint potential on the phosphate potential in succinate-cytochrome c reductase preparations (WILSON *et al.* 1971 a, 1972 a) and the isolated complex containing cytochromes b and c_1 (complex III) (RIESKE 1971) argues against an involvement of cytochrome c. The results can be interpreted also on the basis of a large potential across the mitochondrial membrane produced by the energization (see next paragraph). In the case of cytochrome b they can be interpreted also on the basis of a highly localized H^+ release by cytochrome b oxidation in the membrane (see WIKSTRÖM 1971 c) on the assumption that the coupling is driven by H^+ ions in the membrane (see Section 3 b below).

HINKLE and MITCHELL (1970) carried out potentiometric studies on the cytochrome oxidase part of the cytochrome chain. Ferri-ferrocyanide was used as the redox couple. Presumably, the ferri-ferrocyanide couple acts through cytochrome c which is situated on the surface of the inner membrane, since these reagents do not seem to penetrate and cytochrome c seems to be present at the surface (see Section A 3). When CO was used to remove the spectrophotometric interference of cytochrome a_3, addition of ATP caused cytochrome a to assume an apparent higher state of oxidation. This was interpreted to be the result of the ATP induced generation of a membrane potential, negative inside. The apparent half reduction potential (E_A) was considered to follow the relationship $E_A = E_m + \Delta\psi$, where E_m is the actual half reduction potential and $\Delta\psi$ the potential across the mitochondrial membrane. X is the fraction of the total membrane dielectric width at which the component is fixed. The shift in E_A was produced by the addition of K^- and valinomycin in a manner consistent with this formulation, assuming $\Delta\psi$ to correspond to the K^+ diffusion potential. The shift in redox potential was about half that expected, suggesting that X for this case is approximately $1/2$ (*i.e.*, cytochrome a is approximately in the middle of the membrane and a_3 would then be in the interior). Cytochromes c and c_1 were not affected by the diffusion potential, suggesting that they are on the outer surface. A somewhat more complex explanation can be used for the case of cytochrome b (see DUTTON and WILSON 1974). Cytochrome b can be assumed to have an increase in apparent redox potential by an interaction with an inner component. This component mediates from cytochrome c_1 electroneutrally and cytochrome c interacts with the added dye. The cytochrome b would be located close to the outer surface. As already discussed, other investigators (WILSON and DUTTON 1970 b, LINDSAY and WILSON 1972, LINDSAY 1974) ascribed the changes in E_m to a change of a_3 to a high energy form. CO was found to shift the apparent midpoint potential, an effect which was explained as an indirect effect of heme-heme interaction and the CO preferential binding to reduced cytochrome a_3.

The results obtained with submitochondrial particles (DUTTON *et al.* 1971, LINDSAY *et al.* 1972) were in general agreement with the results obtained with intact mitochondria (although only half of the system seems active). These results were not considered consistent with the effects of a membrane potential since presumably these vesicles are inside-out. However these difficulties for the chemiosmotic mechanism can be surmounted with more complex models (see DUTTON and WILSON 1974).

In summary, according to the chemiosmotic hypothesis, the half reduction potential changes can be explained at least in part on the basis of the nature of the mediating dye, the position of the component in the membrane and the pathway of interaction with the dye (see MITCHELL 1968, HINKLE and MITCHELL 1970).

If a respiratory chain component were involved in energy transduction the presence of two or more species of each of the cytochromes involved in a transducing step would be necessary, *i.e.*, various high energy or low energy forms. Evidence has been obtained for phosphate potential induced spectral changes in an oxidized cytochrome component of cytochrome oxidase (WILSON et al. 1972 b, ERECIŃSKA et al. 1972) and in reduced cytochrome a_3 (WIKSTRÖM and SARIS 1970, LINDSAY and WILSON 1972, LINDSAY 1974) of mitochondria. The changes are prevented by the presence of un-couplers or oligomycin. The shifts in the reduced forms of cytochrome a_3 probably are not the result of an oxidation-reduction reaction (LINDSAY and WILSON 1972).

Three distinct b cytochromes have been detected spectroscopically in mito-chondria and submitochondrial particles (*e.g.*, SLATER et al. 1970 a, b, WIK-STRÖM 1971 b, YU et al. 1972, see WIKSTRÖM 1973 for a review). One and perhaps two of these forms are affected by antimycin (see WIKSTRÖM 1971 b). The antimycin insensitive b cytochrome is reduced by substrates in coupled or uncoupled mitochondria or submitochondrial particles. The antimycin sensitive cytochrome b is readily reduced by substrates only in coupled particles and in the presence of ATP. The antimycin insensitive species has been referred to as cytochrome b_K (see CHANCE et al. 1970). The antimycin sensitive species is thought to be involved in energy transduction and has been referred to as cytochrome b_T. The different b cytochromes may not represent different molecular species but rather reflect differences in their environment or binding. The properties of cytochrome b, as reflected for example in its redox potentials (GOLDBERGER et al. 1962) have been found to be affected drastically by its binding.

Antimycin A is bound preferentially to cytochrome b_T in the energized state. In non-energized particles the binding is cooperative and it becomes non-cooperative in energized particles (BONNER and SLATER 1970, WEGDAM et al. 1970). The results obtained with antimycin A also suggest that more than one molecule of cytochrome b is involved in the energized state.

SLATER et al. (1970 b) and WEGDAM et al. (1970) have reported a red shift in the spectrum of cytochrome b upon energization. It presumably could correspond to the formation of a new species of cytochrome b_T. Other workers attribute these shifts to the combination of the spectral difference and the various redox potentials of the different b-cytochromes (WILSON and DUTTON 1970 b, SATO et al. 1971 a, b, WIKSTRÖM 1971 b, DUTTON 1971, DUTTON et al. 1972 b). Hence there is agreement from spectroscopy of more than one species of a cytochrome (energized and non-energized) only for cytochromes a and a_3.

The redox potential studies are consistent with the presence of high energy forms of cytochromes at sites II and III upon energization. In addition, spectroscopically detectable changes in cytochrome a and a_3 are consistent with the presence of high energy forms of cytochrome oxidase. Similar data are available also for the components associated with site I. This topic has been reviewed recently by OHNISHI (1973). The FeS proteins have been studied by EPR techniques and their characteristic redox potentials have been evaluated (OHNISHI *et al.* 1972 a, b, c). The half reduction potentials are listed in the diagram which illustrates their position in the respiratory chain (Fig. 11). The half reduction potentials show a large gap between center 1, 3, and between 4 and 2. This suggests the presence of phosphorylative site I between these centers. Center 1 a seems to have a potential which depends on the phosphate potential in a manner analogous to that of the cytochromes discussed (OHNISHI *et al.* 1972 b). The absence of at least part of the iron-sulfur proteins coincides with an absence of phosphorylation. Iron-sulfur proteins of site I and site II phosphorylation are absent in *S. cerevisiae* or *S. carlbergensis* unless they have been aerated during their stationary stage (see OHNISHI 1970). In *Candida utilis* (*Torulopsis utilis*) the iron-sulfur proteins are present normally in the stationary phase of growth along with site I, except when grown in media containing a low concentration of iron (LIGHT *et al.* 1968, OHNISHI *et al.* 1969, GARLAND 1970) or sulfur (HADDOCK and GARLAND 1971). Site I function and the iron-sulfur protein signal are re-established by growing the cell in a medium supplemented with sulfur or iron. The FeS signals and the NADH dehydrogenase complex present in the stationary phase are different from those present during the log phase of growth (see COBLEY *et al.* 1973).

2. Dissection of the Respiratory Assemblies and the Components Responsible for Coupling

The process of dissecting out the various components has reached the stage in which the major enzymatic activities can be associated with specific fractions obtained by sodium dodecyl sulfate-polyacrylamide gel electrophoresis (*e.g.*, see CAPALDI 1974).

The mitochondrial respiratory chain can be separated into four enzyme complexes (HATEFI *et al.* 1961 a, b, 1962 a, b, HATEFI 1966, FOWLER *et al.* 1962, ZIEGLER and DOEG 1962, see HATEFI *et al.* 1974 a). These complexes have been numbered I to IV. Complex I transfers reducing equivalents from NADH to ubiquinone, complex II from succinate to ubiquinone, complex III from ubiquinone to cytochrome c and complex IV, from cytochrome c to oxygen. Complex I and III can be recombined to form the NADH-cytochrome c reductase span, and complex II and III to form the succinic dehydrogenase-cytochrome c reductase span. The probable arrangement of the complexes in the mitochondria is represented in Fig. 14 (from HATEFI, unpublished).

Complex I contains $20^0/_0$ lipid. It can be separated into three other fractions which have not been reconstituted (HATEFI and STEMPEL 1967, DAVIS and HATEFI 1969). NADH dehydrogenase (HATEFI and STEMPEL 1967, 1969, HATEFI *et al.* 1969) is composed of FMN, Fe, and acid labile sulfur in a 1 : 4 : 4 stoichiometry. In addition, two other fractions can be isolated, an iron-sulfur protein and a fraction containing the bulk of the solids of complex I, which includes iron and acid labile sulfide. Liquid helium EPR spectroscopy suggests a total of four iron-sulfur centers, centers 1–4 (OHRME-JOHNSON *et al.* 1971) although probably five centers are present. All of these centers are reduced by NADH. Complex I also exhibits NADPH dehydrogenase activity in the absence of NADH. NADPH reduces FeS center 2 and partially 3 and 4, but not center 1 (HATEFI 1973, HATEFI and HANSTEIN 1973).

Complex II contains succinic dehydrogenase. The various components can be separated out and reconstituted (HANSTEIN *et al.* 1971, DAVIS and HATEFI 1972). In addition, it contains a cytochrome b (b_{557}, where the subscript

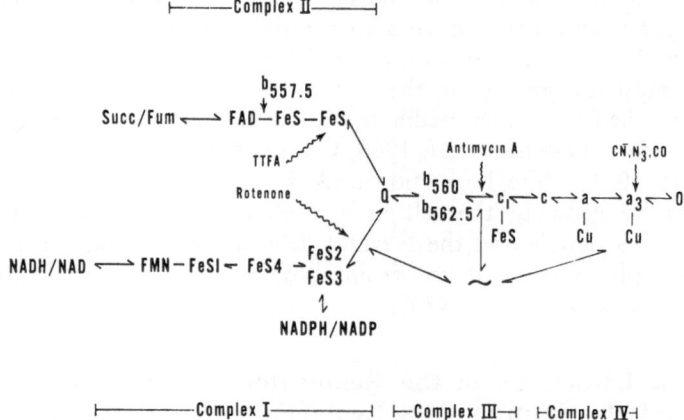

Fig. 14. The complexes of the mitochondrial respiratory chain. (Courtesy of Y. A. HATEFI.)

indicates the major α peak in nm at 77 °K) which is not succinate reducible but can be reduced by dithionite (DAVIS *et al.* 1972).

Two FeS proteins have been demonstrated in the span succinate-ubiquinone (designated S-1 and S-2 by OHNISHI *et al.* 1973, 1974 a, 1974 b; see also BEINERT and SANDS 1960). Recently BEINERT *et al.* (1974) demonstrated a third FeS protein associated with complex II. This FeS protein is of the high potential iron-sulfur protein type. OHNISHI *et al.* (1974 a) also reported on a high potential FeS protein (designated S-3, $E_m = 60 \pm 15$ mv) in soluble succinate dehydrogenase preparations. The concentrations of the S-1 and the S-2 components are approximately in the same concentrations as the flavin component (OHNISHI *et al.* 1974 a). The midpoint redox potentials were found to be -5 ± 15 mv for S-1 and -400 ± 15 mv for S-2.

Complex III contains equimolar amounts of cytochrome c_1 and two different kinds of cytochromes b (b_{560} and $b_{562.5}$) (DAVIS *et al.* 1972, 1973). Cytochrome b_{560} is reduced readily by substrates and cytochrome $b_{562.5}$ is reduced by substrates in the presence of antimycin A. They probably correspond to cytochrome b_K and b_T respectively (CHANCE *et al.* 1970). Another compound (chromophore 558, DAVIS *et al.* 1973) has also been detected spectrophotometrically in this complex.

Complex IV contains cytochrome oxidase, apparently constituted by cytochromes a and a_3 as well as Cu (*e.g.*, GRIFFITHS and WHARTON 1961 a, b).

Probably 2 Cu are present per heme (SLATER *et al.* 1965). Substrates reduce one of the coppers (SANDS and BEINERT 1959, GRIFFITHS and WHARTON 1961 a, b) and this reduction is blocked by cyanide which is equimolar to the heme. These experiments argue for a functional role of the copper in cytochrome oxidase. No signal can be detected for the second copper. The scheme discussed so far conforms to the representation of Fig. 14 and Table 15 (HATEFI *et al.* 1974).

Table 15. *Components of Complexes* I, II, III, and IV
(from HATEFI *et al.* 1974, used by permission)

Complex	Component	Concentration (per mg protein)
I. DPNH-Q reductase	FMN [1]	1.4–1.5 nmol
	nonheme iron	23–26 ng-atom
	labile sulfide	23–26 nmol
	ubiquinone	4.2–4.5 nmol
	lipids	0.22 mg
II. Succinate-Q reductase	flavin [2]	4.6–5.0 nmol
	nonheme iron	36–38 ng-atom
	labile sulfide	32–35 nmol
	cytochrome b	4.5–4.8 nmol
	lipids	0.2 mg
III. QH_2-cytochrome c reductase	cytochrome b	8.0–8.5 nmol
	cytochrome c_1	4.0–4.2 nmol
	nonheme iron	10–12 ng-atom
	labile sulfide	6–8 nmol
	ubiquinone	2–4 nmol
	lipids	0.4 mg
IV. Cytochrome c oxidase	cytochromes a, a_3	8.4–8.7 nmol
	copper	9.4 ng-atom
	lipid	0.35 mg

[1] Complex I contains no FAD.
[2] All the flavin of complex II is succinate dehydrogenase flavin.

Several proteins have been found to restore or enhance phosphorylation or the partial reactions of oxidative phosphorylation when added either individually or together to mitochondrial membrane preparations which can carry out respiration. Because of their probable involvement in the coupling between oxidation and phosphorylation, they have been called coupling factors. Ideally, they should restore activity in membrane preparations from which they have been removed by extraction procedures. A number of coupling factors have been isolated from mitochondria in recent years. Some of the coupling factors have ATPase activity (*e.g.*, F_1 and AD), one has been shown to catalyze ATP-P_i and ATP-ADP exchange reactions (Factor AD), and others have no demonstrable enzymatic activity of their own. The relationship between the various factors and the nature of their involvement in oxidative phosphorylation is not entirely clear (see SENIOR 1973, BEECHEY and CATELL 1973). There are indications that the oligomycin (and rutamycin) sensitive ATPase plays a most fundamental role in ATP synthesis (see TZAGOLOFF 1974, PENEFSKY 1974). For example, it is possible to reconstruct a system capable of carrying out oxidative phosphorylation from vesicles containing elements of the respiratory chain and the ATPase (RACKER and KANDRACH 1971). In addition, oligomycin completely blocks oxidative phosphorylation in intact mitochondria (LARDY et al. 1964, 1965), and anti-bodies to one of the ATPase components (F_1, see below) block phosphoryla-tion. For these reasons the view is beginning to emerge that the four com-plexes of the respiratory chain and the oligomycin sensitive ATPase may well represent the basic unit of oxidative phosphorylation in intact mito-chondria (see, e.g., MacLENNAN 1970 a, SENIOR 1973 a, TZAGOLOFF 1974).

The oligomycin sensitive ATPase is unable by itself to synthesize ATP or to catalyze exchange reactions. When incorporated into lipoprotein vesicles, it becomes capable of carrying out exchange reactions (e.g., ATP-P_i exchange, KAGAWA and RACKER 1971, KAGAWA et al. 1973) and ATP-driven H^+ translocation (KAGAWA et al. 1973).

PULLMAN et al. (1960) isolated a soluble ATPase (F_1) which increased the efficiency of phosphorylation in certain types of submitochondrial particles (PENEFSKY et al. 1960, see PENEFSKY 1974). Unlike mitochondrial phosphoryla-tion or mitochondrial membrane ATPase activity, F_1 was found to be insensi-tive to oligomycin and was inactivated rapidly by cold. Another protein, ex-tracted from the inner membrane of mitochondria confers oligomycin sensitivity on F_1 (RACKER 1964, KAGAWA and RACKER 1966). This protein has been named the oligomycin sensitivity conferring protein (OSCP). The properties of the oligomycin sensitive complex have been studied intensively in the past few years and the results have been reviewed recently (e.g., TZAGOLOFF 1971 a, SENIOR 1973, PENEFSKY 1974). The sensitivity of the complex to oligomycin depends probably on another protein as well (see below).

F_1 is part of the larger oligomycin sensitive liproprotein complex from which it can be extracted (TZAGOLOFF et al. 1968 a). Its involvement in the complex is shown by the fact that antibody against F_1 inactivates the oligo-mycin sensitive ATPase of submitochondrial particles (FESSENDEN and RACKER 1966, SCHATZ et al. 1967). The use of the anti-F_1 antibody also permits demonstrating that F_1 is required for the synthesis of ATP and the exchange reactions of the inner mitochondrial membrane (FESSENDEN and RACKER 1966, HINKLE et al. 1967). F_1 corresponds to a particle with a diameter 80 to 100 Å (RACKER et al. 1965, SCHATZ et al. 1967, RACKER and HORSTMAN 1967) which appears constituted by six subunits in hexagonal array.

Early studies using F_1 from beef heart (PENEFSKY and WARNER 1965) or from yeast (SCHATZ et al. 1967) suggested a molecular weight of about 285,000. Later studies suggest a much larger molecule, about 350,000 to 380,000 in molecular weight for beef heart (LAMBETH et al. 1971, KNOWLES and PENEFSKY 1972), rat liver (LAMBETH and LARDY 1971, CATTERALL and PEDERSEN 1971) and yeast (SCHATZ et al. 1967, SONE et al. 1969, TZAGOLOFF and MEAGHER 1971). Five different polypeptides ranging in molecular weight from approximately 7,000 to 60,000 have been separated out using sodium dodecyl sulfate (SDS) gel electrophoresis (see TZAGOLOFF 1971, SENIOR 1973). These have been numbered 1 to 5 (the lowest number corresponding to the highest molecular weight).

Five subunits are held together firmly in the F_1 complex. A sixth is bound more loosely (see SENIOR 1973 b, 1975). The complex has eight sulfhydryl groups and two disulfide bridges (i.e., twelve sulfhydryl groups when fully reduced). Of these twelve, eight are in subunit 1, two in subunit 2. Subunits 3 and 5 have one each. Subunits 2 and 4 have none. One disulfide bridge is thought to link subunits 3 and 5 and another disulfide bridge is thought to be present in subunit 1 (SENIOR 1975). It has been suggested that the subunits are present in beef heart ATPase in a stoichiometry of two subunits 1, two subunits 3 and two subunits 5, with 2 and 4 still unspecified (SENIOR 1975).

The stoichiometry suggested for rat liver ATPase proposes three subunits each for the two larger polypeptides (equivalent to 1 and 2) and one each for the lower molecular weight polypeptides (CATTERALL 1973, PEDERSEN et al. 1974).

The mitochondrial ATPase from beef heart mitochondria firmly binds three molecules of ATP and two of ADP per ATPase molecule (HARRIS et al. 1973). One of the two ADPs is bound loosely. PEDERSEN et al. (1974) have presented evidence supporting the concept that the high affinity ADP site is involved in phosphorylation and the low affinity site in ATP hydrolysis.

The oligomycin sensitivity conferring protein is about 18,000 in molecular weight (MACLENNAN and TZAGOLOFF 1968). Viewed with the electron microscope, it appears as a cylindrical particle 30 to 50 Å in diameter (MACLENNAN and ASAI 1968). No enzymatic activity has been detected for OSCP. However, as mentioned already it confers oligomycin or rutamycin sensitivity to F_1. OSCP functions as a link between F_1 and other proteins of the complex which are present in the inner membrane (MACLENNAN and TZAGOLOFF 1968). Studies with mutants of S. cerevisiae demonstrate that resistance and sensitivity to oligomycin depend on a mitochondrial membrane fraction other than OSCP. In reconstituted systems from wild type or oligomycin resistant mutants, the membrane fraction determined whether the system was oligomycin resistant (when the mutant membrane fraction was used) or sensitive (when the wild type membrane fraction was used) (SHANNON et al. 1973, GRIFFITHS and HOUGHTON 1974). Therefore, oligomycin resistance or sensitivity does not involve solely OSCP.

Mitochondria possess also an inhibitor of the ATPase. This inhibitor has been isolated from beef heart mitochondria (PULLMAN and MONROY 1963) and it has a molecular weight of about 10,000 (BROOKS and SENIOR 1971, NELSON et al. 1972). The inhibitor masks the ATPase activity of submitochondrial particles (RACKER and HORSTMAN 1967). It is effective in blocking the ATPase activity of either F_1 or the oligomycin sensitive ATPase complex (PULLMAN and MONROY 1963, TZAGOLOFF et al. 1968 a). After combining with the inhibitor, F_1 is no longer cold labile, indicating a stabilization of quaternary structure (PULLMAN and MONROY 1963). The function of the ATPase inhibitor is unknown. It may play a role in respiratory control (PULLMAN and MONROY 1963, HORSTMAN and RACKER 1970) or in the actual coupling to phosphorylation. The inhibitor has been isolated from beef heart. It inhibits the ATPase activity of beef heart, yeast and liver F_1. However, TZAGOLOFF (1971) reports being unable to isolate it from yeast and there are no reports of its isolation from liver mitochondria. The ATPase inhibitor dissociates from the ATPase when the ATP/ADP ratio is low and when electron transfer is taking place (VAN DE STADT et al. 1973) suggesting an involvement in the energy coupling mechanism.

Another protein, still unidentified, is required to reconstitute oligomycin sensitive-ATPase (BULOS and RACKER 1968, TZAGOLOFF 1970). It has been isolated but not purified (MACLENNAN and TZAGOLOFF 1968). It is thought to correspond to the component responsible for the attachment of the complex to the inner mitochondrial membrane. This protein may correspond to the factor which confers oligomycin sensitivity or resistance in wild type yeast or the mutants discussed above.

Two factors probably related to the oligomycin sensitive ATPase complex deserve some discussion. Factor AD (SANI et al. 1970, FISCHER et al. 1971) has a low ATPase activity and it catalyzes a low level of ATP-P_i exchange which is sensitive to oligomycin, 2,4 dinitrophenol and mercurials. Although the claim has been made that the factor is truly soluble (FISHER et al. 1972) this has been challenged by other workers who consider a small portion of the preparation vesicular. This vesicular portion could be responsible for the activity of the preparation which is relatively low (KAGAWA et al. 1973).

A complex catalyzing ATP-P_i exchange in the presence of phospholipid has been isolated from beef heart mitochondria (HATEFI et al. 1974 b) and has been named complex V. It resembles in polypeptide composition the oligomycin-sensitive ATPase. The ATP-P_i exchange is uncoupler sensitive and can be blocked by antibiotics known to inhibit phosphorylation (e.g., rutamycin).

3. Mechanisms of Oxidative Phosphorylation

The discussion of the coupling of the electron flow in the cytochrome chain to phosphorylation has been dominated in the past few years by the debate centered in part on the chemiosmotic model of oxidative phosphorylation. The arguments in favor of the model have been presented in detail in the review of GREVILLE (1969) to which the reader is referred. This model will be discussed in the section which follows (3 a) which examines the general question of the coupling of phosphorylation to the flow of ions in the direction of the electrochemical gradient. Alternative models have been currently considered by many investigators. Some of these involve a high energy state (Section 3 b), others involve the formation of high energy chemical intermediates, either in the formation of high energy covalent bonds or a high energy conformational state of protein components. The subject of oxidative phosphorylation has been thoroughly reviewed recently (SLATER

1974, BALTSCHEFFSKY and BALTSCHEFFSKY 1974). The chemical intermediate models together with the chemiosmotic model have been discussed in the reviews of SLATER (1971, 1974) (see Section 3 c).

a) Coupling by Ion Fluxes in the Direction of the Electro-Chemical Potential Gradient

The feasibility of coupling ionic flows in the direction of their electro-chemical gradient to phosphorylation is unquestionable. Much experimental evidence in a number of systems is consistent with this view. This evidence

Table 16. *ATP Synthesis by Ionic Flow*

System	References
Sarcoplasmic vesicles: Ca^{2+} efflux	KANAZAWA et al. 1970
	BARGOLIE and MAKINOSE 1971
	MAKINOSE 1971
	MAKINOSE and HASSELBACH 1971
	MAKINOSE 1972 a, b
	PANET and SELINGER 1972
	DEAMER and BASKIN 1972
Mitochondria: valinomycin induced K^+ efflux	COCKRELL et al. 1967
	MASSARI et al. 1972
Chloroplast fragments: H^+ flux	JAGENDORF and URIBE 1966
Bacteriorhodopsin and mitochondria ATPase vesicles	RACKER and STOECKENIUS 1974
Red blood cells K^+ efflux	GLYNN and LEW 1970
Thiobacillus novellus H^+ flux	COLE and ALEEM 1973

includes studies carried out with chloroplasts, isolated mitochondria, vesicles derived from the sarcoplasmic reticulum, red blood cells and a bacterial membrane system. These are listed in Table 16 with the appropriate references. Two of the systems, the sarcoplasmic reticulum and the reconstituted bacterial purple membrane system may be of particular significance for the understanding of mechanisms because of their simplicity. The sarcoplasmic reticulum enzyme, probable a single molecular species, is thought to correspond to 70 percent of the total membrane protein (INESI et al. 1973) although other estimates have ranged from 18 to 90 percent (MARTONOSI 1968, SELINGER et al. 1969, MACLENNAN 1970 b, McFARLAND and INESI 1971, MACLENNAN et al. 1971, MEISSNER and FLEISCHER 1971). The enzyme can be isolated and identified during fractionation procedures, either by its enzymatic activity [*i.e.*, Ca^{2+} dependent ATPase (see INESI et al. 1973)] or by its P^{32} label if incubated in the presence of labelled ATP (MARTONOSI and HALPIN 1971, MACLENNAN et al. 1971, MEISSNER and FLEISCHER 1971). The molecular weight appears to be in the neighborhood of 100,000 as shown by SDS gel electrophoresis (see INESI et al. 1973, HASSELBACH et al. 1973). The Ca^{2+} transport system can be reconstituted from the Ca^{2+}-ATPase and phospholipids (RACKER 1972, RACKER and EYTAN 1973, WARREN et al. 1974) or from disrupted vesicles (THE and HASSELBACH 1972, MEISSNER and FLEISCHER 1973, 1974). A number of experiments have shown that the Ca^{2+} pump can be run in reverse with the phosphorylation of the ATPase (KANAZAWA et al. 1971, YAMADA and TONOMURA 1972, YAMADA et al. 1972) or the synthesis of ATP from ADP and P_i (KANAZAWA et al. 1970, BARGOLIE and MAKINOSE 1971, MAKINOSE and HASSELBACH 1971, MAKINOSE 1972 a, b, PANET and SELINGER 1972, DEAMER and BASKIN 1972, HASSELBACH et al. 1973). Preliminary results with an apparently solubilized form of Ca^{2+}-ATPase of the sarcoplasmic reticulum suggest that ATP may be formed in vitro by an interaction of the enzyme with phosphate in the presence of Mg^{2+}, followed by Ca^{2+} treatment in the presence of ADP (KNOWLES and RACKER 1975). These findings suggest that the energized form of the enzyme has characteristic conformations corresponding to their energy state (in this case obtained with the Mg^{2+} and Ca^{2+} treatments). Similar results were obtained previously with a Na^+-K^+ ATPase preparation from guinea-pig liver. In this case, treatment with a low Na^+ concentration followed by high Na^+ and ADP results in the synthesis of ATP (TANIGUCHI et al. 1974).

The reconstitution of membrane vesicles from Holobacterium halobium with the oligomycin sensitive mitochondrial ATPase has more direct pertinence to the chemiosmotic model. The purple membrane appears to contain only one protein, bacteriorhodopsin (OESTERHELT and STOECKENIUS 1971). The reconstituted system picks up H^+ upon illumination. When it is reconstituted with the mitochondrial ATPase, the system is capable of photophosphorylation (RACKER and STOECKENIUS 1974).

Experiments carried out with vesicles derived from these bacteria suggest that illumination gives rise to membrane potentials detectable by the use of an electrofluorimetric cyanine dye (RENTHAL and LANYI 1975). The involvement of a membrane potential in photophosphorylation has been proposed for some time. A good deal of evidence has been presented in support of this point of view based on absorption changes of photosynthetic vesicles thought to correspond to electrochromic shifts (e.g., see JACKSON and CROFTS 1969, WITT 1971) and changes in potential in whole suspensions of vesicles monitored by macroelectrodes placed in different parts of the suspension (WITT and ZICKLER 1973, 1974, FOWLER and KOK 1974). Apart from the evidence collected in photosynthetic systems, in Neurospora there is evidence for electrogenic pumps powered by ATP (and hence the possibility of carrying out the reverse reaction) (see SLAYMAN et al. 1973).

These various experiments leave no doubt that ATP synthesis can take place by the transfer of ions from one compartment to another in the direction of their electrochemical gradient. Nevertheless, there is little evidence that this mechanism of phosphorylation plays a significant role in intact mitochondria.

The chemiosmotic hypothesis proposes a primary role for such a transducing system where the electrochemical gradient is constituted by a H^+ ion concentration gradient and a potential across the semipermeable membrane, the so-called *protonmotive force.* The model has been presented in detail in a series of articles (MITCHELL 1961, 1966 a, c, 1967, 1969 a, b, MITCHELL and MOYLE 1967 a, b, c) and monographs (MITCHELL 1966 b, 1968). A possible chemiosmotic molecular mechanism for the ATPase has been recently detailed (MITCHELL 1974, see also MITCHELL 1975, BOYER 1975). The electron transport is postulated to be responsible for the gradient in mitochondria by producing an efflux of protons. This is the consequence of an asymmetric

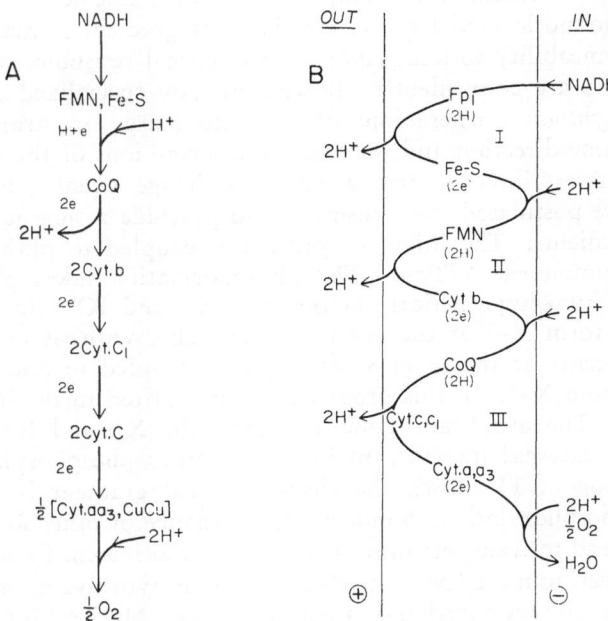

Fig. 15. Schemes for the arrangement of the various components of the respiratory chain. *A.* The generally accepted sequence. *B.* The sequence postulated by the chemiosmotic hypothesis. (From SLATER 1971, used by permission.)

proton discharge in the steps in which reduced H-carriers (*e.g.*, reduced CoQ or NADH) are oxidized by the electron carrying cytochromes. Presumably, there are three such steps or *loops* per cytochrome chain. In this way, 6 H$^+$ are separated between the internal and the external phase by the transfer of an electron pair from NADH to oxygen. The loops are represented diagrammatically in Fig. 15 *B*. The experimental evidence supports the possibility of producing protons in this manner. 6 H$^+$ have been reported to be released from rat liver mitochondria when β-hydroxybutyrate is used as a substrate and 4 H$^+$ when succinate is used, corresponding to 2 H$^+$ per ATP formed by coupled mitochondria (MITCHELL and MOYLE 1967 b). Similar results have been obtained with submitochondrial particles (HINKLE and HORSTMAN 1971). However, the stoichiometry may also be coincidental. The net influx of cations (*e.g.*, Ca^{2+}, Mg^{2+}, K$^+$ etc.) under the conditions used may well require the energy from three energy conserving sites in the appropriate stoichiometry (*i.e.*, 2 K$^+$/$\sim$ P or 1 Ca^{2+}/$\sim$ P). In the absence of sufficiently permeable anions the H^+ would have to leave the internal compartment to maintain electroneutrality (or alternatively a cationic pump may result in a H^+-cation exchange see Section C 4). Present evidence does not support the details of the sequence of the respiratory chain proposed in the chemiosmotic hypothesis (see SLATER 1971). Rather it is in agreement with the scheme presented in Fig. 15 A. The hypothesis could be modified easily to meet the proper sequence and satisfy the chemiosmotic requirement as well by intercalating other hypothetical redox components into the scheme.

In the chemiosmotic model the electrochemical gradient is maintained by a virtual impermeability to ions, i.e., a high electrical resistance of the membrane. Transfers are conveniently allowed only by specialized mechanisms, the so-called *symports*, where ions of opposite charge are transferred together in the same direction and the *antiports*, where ions of the same charge in the two phases, internal and external, exchange equally by exchange diffusion. These postulated mechanisms would preclude a significant dissipation of the gradients. The influx of protons is coupled to phosphorylation through an asymmetric ATPase. The phosphorylation takes place by the dehydration of two hypothetical components, X^- and IO^- (in conjunction with $2 H^+$) to form $X-I$ at the outer surface. The synthesis of ATP from ADP and P_i occurs at the inner surface and is coupled to and regenerates X^- and IO^- from $X-I$. In this process $2 H^+$ are shifted to the inside of the mitochondrion. The membrane potential forces the X^- and IO^- from the internal to the external interface to initiate another phosphorylative cycle. The translocation of H^+ down the electrochemical gradient is the driving force for the phosphorylation. Similarly, the exchange of other ions (e.g., K^+) for H^+ would lead to transport into the mitochondrial lumen. Experimentally, two H^+ have been found to be transferred per ATP hydrolyzed in the reverse reaction either by intact mitochondria (MITCHELL and MOYLE 1968) or by submitochondrial particles produced by sonication (THAYER and HINKLE 1973). In the submitochondrial particles the synthesis of ATP would involve the same stoichiometry presumably, but the protons would be transferred in the opposite direction since the particles behave as if they were inside out. This matter is discussed in Sections A 3 and C 4. Again, the transport of ions energized by the ATP hydrolysis by another mechanism could result in the same stoichiometry, in relation to H^+. The rate of oxidation of substrates is regulated by the magnitude of the *protonmotive force*. Dissipation of the *protonmotive force* (e.g., by uncouplers, which are presumed to increase the permeability to H^+, or by phosphorylation, which presumably transfers H^+ to the internal space) increases the respiratory rate. Conversely, the translocation of H^+ will stop when matched by a sufficiently high electrochemical gradient. Evidence against this portion of the chemiosmotic model will be discussed later in this section (p. 84–85).

The evidence pertinent to the presence of loops is still fragmentary. However, some of the components of the mitochondrial electron transport chain are thought to be localized in opposite sides of the inner mitochondrial membrane (e.g., KLINGENBERG and VON JAGOW 1970, LEE 1970, RACKER et al. 1970, SCHNEIDER et al. 1972, TINBERG et al. 1974, also see Section A 3) which may function as the postulated loops. The production of a proton gradient concomitant to the electron transport in the respiratory chain has been reported. Presumably, the H^+ leaving the mitochondria exchanges for other ions (MITCHELL and MOYLE 1967 b, c, MITCHELL 1967, 1969 a, b). The estimated H^+ gradient is not sufficient to support phosphorylation in exchange for H^+ influx. For this reason, it has been proposed that a potential across the mitochondrial membrane is responsible in part, for the electrochemical gradient. The membrane potential is the result of the charge imbalance caused by the H^+ efflux accompanying metabolism. Presumably, in intact mitochondria the inside phase would be negative. The steepness of the gradient, whether resulting from a membrane potential or a H^+ concentration gradient, can be expressed as an electric potential, and is shown in Equation 9 as done by MITCHELL. In his equation ΔP is the *protonmotive force*, $\Delta\Psi$ the membrane potential, R is the gas constant, T the temperature and F the Faraday.

$$9. \quad \Delta P = \Delta \Psi + 2.3 \frac{R\,T}{F} \Delta \mathrm{pH}$$

MITCHELL and MOYLE (1969 b), have estimated the total *protonmotive force* to be approximately 230 mv (see also NICHOLLS 1974). Much lower values have been derived by other authors (see below). The actual *protonmotive force* which would be needed for phosphorylation depends on the concentration of the various components. Under state 4 conditions (in which ATP, ADP, and P_i have equilibrated with the system) it has been estimated to be between — 370 and — 380 mv (SLATER 1971). Calculations based on more up-to-date ΔG^c for ATP synthesis (ROSING and SLATER 1972) estimate the required force to be in the neighborhood of — 320 mv. Values calculated from the ATP, ADP and P_i concentrations determined experimentally under conditions used to estimate the *protonmotive force* arrive at somewhat lower figures (NICHOLLS 1974). Since the pH component is necessarily limited, a large portion of the protonmotive force would have to correspond to the membrane potential. However, biological membranes generally are not able to support a potential much in excess of 200 mv. The membranes of squid and lobster axons break down at a potential of approximately — 150 to — 200 mv (COLE and MOORE 1960, JULIAN et al. 1962). *Chara* and *Nitella* cells exhibit a similar effect at approximately — 300 mv (COSTER 1965). This effect is probably a general property of lipid containing membranes since lipid bilayers (phosphatidyl choline$^+$ in tetradecane) also break down at approximately — 200 mv (HUANG et al. 1964, MIYAMOTO and THOMPSON 1967).

Evidence for a potential across the mitochondrial semi-permeable membrane is scant. Perhaps the most convincing evidence stems from experiments using the electrofluorometric dye 3,3'-dipropylthiodicarbocyanine (LARIS et al. 1975, see discussion below). Some data have been presented on the influx or efflux upon energization of highly permeable organic cations or anions present in very low concentrations (GRINUS et al. 1970, BAKEEVA et al. 1970). The expulsion of a cation (*e.g.*, in inside-out submitochondrial particles) is interpreted as the consequence of a potential, inside positive. Similarly, the expulsion of an anion (*e.g.*, in mitochondria) is interpreted as the result of the development of a membrane potential, inside negative. Exchanges of cations and anions are expected as the consequences of the H^+ ion exchanges and in fact are considered part and parcel of the exchange in the MITCHELL hypothesis even when no membrane potential is developed. In addition, in at least some experiments (see MASSARI *et al.* 1972) the results are consistent with the notion that the organic anions are transferred together with a cation. The data presently available from these exchanges cannot be construed as evidence for a membrane potential.

MITCHELL and MOYLE (1969 b) estimate the membrane potential from the distribution of K^+ induced by valinomycin. The calculation is based on the assumption that the distribution of K^+ is the consequence of a large increase in the permeability of K^+ induced by the valinomycin. Presumably, this results in a Donnan distribution of the K^+, imposed by the large potential across the mitochondrial membrane (assumed to be negative inside). These estimates are the result of faulty application of theory since the data can be quantitatively explained in the absence of an electrogenic process. In the presence of valinomycin, K^+ exchanges stoichiometrically for H^+ in a metabolically dependent process (MITCHELL and MOYLE 1969 b). The increase in internal non-diffusible negative charges which is neutralized by the K^+ correspond to the fixed charges of the Donnan formulation. Hence the K^+ distribution should follow a Donnan ratio quantitatively without an electrogenic pump. Under conditions of high K^+ permeability (*e.g.*, in the presence of valinomycin), a diffusion potential determined by the internal and external K^+ concentrations and following the Nernst equation is likely to be present. However, this should not express itself under normal *in situ* conditions.

Other assumptions are also questionable. For example, the results seem identical regardless of the coupling state of mitochondria. In the experiment reported in Fig. 6 of MITCHELL and MOYLE (1969 b) the respiratory rate of the mitochondria in the presence of 100 µg valinomycin gm protein^{-1} is 60 natoms min^{-1} (mgm protein)$^{-1}$. This rate is about 5 times the control rate shown in the figure, a rate greater than in the presence of the uncoupler, carbonylcyanide p-trifluoromethoxyphenylhydrazone (FCCP), in other experiments (*e.g.*, Fig. 7 of MITCHELL and MOYLE 1969 b). Despite this high degree of uncoupling the results are comparable to those obtained in other experiments where the rate of respiration was much lower.

The effect of the valinomycin and the mechanism controlling the distribution of ions is likely to be more complex. The net passage of K^+ induced by valinomycin is accompanied by either anions (*e.g.*, HARRIS and PRESSMAN 1969, ROSSI *et al.* 1967, BRIERLEY 1970) or by a counterflow of H^+ (*e.g.*, MITCHELL and MOYLE 1969 a). Therefore, the findings are not in agreement with a mechanism by which valinomycin simply increases the permeability of K^+. In fact, there are some indications that the effect of valinomycin in biological systems may be complex (TELFER and BARBER 1974). A simple non-specific interaction of valinomycin with the lipid component of the membrane suggested by the model of MITCHELL and MOYLE (1969) also appears rather unlikely from the finding of valinomycin-resistant mito-chondrial mutants (GRIFFITHS et al. 1974). Other results are also in dis-agreement with some of the assumptions used in the calculations of membrane potential. The proposed mechanism of distribution requires that in the steady state the K^+ concentration ratios between the inside and outside phases be solely dependent on the hypothesized membrane potential and independent of valinomycin concentration. This independence has been, in fact, reported by MITCHELL and MOYLE (1969 b; see Fig. 6 of reference) and ROTTENBERG (1973). Other results, however, are not in agreement with this interpreta-tion (ROTTENBERG and SOLOMON 1969, MASSARI et al. 1972 b) which is a basic assumption of this approach (see also discussion on p. 97–100).

The assumptions used to calculate membrane potentials in mitochondria by the use of valinomycin are questionable. In addition, studies carried out with the same approach are not in agreement. MITCHELL and MOYLE (1969 b) estimated in intact mitochondria by measurement of H^+ efflux and the K^+-induced valinomycin uptake, a total *protonmotive force* of — 230 mv in state 4. This gradient would not be sufficient to produce 1 ATP per 2 H^+ transferred in the direction of the gradient. Recent estimates of *protonmotive force* using similar methods are in agreement with a value of about — 230 mv (NICHOLLS 1974). This is below the size of the phosphate potential estimated under conditions identical to those used to estimate the *protonmotive force* (NICHOLLS 1974).

With the exception of the recent study of NICHOLLS (1974) mentioned already, results obtained after those of MITCHELL and MOYLE generally support much lower estimates of *protonmotive force*. The *protonmotive force* was estimated by a similar approach by PADAN and ROTTENBERG (1973), to be approximately — 130 to — 150 mv in state 4. Similarly, an earlier study of ROTTENBERG (1970), under somewhat different conditions, estimates an electrochemical potential across the mitochondrial membrane of about — 63 mv. Under these latter conditions, according to ROTTENBERG, about — 105 mv would be required for the synthesis of 1 ATP for each transfer of 2 H^+.

The data do not fit the theory quantitatively even accepting the question-able assumptions proposed by MITCHELL and MOYLE. Similar low estimates of presumed *protonmotive force* have been presented by MASSARI and AZZONE (1970). For these reasons, it becomes necessary to consider whether the apparent agreement between the data of MITCHELL and MOYLE (1969 b) and the chemiosmotic hypothesis may be coincidental. The quantitative dis-agreement between their estimates and that of others using similar assump-tions (e.g., ROTTENBERG 1970) suggests that this might well be the case. Perhaps this problem could be clarified using some disrupted preparation derived from mitochondria. It should be noted that if valinomycin induces the active transport of K^+ by a carrier mechanism as proposed by others the equations governing the steady state may well be directly related to the parameters expressed by the equation used to calculate the presumed mem-brane potential. The energy requirement of transport per mole transported is also expressed by the log of the (K^+) concentration gradient [*i.e.,* $\Delta G = 2.3\,RT\,\Delta \log(K^+)$ or, expressed as an electric potential, $\Delta E = 2.3\,RT/F\,\Delta \log(K^+)$]. Although the valinomycin experiments cannot be considered evidence for a membrane potential, it should be noted that a carrier mechanism would find it difficult to explain the relationship between the K^+ gradient (presumably corresponding to a diffusion potential) and the

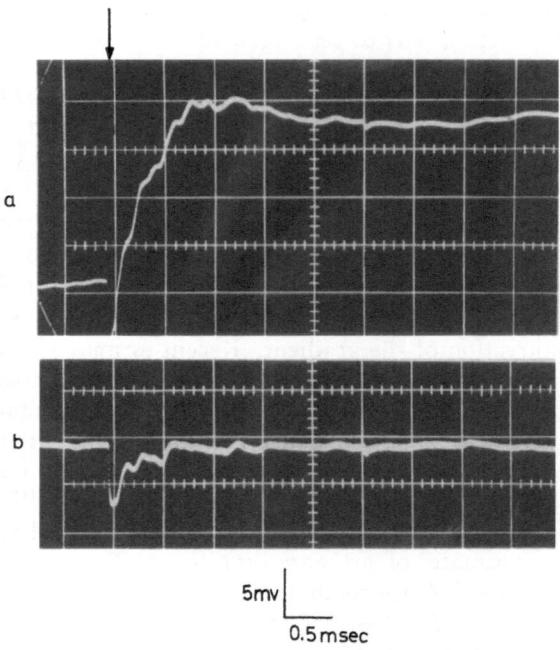

5mv
0.5 msec

Fig. 16. Oscilloscope tracing of a piezoelectrically controlled impalement of a giant *Drosophila* mitochondrion. Experiments of J. T. Tupper and H. Tedeschi. Part a. A record of the potential as a function of time. Part b Control: activation of the device without impalement. The arrow indicates the activation of the piezoelectric device used to advance the microelectrode. (From Tedeschi 1971 a.)

capacity to phosphorylate in the presence of valinomycin found by Rotten-berg (1970). However uncoupling effects of K^+ in the presence of valinomycin have been reported at similar concentrations (see Mitchell and Moyle 1969 b, p. 479), independently of its presumed effects on *protonmotive force*.

Other approaches have led to entirely different estimates of membrane potentials. Harris and Pressman (1969), have calculated membrane potentials in liver mitochondria from the anion concentrations assuming a Donnan distribution of the anions. These potentials are much smaller than those predicted from the Mitchell hypothesis. In addition they are of reversed polarity (inside positive) and relatively independent of metabolism. They correspond closely to those estimated with microelectrodes in *Drosophila* mitochondria (see below). Similar calculations can be made from the distribution of the permeant cation methylamine (Harris and Bassett 1972). In addition to providing evidence for a membrane potential, positive inside, these distributions are difficult to explain with the chemiosmotic model.

Tupper and Tedeschi (1969 a, b, c), using microelectrodes in giant *Drosophila* mitochondria, have observed potentials in the range of 10 to 20 mv, with the inside positive. A fast sweep oscilloscope tracing is shown in Fig. 16 (from Tedeschi 1971 a, data of Tupper and Tedeschi). The piezoelectric

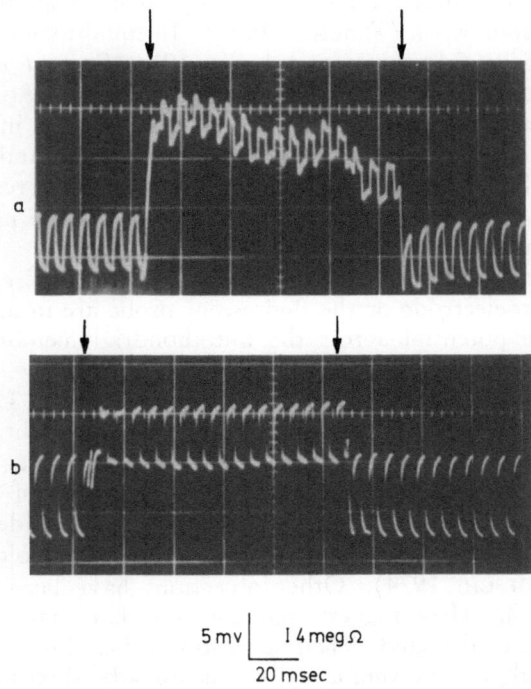

5 mv   1 4 meg Ω

20 msec

Fig. 17. Oscilloscope tracings of mitochondrial impalements. The arrows indicate first the activation of the piezoelectric device advancing the microelectrode. The second arrow indicates the withdrawal of the electrode. The faster deflections correspond to current pulses used to estimate the membrane resistance. (From Tupper and Tedeschi 1969 a.)

device which moves the microelectrode was triggered at the arrow. Trace a of the figure represents the record from the impalement of a mitochondrion. Trace b of the figure corresponds to a control in which the electrode is advanced without impalement. After impalement, the potential (about 20 mv, inside positive) did not decay significantly with time. A decay can be detected however with repeated impalements (Tedeschi 1971, data of Tupper and Tedeschi) and a potential is recorded until the mitochondria appear with phase contrast microscope to be damaged. A record of an impalement for both the membrane potential and the resistance is shown in Fig. 17. The heigths of the pulses in the record are inversely proportional to the resistance. The results show that the resistance and the potential increase as a result of the empalement (first arrow). They return to their original values upon withdrawal of the electrode (second arrow). The potentials do not vary significantly with metabolic conditions (Tupper and Tedeschi 1969 b). They are quantitatively predictable from the ratio of internal to external organic anions (Tupper and Tedeschi 1969 c and Tedeschi 1971 a) and they vary predictably with osmotically active volume (Tupper and Tedeschi 1969 a). For these reasons they are likely to reflect closely the potentials across the mitochondrial membrane. Results of experiments carried out with *Drosophila* mitochondria using the fluorescent probe 3,3′-dihexyl-2,2′-oxacarbocyanine (CC_6) are in agreement with the microelectrode work (Tedeschi 1974). In squid axons (Cohen et al. 1974), red blood cells (Hoffman and Laris 1974, Sims et al. 1974) and synaptosomes (Goldring and Blaustein 1973) the fluorescence of cyanine dyes reflects the membrane potentials. The fluorescence of CC_6 in the presence of the mitochondria is affected by anion concentration and the osmotic pressure of the medium in a way which closely parallels the results observed with microelectrodes. It is not significantly affected by the metabolic state of the mitochondria.

Therefore in mitochondria isolated from *Drosophila*, the results obtained with either the microelectrode or the fluorescent probe are in agreement with the notion that the potential across the mitochondrial membrane plays no role in phosphorylation.

The microelectrode findings have been questioned by Liberman and Skulachev (1970) on the grounds that the measured membrane resistance of the mitochondria is too low compared to that postulated by them and Mitchell. However, as previously noted the magnitude of the resistance (minimally estimated as 1–2 Ω cm² calculated without considering the convolutions as part of the surface area) is not unusual in biological systems (see discussion, Tedeschi 1974). Other objections have been presented by Lassen et al. (1971). They suggest that the mitochondrial potential must decay too rapidly to be detected. Their suggestion is based on the rapid decay they find in Ehrlich ascites tumor cells. As already discussed (Tedeschi 1974) the rapid decay has not been found in other studies and may represent an artifact of their experiments. We do not find a rapid decay at least in the time scale we have examined (see Fig. 16).

Laris et al. (1974) observed changes in the fluorescence of the dye 3,3′-dipropylthiocarbocyanine [diS-C_3(5)] accompanying changes in metabolic states in hamster liver mitochondria. The changes in fluorescence accompany energization with succinate or ATP and can be inhibited with the appropriate uncoupler or metabolic block. The system was calibrated using the fluorescence in the presence of valinomycin at various external concentrations of KCl. The conclusion was reached that energization induces potentials of the order of 150–180 mv, inside negative. This study is important because it is the first estimate of a negative membrane potential using an indirect technique which does not use valinomycin in the experimental suspensions. As already discussed, in the presence of valinomycin the results can be interpreted without invoking a metabolically induced membrane potentials. The results of Laris et al. (1975) do conflict with those obtained by Tedeschi (1974) with *Drosophila* mitochondria using a similar dye. Undoubtedly further studies will clarify this contradiction. It should be noted, however, that an interpretation of these results also does not require the assumption of a membrane potential. The mechanism of the fluorescence change is thought to correspond to a quenching dependent on the internal concentration of the dye (SIMS *et al.* 1974). One possible interpretation of the data would invoke a redistribution of the dye imposed by a metabolically induced membrane potential, as done with lipid soluble ions by other investigators (*e.g.*, see LIBERMAN and SKULACHEV 1970) and proposed by LARIS *et al.* However, the redistribution could occur as an exchange of the cation for H$^+$ without the involvement of either a change in the potential across the mitochondrial membrane or by an anionic pump. Non-specific cation transport can occur as the consequence of anion translocation (*e.g.*, see BRIERLEY 1974, LEHNINGER 1974) as discussed in Section C 4 a.

Aside from the observations already discussed a number of others are not consistent with the chemiosmotic model. In the presence of valinomycin, as many as 3 to 4 K$^+$ are transported per high energy bond (COCKRELL *et al.* 1966, ROSSI and AZZONE 1969, 1970, AZZONE and MASSARI 1971) or per 2 H$^+$ exchanged (AZZONE and MASSARI 1971) rather than the 2 required by the chemiosmotic model. This point will be discussed in more detail in the section on transport of ions (C 4).

The chemiosmotic hypothesis (MITCHELL 1961, MITCHELL and MOYLE 1965) predicts that uncouplers produce a collapse of the electrochemical gradient by acting as proton carriers. There are in fact indications that uncouplers such as FCCP accelerate the decay of the H$^+$ gradient in mitochondria at least under some conditions (*e.g.*, MITCHELL and MOYLE 1967 a, b, c, 1968). In addition, uncouplers appear to increase the conductivity of artificial bimolecular lipid membranes (BIELAWSKI *et al.* 1966, SKULACHEV *et al.* 1967, 1968, LIBERMAN and TOPALY 1968, HOPFER *et al.* 1968). The results agree with the notion that the increase in conductivity is primarily the result of an increase in the flow of H$^+$ or OH$^-$ ions (HOPFER *et al.* 1968). However, the uncoupling activity of a variety of uncouplers at various pHs does not match their ability to increase the conductivity of artificial lipid layers (WILSON *et al.* 1971 b). Similarly, at least in the case of 2,4-dinitrophenol and trinitrophenol, the uncoupling ability does not parallel their effect on the H$^+$ conductivity of submitochondrial particles (HANSTEIN and HATEFI 1974 b). In these experiments the H$^+$ gradient is generated by introducing a pulse of substrate (NADH) and the H$^+$ conductivity is estimated by the time course of the equilibration of the H$^+$. The ability of uncouplers to increase H$^+$ conductivity does not seem to be a suitable explanation for their effect in the uncoupling of oxidative phosphorylation. In addition, there is considerable evidence that uncouplers act on the protein components of mitochondria and not lipids. The binding of substituted phenols to mitochondria is not altered significantly by extraction of the lipid components. Furthermore, the protein residue binds the uncouplers in a manner entirely similar to intact mitochondria (WEINBACH and GARBUS 1965). In addition, photoaffinity labelling of the uncoupler, 2-azido-4-dinitrophenol, results in covalently binding the uncoupler to a protein component of the mitochondria inner membrane

(HANSTEIN and HATEFI 1974 a, HATEFI *et al.* 1974 b) of a molecular weight of about 29,000. The complex isolated by HATEFI *et al.* (1974 b), complex V, which catalyzes ATP-P$_i$ exchange is enriched in binding sites for the uncoupler 2-azido 4-nitrophenol, again suggesting that uncoupling is not the result of an unspecific interaction of the uncouplers with the lipid components of the membrane. Similar results have been obtained labelling with the uncoupler, 2,4-dinitrophenol-5-(bromoacetoxyethoxy) phenol which covalently binds to sulfhydryl groups (COPELAND *et al.* 1974). The probable involvement of protein components in the action of uncouplers is also supported by the finding of uncoupler resistant mitochondria in yeast mutants (GRIFFITHS *et al.* 1972).

These results support the notion that uncouplers interact with protein components on mitochondria and that the action of the uncouplers is intimately involved with the formation of high energy intermediates and not some indirect effect on the mitochondrial internal membrane. The results of other studies are less clear.

Uncouplers may have effects on soluble systems. 2,4-dinitrophenol has been reported to increased the activity of soluble ATPase from mitochondria (*e.g.*, PENNIAL 1960, PULLMAN *et al.* 1960, SELWYN 1967, AKIMENKO 1971, CANTLEY and HAMMES 1973). The revelance of the effect of uncouplers on the ATPase in relation to the chemiosmotic model is difficult to evaluate and the results of the various experiments are difficult to compare. The activation is generally but not always small and the concentrations of DNP used vary significantly from one study to another. AKIMENKO (1971) present data suggesting that the DNP effect is the result of the release of an inhibition of the ATPase by ADP. They infer that the effect of DNP is unrelated to its uncoupling action in agreement with recent results (PEDERSEN 1974), which show that other uncouplers do not activate purified ATPase, suggesting that the DNP activation is unrelated to its uncoupling activity.

The effects of uncouplers on a soluble preparation [a combination of factor A and D of SANADI catalyzing ATP-P$_i$ and ATP-ADP exchange (FISHER *et al.* 1971)] have been studied in this respect. The ATP-P$_i$ exchange is inhibited by uncouplers and oligomycin. However, the absence of membranes from these preparations has been challenged (KAGAWA *et al.* 1973).

The synthesis of ATP has been claimed to occur in disrupted or soluble systems either on the basis of the occurrence of actual ATP synthesis from ADP and P$_i$ (COLE and ALEEM 1973, HUNTER *et al.* 1974) or the presence of exchange reaction thought to be part of the ATP synthesizing system. The ADP-P$_i$ exchange in chloroplast coupling factor (*e.g.*, FORTE *et al.* 1972) or the ATP-P$_i$ exchange have been reported in lysolecithin treated mitochondrial preparation lacking vesicles (KOMAI *et al.* 1973) or in soluble mitochondrial factors (FISHER *et al.* 1971). These data have been considered by some investigators to be incompatible with the chemiosmotic hypothesis (*e.g.*, GREEN 1974). However, the presence of exchange reactions in the absence of membranes does not invalidate the chemiosmotic model. For example, the formation of ATP itself may not require energy (see p. 88

below), but its release might. Hence, the exchange reactions may not be pertinent in this respect. Similarly, the presence of high energy intermediates does not necessarily contradict the chemiosmotic model which is only concerned with the primary mechanism of energy conservation. In contrast, any observation of the synthesis of free ATP by soluble factors, or in the absence of vesicular elements would indeed invalidate the hypothesis. However, it is difficult to establish beyond reproach the absence of vesicles by indirect methods. The results of electron microscopy are too dependent on preparatory procedures. It would not be surprising that some membranes survived the extensive disruptive procedures and in addition, were labile in relation to the fixatives used. The preparation derived from *Thiobacillus novellus* (COLE and ALEEM 1973) was deemed soluble because some of the ATP synthesizing system would not sediment when centrifuged at 300,000 G for 3 hours. However, the published electron micrograph (for the particles not sedimentable at 144,000 for 3 hours) does not permit excluding the presence of large particles or vesicles. The lack of sedimentation could be the result of the association of the phosphorylating system with lipid components of low density.

Similar objections can be raised in the case of lysolecithin treated electron transport particles (HUNTER *et al.* 1974), although when viewed with the electron microscope the particles do not seem to show vesicular elements. The preparation is not uncoupled by valinomycin added in the presence of nigericin. The lack of uncoupling in the presence of both antibiotics suggests at least malfunction of the membrane but does not necessarily prove its absence.

In experiments with mitochondria (MASSARI and AZZONE 1972 b) and submitochondrial particles (AZZONE and MASSARI 1972) the permeability of the semi-permeable membrane has been altered by experimental treatment (*e.g.*, hypotonicity and calcium phosphate treatment in the case of mitochondria and sonication in the case of submitochondrial particles). These studies claim that the energy linked functions of these treated particles remain. In the case of the mitochondria, this claim is based on the ability of mitochondria to shrink in the presence of ATP. In the case of the submitochondrial particles it is based on the retained capacity to respond appropriately during energization in the presence of dyes (*e.g.*, to exhibit a change in fluorescence during energization in the presence of ANS). However, the energization data is not presented in the reports, and the shrinkage induced by ATP in the treated mitochondria may well be unrelated to energy coupling. In the absence of more direct or detailed data a critical evaluation will have to wait further developments.

However, other data on the coupling of energy to various reactions can be marshalled to argue against the chemiosmotic hypothesis. The obligatory dependence on an electrochemical gradient for the coupling would necessarily make each coupling site completely equivalent. In the chemiosmotic model, phosphorylation does not take place in specific locations associated with the cytochrome chain. Indeed, experiments have demonstrated that the energy captured at one site in the cytochrome chain can be used to drive a reaction in another portion of the cytochrome chain (see ERNSTER and LEE 1964). However, there are indications of specific coupling sites in specific locations in the cytochrome chain as shown by the differences in the coupling at the different sites. For example, 2,4-dinitrophenol (KATYARE et al. 1971) as well as chlorophenoxyisobutyrate (PANINI and KURUP 1974) have a differential uncoupling effect on the three phosphorylative sites. The inhibitor hydroxylamine (WIKSTRÖM 1971) preferentially inhibits site III in submitochondrial particles derived from beef heart. Similarly, iron sulfur deficient mitochondria lack site I phosphorylation which can be readily restored by adding the missing sulfur or iron in the culture medium. The deficient mitochondria are unable to reduce NAD using glycerophosphate as a substrate (GARLAND 1970). The non-equivalence of the various phosphorylative sites is also supported by experiments on the kinetics of state 4 to 3 transition (VELDSEMA-CURRIE and SLATER 1970). Ubiquinone becomes more reduced first, then more oxidized, indicating that the reactivity of site I is probably greater than site II or III.

Similar implications come from studies of ATP driven succinate linked NAD^+ reduction and nicotinamide nucleotide transhydrogenase reactions carried out with submitochondrial particles. 2,4-dinitrophenol (DANIELSON and ERNSTER 1963), FCCP, oligomycin (ERNSTER et al. 1973) and aurovertin (LENAZ 1965, ROBERTON et al. 1968) inhibit the NAD reduction more effectively than the transhydrogenase reaction. This is to be expected since the energy requirement for the former is greater. However, the ATPase inhibitor used inhibits the two equally. The complexing of the inhibitor seems to be tight and can be varied by increasing its concentration (ERNSTER et al. 1973). In the chemiosmotic hypothesis a graded inhibition with these characteristics should affect the less favorable reaction more. Aurovertin affects ATP requiring reactions, differently from those of oxidative phosphorylation. This differential effect is difficult to explain on the basis of the chemiosmotic hypothesis. Aurovertin binds to F_1 on a one to one basis (BERTINA et al. 1973). It has effects similar to oligomycin in blocking oxidative phosphorylation, ATP-P_i exchange and O^{18} exchange between P_i, and H_2O (LARDY et al. 1964). The effects of aurovertin also have several other distinct features. Oligomycin inhibitors the ATP protection against P_i swelling, the shrinkage of mitochondria induced by ATP and the swelling induced by ATP under some conditions. In contrast, aurovertin does not affect these activities at concentrations at which oxidative phosphorylation is inhibited (CONNELLY and LARDY 1964), nor does it block the transport of Ca^{2+} (LENAZ 1965). The swelling of the mitochondria is presumed to be the consequence of the transport of ions (see ANAGNOSTI and TEDESCHI 1970, IZZARD and TEDESCHI 1970, IZZARD and TEDESCHI 1973). The chemiosmotic model would predict equal interference for oxidative phosphorylation and transport, since both depend on the *protonmotive force*.

As already mentioned, in the chemiosmotic model the driving force for respiration is the dissipation of the electrochemical gradient (*i.e.*, the dissipation of the *protonmotive force*) by the energy utilizing reactions. Accordingly, an increase in phosphorylation or a dissipation induced by an uncoupler should increase respiration by decreasing the electrochemical gradient. The independence of the respiratory rate on the presumed *protonmotive force* under phosphorylating conditions does not support the chemiosmotic concept. ROTTENBERG (1970) exposed mitochondria to various concentrations of K^+ in the presence of valinomycin and under phosphorylative conditions. If valinomycin makes the system much more permeable to K^+ than to other ions, the procedure should produce a K^+ diffusion potential predictable by the use of the Nernst equation. In this study the H^+ concentration gradient was calculated from the distribution of 5,5-dimethyl-2,4-oxozolidinedione (DMO). The decrease in the apparent electrochemical gradient produced by increasing the external K^+ results in a decrease in phosphorylative capacity, qualitatively consistent with the chemiosmotic hypothesis. As already discussed the presumed *protonmotive force* is about half what is needed for phosphorylation. In addition, there is no increase in respiration regardless of the reduction of the electrochemical gradient. These two findings are irrevocably inconsistent with the chemiosmotic hypothesis. In a similar study, PADAN and ROTTENBERG (1973), estimate the total presumed *protonmotive force* under phosphorylative conditions (state 3) in the presence of valinomycin. The H^+ concentration gradient was calculated from the distribution of 5,5-dimethyl-2,4-oxozolidinedione and the membrane potential calculated from the valinomycin induced potassium distribution. The expected dependence of respiration on the calculated *protonmotive force* was found for the uncoupling effects of 2,4-dinitrophenol and valinomycin plus gramicidin but not for the case of phosphorylation (state 3). The authors conclude that the results are not compatible with the chemiosmotic hypothesis in its present form. However the reported results are not in agreement with two other studies (MITCHELL and MOYLE 1969 b, NICHOLS 1974).

b) Other Models of Coupling Involving High Energy States

The previous section examined the possibility that the flow of ions in the direction of their electrochemical gradient is coupled to the phosphorylative process. In particular the discussion focused on the chemiosmotic model of MITCHELL. Other proposals not involving the formation of high energy intermediates have also been presented and they will be briefly examined in this section. WILLIAMS (1961, 1969, 1972, 1974) proposes a separation of H^+ and OH^- brought about by respiration similar to that of the chemiosmotic hypothesis. However, the H^+ is formed in the membrane phase. The phosphorylation of ADP can be regarded as a dehydration, as follows:

$$ADP - OH + HOP \rightleftharpoons ADPOP + H_2O$$

H^+ intervenes in the phosphorylation by removing H_2O already present in low concentrations in the membrane phase (to form H_3O). Actually since the reaction shown above takes up H^+ (not shown in the equation), the accumulation of H^+ in a hydrophobic phase could also push the reaction toward ATP synthesis.

AZZONE (1972) proposes an ill defined activated membrane state. GREEN and JI (1972 a, b, 1973) and GREEN (1974) in their *electromechanochemical* model link phosphorylation to the separation of charges across the mitochondrial membrane caused by a proton flow resulting from respiration. These shifts lead to the formation of P_i^+ (bound to an hypothetical protein component) and $ADPO^-$. The combination of P_i^+ and $ADPO^-$ leads to ATP synthesis. Similar exchanges can lead to ion transport. The mechanism is accompanied by conformational changes of the molecules constituting a single functional unit of electron transport and phosphorylation. The model attempts to coordinate most of the recent observations on mitochondrial behaviour. However, several features of the model are vague, at times unnecessarily detailed and in part contradictory. Generally, it does not further understanding or provide a useful framework for formulating new experiments. The contradictions make it very difficult to evaluate. For example, GREEN and JI (1972 b) state, "The substrate oxidation leads to a separation of electrons and protons in the electron transfer complexes that gives rise to an electric field in the direction perpendicular to the surface of the inner membrane". However, GREEN (1974) presents the following: "The notion of membrane potential is implicit in the chemiosmotic model of MITCHELL ... but it has no counterpart in the electromechanochemical model". Perhaps the contradictions are actually modifications of the original models not clearly spelled out in the more recent articles.

In their "paired moving charges" model, GREEN and REIBLE (1974, 1975) propose a direct coupling between the electron flow across the membrane and the translocation of ions to maintain electroneutrality. This process results in the net transport of ions or the phosphorylation of ADP. The model allows for the H^+ effluxes accompanying metabolism as the consequence of the electron shifts and does not invoke the presence of a membrane potential. It differs basically from the chemiosmotic model in that the electron flow is directly involved in transduction.

Several investigators propose a mechanochemical coupling between oxidation and phosphorylation (e.g., HACKENBROCK et al. 1971 b, GREEN 1974). Mitochondria, whether in situ or isolated, exhibit distinct configurations characteristic of their metabolic state (e.g., HACKENBROCK 1966, 1972, HACKENBROCK et al. 1971 a, b, PENNINSTON et al. 1968, HARRIS et al. 1968, GREEN et al. 1968). These configurations can be recognized either with electron microscopy (thin sections, freeze-cleavage or negative staining) or by the light scattered by mitochondrial suspensions (e.g., PACKER 1960, 1961, HACKENBROCK 1966). The appearance of mitochondria differs depending on the study or the tissue used. Generally, however, the various observations can be interpreted in the same way. The inner mitochondrial space appears enlarged in the presence of substrate, or substrate and P_i and it appears shrunken under phosphorylating conditions or in the presence of respiratory inhibitors or uncouplers. This interpretation is supported by the fact that these configurations can be mimicked by appropriate osmotic swellings or shrinkages (ASAI et al. 1969, STONER and SIRAK 1969, PACKER et al. 1968, HUNTER et al. 1969).

The configurational changes have been interpreted as evidence for a mechanochemical coupling involved in oxidative-phosphorylation and this interpretation persists in the more recent electromechanochemical model of energy coupling of GREEN (*e.g.*, see GREEN 1974). A mechanochemical inter-pretation is challenged by the findings that the appropriate configurational changes and changes of light scattered by mitochondrial suspensions coincide with the swelling brought about by the uptake of ions (PACKER *et al.* 1966, UTSUMI and PACKER 1967, HUNTER *et al.* 1969, BLONDIN and GREEN 1969, ANAGNOSTI and TEDESCHI 1970, IZZARD and TEDESCHI 1970, 1973). In at least some cases, the amount of light scattered by the suspensions in various metabo-lic states can be accounted for quantitatively by the osmotic volume changes brought about by the uptake of ions [*e.g.*, in the presence of phosphate (P_i) ANAGNOSTI and TEDESCHI 1970, IZZARD and TEDESCHI 1970, 1973], or by their net efflux (*e.g.*, under phosphorylating conditions, IZZARD and TEDESCHI 1970, 1973). There is an inverse relationship between the P_i induced transport and phosphorylation so that there is a net efflux of ions following the onset of phosphorylation. A similar inverse relationship has been observed in the study of K^+ and Mg^{2+} transport induced by mercurials (SOUTHARD and GREEN 1974 b). The claim of HACKENBROCK *et al.* (1971 b) that the uptake of various ions is compensated by the release of Mg^{2+} (HACKENBROCK *et al.* 1971 b, Fig. 3 of reference) is contrary to our experience (IZZARD and TEDESCHI 1973).

In addition to the evidence just cited for an osmotic basis for the configura-tional changes, these changes do not correspond invariably to the appropriate metabolic state, as would be necessary for the mechanochemical model (*e.g.*, HACKENBROCK 1966, SORDAHL *et al.* 1969, WEINBACH *et al.* 1967, KUNER and BEYER 1970, WEBER and BLAIR 1969).

c) Chemical Intermediate and Conformational Models in Phosphorylation

Chemical-intermediate models of oxidative phosphorylation involve as the primary energy capturing device, the synthesis of a high energy form of a respiratory chain carrier. Some of these models focus on the prosthetic group of the cytochromes. Formally similar models involve conformational changes in the folding of the protein chains of the cytochromes or the ATPase (see SLATER 1971, 1974, SLATER *et al.* 1974 for detailed formulations). Although these two kinds of models are significantly different, they can be represented in the same general conceptual framework.

There is some evidence for a conformational change in at least two cyto-chromes. In the case of cytochrome c oxidase there is evidence that binding of one heme by CO or azide increases the extinction coefficient of the other (see WILSON *et al.* 1972 b, LEIGH *et al.* 1974). The reduction of one heme produces a high spin electron state on the other heme iron (see VAN GELDER and BEINERT 1969, LEIGH *et al.* 1974). There are also indications of inter-actions from circular dichroism studies (VAN GELDER and TIESJEMA 1973), the reactivity of the hemes to cyanide (VAN BUREN and SCHILDER 1973) and from other spectroscopic data on anaerobic-aerobic transitions (NICHOLLS and PETERSEN 1974, OSHINO *et al.* 1974).

The binding of antimycin to cytochrome b in complex III also shows a cooperative behavior (BERDEN and SLATER 1972) as does the aurovertin binding sit in the ATPase of rat liver mitochondria (BERTINA *et al.* 1973,

YEATES 1974). In addition, the fluorescence of the aurovertin-ATPase complex increases during oxidative phosphorylation (BERTINA et al. 1973, CHANG and PENEFSKY 1973, 1974) suggesting a conformational rearrangement. In fact, cooperativity may be a general property of mitochondrial systems (see PANINI and KURUP 1974). In addition to the systems already mentioned, cooperative behavior has been shown for rotenone and piericidin inhibition of glutamate oxidation (GARLAND et al. 1969), oligomycin inhibition of state 3 succinate oxidation (SLATER and TER WELLE 1969), dinitrophenol stimulation of ATPase (KATYARE et al. 1971) and the effect of bongkrekic acid, presumably on the adenine nucleotide tranlocase (HENDERSON and LARDY 1971).

The evidence for high energy forms of the cytochromes has been discussed in part in Section 1 b. Some of the considerations leading to the formulation of these models have been discussed as alternatives to the chemiosmotic model (Section 3 a). For the purpose of discussion a scheme is presented below primarily following the conventions of SLATER (1971). Except for the primary coupling reaction (reaction 10), the points to be discussed are equally applicable for the chemiosmotic model which also has found the need for postulating chemical intermediates.

10. $AH_2 + B + C \rightleftharpoons A \sim C + BH_2$

11. $A \sim C + X \quad \rightleftharpoons X \sim C + A$

12. $X \sim C + P_i \quad \rightleftharpoons X \sim P_i + C$

13. $X \sim P_i + ADP \rightleftharpoons ATP + X$

In this formulation A and B are components of the respiratory chain and C and X are ligands (which would not be present in a conformational model). C and $C \sim X$ have the capacity to be used in each one of the three coupling sites (see ERNSTER and LEE 1964). $X \sim P$ is a phosphorylated intermediate. ATP-ADP exchanges would be a reflection of reaction 13, ATP and P_i exchanges a reflection of reactions 12 and 13. H_2O, P_i exchanges involve reaction 12. Similarly, ATP-H_2O exchanges reflect 12 and 13.

Oligomycin inhibits the P_i-H_2O, suggesting a block in reaction 12. Uncouplers (e.g., S-13) have a differential effect (BOYER et al. 1973). When ATP-H_2O and the P_i-ATP exchanges are inhibited significantly, the P_i-H_2O exchange is not. In addition, the P_i-H_2O exchange requires ADP (JONES and BOYER 1969). These observations suggest that the scheme represented above (equations 10 to 13) is not correct. BOYER et al. (1973) suggest an entirely different scheme to explain these differential effects. The energy requiring step during the formation of ATP is the release from the membrane phase rather than its synthesis. This can be represented as follows:

$$\text{membrane phase:} \begin{cases} P_i + ADP \rightleftharpoons H_2O + ATP \text{ bound} \\ ATP \text{ bound} + \text{energy} \rightleftharpoons ATP_{\text{free}} \end{cases}$$

This sequence would then explain the P_i-H_2O data and its insensitivity to the presence of uncouplers. The exchanges could then be less sensitive to the presence of uncouplers than the actual formation of soluble ATP.

The mitochondrial ATPase isolated from heart mitochondria firmly binds three molecules of ATP and two of ADP (HARRIS et al. 1973). Another ADP is thought to be loosely bound. Treatment with salts at 0° dissociates the ATPase into its subunits (PENEFSKY and WARNER 1975) and also releases the bound nucleotides. This evidence has been woven into a model in which the firmly bound ATP and ADP are involved in producing an active, restrained conformation of ATPase. The loosely bound ADP is considered to be involved in the phosphorylation reaction. The latter does not require energy. The detachment of the newly formed ATP, however, is linked to the transfer of electrons in the respiratory chain, resulting in the liberation of all the bound nucleotides and with the net synthesis of 1 ATP from ADP and P_i. This model is in general harmony with the model proposed by Boyer (see SLATER 1974).

4. Permeability and Transport

a) The Transport of Cations and General Models of Transport

The mitochondrial membrane permeability, the transport of ions and the related topics of osmotic behavior and the binding of ions have been repeatedly reviewed in recent years (LEHNINGER et al. 1967, CHANCE and MONTAL 1971, AZZONE and MASSARI 1973, AZZONE et al. 1974, PRESSMAN 1970, KLINGENBERG 1970 a, b, BRIERLEY 1974).

Isolated mitochondria behave as almost perfect osmometers when suspended in a medium containing solutes to which they are relatively impermeable (TEDESCHI and HARRIS 1955, 1958, ROSSI and AZZONE 1969, MASSARI et al. 1972 b, MUSCATELLO et al. 1972). The permeability of the mitochondrial semi-permeable membrane to water is extremely high (TEDESCHI and HARRIS 1955, 1958, MASSARI et al. 1972 b) and consequently for all intents and purposes the mitochondria can be considered in osmotic equilibrium at all times. Generally, their permeability to non-electrolytes is of the same order of magnitude as that of cell membranes (TEDESCHI and HARRIS 1955, TEDESCHI 1959, JACKSON and PACE 1956, MASSARI et al. 1972 b). Despite statements to the contrary in the literature, the permeability of mitochondria to sucrose, mannitol and salts is significant and probably higher than that of cells such as erythrocytes (e.g., see JACKSON and PACE 1956, AMOORE and BARTLEY 1958, AMOORE 1960, ULRICH 1959, TEDESCHI 1959, 1965, see TEDESCHI 1971 b).

Mitochondria are enclosed by two membranes. The semipermeable membrane studied in isolated mitochondria corresponds to the inner mito-chondrial membrane (TEDESCHI 1959). This is evidenced by the fact that the swelling over a wide range of mitochondrial volume does not seem to alter significantly the osmotic behavior and the permeability of isolated mito-chondria to non-electrolytes. Furthermore the results are consistent with the interpretation that the surface area available to small molecules remains constant during swelling. These results indicate that the semi-permeable membrane of isolated mitochondria is convoluted and hence corresponds to the internal mitochondrial membrane. The outer mitochondrial membrane does not seem to play a role in isolated preparations. However, it is entirely possible that it may be functionally significant in vivo.

Mitochondria can transport actively ions since these are transferred against an electrochemical gradient. Mitochondria are also thought to translocate ions in the direction of the electrochemical gradient in a process which is dependent on the expenditure of energy. The term active transport is generally applied to this form of translocation as well (AZZONE and MASSARI 1973), although it may not be active in the thermodynamic sense. The transport of several ions depends on metabolism. The adenine translocator, for example, favors ATP exit during metabolism (KLINGENBERG 1970 b). The glutamate translocator (indicated by the swelling in isoosmotic ammonium salt) seems also to depend on metabolism (e.g., BROUWER et al. 1973) as does the ornithine transport system (GAMBLE and LEHNINGER 1973) and the efflux of aspartate from rat heart mitochondria (LaNOUE and WILLIAMSON 1971, BROUWER et al. 1973). In the case of glutamate, however, other results suggest that no energy is required in establishing a glutamate steady state consistent with a Donnan distribution of the anions (KING and DIWAN 1972).

The study of solutes exchanged by isolated mitochondria has been carried out in a variety of ways. An indirect method for following the penetration of substrates uses the redox state of pyridine nucleotides as an indicator of their entry into the mitochondrial interior (e.g., CHAPPELL and CROFTS 1965 b, KLINGENBERG 1967). The permeability and active transport of mitochondria can also be followed indirectly by monitoring the light scattered or transmitted by mitochondrial suspensions. The scatter (or the optical density of the suspensions) varies inversely with mitochondrial volume (see TEDESCHI and HARRIS 1955, 1958). Since mitochondria approximate perfect osmometers (e.g., TEDESCHI and HARRIS 1955), the uptake of osmotically active components is reflected quantitatively in osmotic volume changes. The method has been used qualitatively by many workers (e.g., CHAPPELL and CROFTS 1966, see also BRIERLEY 1974). However, its full potential is realized only when it is used quantitatively. The photometric method has been developed as a quantitative tool for following mitochondrial volumes and to estimate the uptake of solutes (TEDESCHI and HARRIS 1958) and it has been used successfully in at least two different laboratories (e.g., see TEDESCHI 1959, TUPPER and TEDESCHI 1967, IZZARD and TEDESCHI 1970, 1973, MASSARI et al. 1972 c).

Ion specific electrodes and in particular cationic electrodes highly sensitive to K^+ or Na^+ permit monitoring the concentration of these cations in the medium (e.g., PRESSMAN 1968). Although Ca^{2+} sensitive electrodes are also available, the external concentration of Ca^{2+} can be monitored accurately and rapidly with the Ca^{2+} indicator dye, murexide (e.g., SCARPA and GRAZIOTTI 1973). A number of electrodes can be used to monitor the net exchange of SCN^- (e.g., see PAPA et al. 1973 b), chloride, carbonate (HERMAN and RECHNITZ 1974) and other anions (e.g., see GRINIUS et al. 1970).

Cations and anions can also be estimated by radioactive tracer techniques or analytical techniques after separation of the mitochondria from the suspending medium. This can be done by centrifugation in which the mitochondria are sedimented to form a pellet. One of the most rapid centrifugation techniques sediments the mitochondria through one or more silicon layers into acid (WERKHEISER and BARTLEY 1957, KLINGENBERG and PFAFF 1967, HARRIS and VAN DAM 1968). Alternatively, the mitochondria can be filtered out in a few seconds (KLINGENBERG and PFAFF 1966, TEDESCHI and HEGARTY 1966, PFAFF and KLINGENBERG 1968). The rapid kinetics of uptake of anions which seem to be translocated by specific transporters can be followed most accurately by blocking the exchange by means of inhibitors before separations (e.g., phenylsuccinate to block succinate transport, QUAGLIARIELLO et al. 1969; Bromocresol Purple for glutamate, BRADFORD and McGIVAN 1973).

Several distinct preparations have been used in the study of mitochondrial transport and mitochondrial biochemistry. As already discussed (Section A 3), several different submitochondrial particles have been prepared. Submitochondrial particles obtained by sonication are usually thought to correspond to vesicles made up of inner mitochondrial membrane which has been turned inside-out by the preparatory procedure. Presumably, they have originated by a pinching off of the membrane infoldings by a process represented diagrammatically in Fig. 5. In contrast, the orientation of the membranes of submitochondrial particles prepared with digitonin is thought to correspond to that of the mitochondrial inner membrane. Submitochondrial particles obtained by the two procedures are most likely a mixture of vesicles possessing either orientation (ASTLE and COOPER 1974). The weight of evidence however, favors the view that the particles derived by sonic radiation have an inside-out orientation predominantly. This is indicated by the biochemical properties of the preparations. For example, the particles oxidize mostly exogenous cytochrome c during reversal of electron transfer (e.g., CHANCE and FUGMAN 1961) whereas mitochondria oxidize endogeneous cytochrome c. In addition, the difference in electrophoretic mobility between mitochondria and sonicated particles is consistent with this notion (THOMPSON and McLEES 1961). The reactivity of the various components with specific antibodies (e.g., to F_1 DI JESO et al. 1969, LEE 1971) or with non-penetrating reagents such as diazobenzene sulfonate or cross-linking with polylysine (SCHNEIDER et al. 1972, TINBERG et al. 1974) is also in agreement with this postulated orientation (see Section A 3 for further discussion).

Except for the cases in which the ions transported form an insoluble precipitate (as in the case of Ca^{2+} phosphate) or are bound to mitochondrial components, it is now generally recognized that ions are taken primarily in an osmotically active form, since the swelling accompanying transport can be quantitatively accounted for by the ions in the mitochondrial matrix. This is the case, for example, for the Ca^{2+} accumulated in mitochondria in the presence of acetate (TUPPER and TEDESCHI 1967), the K^+ accumulated in the presence or absence of valinomycin (ROTTENBERG and SOLOMON 1969, MASSARI et al. 1972 c) or the uptake of Na^+ or K^+ induced by P_i (ANAGNOSTI and TEDESCHI 1970, IZZARD and TEDESCHI 1970, 1973). In fact, the quantitative osmotic reversal of many of the mitochondrial swellings observed so far (TEDESCHI 1959, 1961, TEDESCHI et al. 1965, TEDESCHI and HEGARTY 1965) suggests that they are invariably the result of underlying osmotic effects.

The data accumulated from a variety of experiments have been interpreted primarily from the point of view of four models. It should be noted that these are not necessarily mutually exclusive. Several of the mechanisms might be involved simultaneously. Alternatively under specific conditions only one mechanism of several possible ones may be observed. In addition, mitochondria from different sources may differ significantly in relation to transport mechanisms as found in the case of anionic transporters (see KLINGENBERG 1970 a, b, BROUWER et al. 1973). A complication may also be the consequence of the fact that mitochondria prepared in different laboratories may unaccountably differ in some of their transport properties (e.g., compare CHAPPELL et al. 1968 to LÊ-QUÔC-BRUGUERA and GUADEMER 1973 in relation to maleate transport).

The cation pump model (using K^+ as an example) is represented in diagram 1 of Fig. 18. Presumably, the translocation of cations by means of this model requires a carrier. The transport of K^+ could result in a membrane potential (positive inside) as shown in part B. However, this need not be the case (Part A) depending on the rate of influx of other ions (e.g., anions going in the same direction to maintain electroneutrality). Diagram 2 represents the mechanism of ion transport of the chemiosmotic hypothesis, i.e., an electrogenic H^+ pump stoichiometrically coupled to the respiratory chain. Diagram 3 illustrates a H^+ pump which is not stoichiometrically coupled to the respiratory chain. Again the transport need not be responsible for a potential across the mitochondrial membrane (3 A), although it could produce a membrane potential (3 B). Diagram 4 represents a H^+-cation carrier mediated pump where H^+ and cation transports are coupled and in opposite directions. Transport of cations could also follow a primary anion pump (e.g., see BRIERLEY et al. 1973, BRIERLEY 1974). This could occur, for example, when the anion is carried in an undissociated form. Upon dissociation in the mitochondrial interior (favored by the high internal OH^-), cation transfer would follow to maintain electroneutrality. These models and various experimental findings will be discussed in some detail in the rest of this section.

It has been proposed that the cation (in this case K^+) is the transported species and that H^+ ions or anions exchanges would occur to maintain electroneutrality (e.g., COCKRELL et al. 1966, HARRIS and PRESSMAN 1969). The uptake of K^+ exhibits saturation kinetics, suggesting the presence of a carrier mediated transport directly involving K^+ (see HARRIS et al. 1967, MASSARI and AZZONE 1970 a, b, AZZONE and MASSARI 1971, MASSARI et al. 1972 a). The results of experiments in which the influence of metabolism on the influx of K^+ has been measured also suggest a direct involvement of K^+ in the transport mechanism (DIWAN 1973). The unidirectional influx depends on metabolism, whereas the unidirectional efflux does not. Hence the transport of K^+ cannot involve a passive redistribution of K^+ in response to an electric potential across the mitochondrial membrane.

There are other indications which implicate a cation pump under at least some conditions. Orthophosphate (P_i) induces the accumulation of ions inside mitochondria (ANAGNOSTI and TEDESCHI 1970, IZZARD and TEDESCHI 1970, 1973). The P_i acts primarily as a trigger since it is transported in small amounts compared to the other ions (ANAGNOSTI and TEDESCHI 1970).

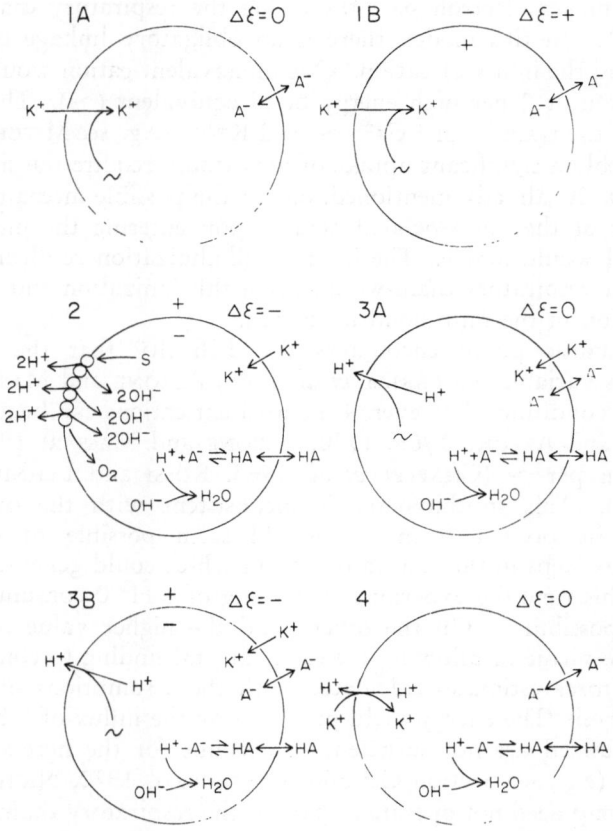

Fig. 18. Models of transport. 1. Primary transport of cations, the anions following passively. Part A indicates a transport not generating a membrane potential. Part B indicates a process generating a membrane potential. 2. The chemiosmotic model. 6 H$^+$ are translocated per electron pair traversing the chain. This transfer results in a membrane potential. The protonmotive force can be coupled to the transport of cations. The transport of anions occurs by the transfer of the undissociated acid. 3. The translocation of H$^+$ by an energy requiring reaction not directly dependent on the respiratory chain. Part A and Part B represent processes which do not and do result in membrane potentials, respectively. 4. An energy requiring translocation in which the influx of 1 K$^+$ is obligatorily linked to the efflux of H$^+$.

The system transports Na$^+$ or K$^+$ (although many other cations were not examined). NH$_4^+$ (or tris$^+$) which has been found to penetrate mitochondria cannot replace these ions (IZZARD and TEDESCHI 1973). The data suggest a limited specificity of the transport system which would be absent if the cations were transferred passively. In addition, some cations are unable to enter mitochondria in the absence of metabolism (BRIERLEY *et al.* 1970) even when present together with the permeant anion, acetate.

The chemiosmotic model proposes that the transport of ions is driven by the proton pump which operates as a consequence of the asymmetric functioning of the respiratory chain. Thus 6 H$^+$ would be transferred to the external medium per electron pair traversing the respiratory chain between NADH and O_2. In this model, there is an obligatory linkage between the efflux of H^+ and the influx of cation. One monovalent cation would be transferred per proton or 2 per high energy bond equivalent ($\sim$). This exchange would result in the transfer of 1 $Ca^{2+}/\sim$ or 2 $K^+/\sim$ (e.g., see MITCHELL 1966 a, 1968). Presumably a significant uptake of ions would require the simultaneous entry of anions. As already mentioned, one of the possible mechanisms would be the transfer of the undissociated acid. Upon entering the mitochondrial lumen, the acid would ionize. The internal alkalinization resulting from the operation of the respiratory chain would favor this ionization and would tend to trap the anion in the mitochondrial lumen.

The chemiosmotic pump encounters the difficulty that the cation /$\sim$ stoichiometry is variable (COCKRELL et al. 1966, AZZONE and MASSARI 1971). Under optimal conditions, however, 4 monovalent cations can be accumulated per $\sim$ (ROSSI and AZZONE 1969, 1970, AZZONE and MASSARI 1971) or two divalent cations per $\sim$ (CHAPPEL et al. 1963, ROSSI and LEHNINGER 1964, CHANCE 1965). This stoichiometry is inconsistent with the chemiosmotic hypothesis in its present form. It would seem possible to hypothesize additional redox steps in the respiratory chain which could generate more H^+. However, at this time the experimental finding of 6 H^+/O consumed seems to preclude this possibility. On the other hand the higher value of this ratio would have the virtue of allowing the experimental finding to conform to the protonmotive force estimates calculated with the assumptions of the chemiosmotic hypothesis. The energy yield provided by the influx of 2 H^+ per mole of ATP synthesized are not sufficient to account for the necessary ΔG for ATP synthesis (e.g., see Section C 3 and ROTTENBERG 1970, NICHOLLS 1974).

A proton pump need not operate as part of the respiratory chain. Hence H^+ could be translocated into the external medium without the stoichiometric restrictions discussed above. The energy required for the transfer could be supplied by ATP hydrolysis or by the oxidative reactions of the respiratory chain. Several proposals of this kind have appeared in the literature (CHAPPELL and CROFTS 1965 a, COCKRELL and RACKER 1969, MONTAL et al. 1970, LIBERMAN and SKULACHEV 1970, ROTTENBERG 1970, 1973, PAPA et al. 1970, 1973 a, b, CARAFOLI et al. 1971, GREEN and JI 1972 a, MASSARI and AZZONE 1970 a, b, AZZONE and MASSARI 1971, AZZONE et al. 1974).

In one kind of proposal the pump is considered to function without the production of a membrane potential. It presumes the presence of a carrier molecule exchanging H^+ for K^+ (MASSARI and AZZONE 1970 a, b, AZZONE and MASSARI 1971, AZZONE et al. 1974) or coupling of the inward movement of K^+ to the influx of OH^- (DIWAN 1973). In another kind of proposal, an electrogenic proton pump is considered to function by producing a membrane potential (CHAPPEL and CROFTS 1965 a, COCKRELL and RACKER 1969, MONTAL et al. 1970, LIBERMAN and SKULACHEV 1970, ROTTENBERG 1970, 1973, PAPA et al. 1970, 1973 a, b, CARAFOLI et al. 1971, GREEN and JI 1972 a).

The presumption that a transport mechanism translocating either a cation or an anion alone would invariably result in a membrane potential is not correct. For example, a proton or cationic pump followed by a passive re-distribution of other ions to maintain electroneutrality has been presumed electrogenic. However, the pump may not create a steady state membrane potential. The rapid, passive redistribution of other ions could result in a negligible membrane potential (*e.g.*, the active transport of K⁺ together with the passive entry of a highly permeable anion). Conversely, the electroneutral accumulation of a cation and anion pair could result in the production of a membrane potential because of the tendency toward back diffusion of either one of the ions in the directions of its concentration gradient. This point may be responsible for a good deal of the confusion and disagreements in the presently formulated models which use the term "electrogenic" indiscriminately.

The most significant evidence for the H⁺-cation pump (for both monovalent and divalent cations) stems from experiments in which the pump is run backwards with the synthesis of ATP from ADP and P_i (Azzone and Massari 1971, see Massari and Azzone 1972 a). The observed passage of both H⁺ and K⁺ in the direction of their respective electrochemical gradients needs to be considered to account for the energy required for the ATP synthesized under these conditions. The involvement of a carrier system for the uptake of K⁺ is also supported by the kinetics (Rossi and Azzone 1969, Massari and Azzoni 1970 a, b). In this model, the carrier would be energized at the inner surface where it would acquire an increased proton affinity. The passage of the proton to the outer surface would result in the de-energization of the carrier. The carrier would act in conjunction with the ion-carrying ionophores and uncouplers since it would have limited accessibility to the membrane interfaces.

The kinetics of the system are in agreement with this model. The uptake of K⁺ in the presence of valinomycin exhibits Michaelis-Menten kinetics in relation to K⁺ concentration. Hence the transport system is saturable in agreement with the notion that a carrier is involved (see Harris *et al.* 1967, Massari and Azzone 1970 a, b, Azzone and Massari 1971, Massari *et al.* 1972 c). Similar saturations appear also in the absence of valinomycin (Harris *et al.* 1967). H⁺ acts as a competitor of K⁺ uptake and valinomycin changes the V_m of the uptake but not the K_m. The same transport system may be involved, at least partly, in both K⁺ and Ca²⁺ transport since the Ca²⁺ uptake can be driven by the valinomycin induced exit of K⁺ (Rossi *et al.* 1967 a, Scarpa and Azzone 1970).

A similar model postulates the inward transport of K⁺ accompanied by OH⁻ (Diwan 1973). Such a mechanism is supported by the observation that the unidirectional K⁺ influx requires both metabolic energy and an alkaline pH in the external medium (Diwan 1973).

Arguments have been presented for a H⁺ pump operating as the primary event in ion transport. In this mechanism, the driving force would be the H⁺ pump itself. The anions and cations would distribute passively in a non-specific exchange not involving the pump. Generally, these models assume the need for a membrane potential. However, as already discussed a potential need not be set up by the H⁺ pump. Since any significant net uptake would require a concomitant transfer of anions, the translocation mechanism of the anion would play a significant role in the net uptake (see Papa et al. 1973 a, Lehninger 1974, Brierley 1974).

In beef heart mitochondria neither potassium acetate nor potassium phosphate in isosmotic concentrations produce swelling in the absence of the oxidation of substrates or the hydrolysis of ATP (Brierley et al. 1968 b, 1971 a, Blondin et al. 1969, Young et al. 1971). The swelling and the accumulation of ions seem to be proportional to the number of phosphorylative sites traversed by electron transport (Brierley et al. 1971 a). Respiratory inhibitors and uncouplers or, alternatively, inhibitors of ATP hydrolysis inhibit the uptake of K+ and anions. The transport system is not specific in relation to the cation. In beef heart mitochondria, in addition to K+, other ions such a choline+, tris+, tetramethyl ammonium (TMA+) can support swelling and are accumulated in the presence of respiration (Brierley et al. 1968 b, 1971 a). A penetrant anion such as acetate or phosphate is required. An inhibitor of phosphate transport, N-ethylmaleimide (NEM) inhibits the phosphate uptake. It has been proposed that the accumulation of weak acids (such as acetate depends on the concentration of the undissociated acid. Data have been presented showing a correlation between the pK of the acids and their permeability (e.g., Crofts 1969, Blondin et al. 1969, Brierley et al. 1970, 1971 a). Since not all weak acids show this correlation, the results suggest that other factors may well be significant. In addition, the uptake of certain anions (e.g., citrate, see Gamble 1973) does not depend on the pH of the medium as would be expected with this model.

The results just discussed can be explained most readily by invoking a H+ pump. Brierley (see 1974) favors a pump where the cation exchange is non-specific and passive since (a) the uptake of the cation seems to be non-specific and (b) the uptake is not favored by the presence of a permeant anion such as NO_3^-, which would not be directly favored by the H+ pump. Results of studies with submitochondrial particles are roughly in agreement with htis mechanism. This mechanism has also been invoked by Lehninger (1974) for Ca^{2+} transport in rat liver mitochondria to explain why not all anions support the Ca^{2+} uptake. P_i, arsenate, butyrate, hydroxybutyrate, lactate and $HCO_3^- + CO_2$ support the Ca^{2+} uptake. On the other hand other anions presumed to penetrate such as NO_3^-, SCN^-, chlorate and perchlorate do not. The conclusion was reached that anions can be taken up only as undissociated weak acids by the mitochondria in a mechanism which depends on the internal alkalinization of the mitochondrial lumen. Presumably the cations are picked up passively (Lehninger 1974).

One of the most meaningful pieces of evidence for a H+ pump mechanism is the increased uptake of ions with a variety of agents, at least some of which can be presumed to increase the passive permeability of cations. The H+ pump allows for the accumulation of cations with increased permeability. These agents are, for example, charged ionophores (Henderson et al. 1969, Pressman 1970) which form complexes with K+, and possibly non-ionic detergents such as Triton X-100 which may act by the same mechanism (van Zutphen et al. 1972, Brierley et al. 1972). Other agents with a similar effect include gramicidin which is thought to form channels across lipid membranes (URRY 1972), heavy metals such as Zn^{2+} (BRIERLEY and SETTLEMIRE 1967), Cu^{2+} (HUANG et al. 1972), Pb^{2+} (SCOTT et al. 1971), mercurials (BRIERLEY et al. 1968 a, SCOTT et al. 1970, and BRIERLEY et al. 1971 b, 1973) and N-ethyl-maleimide (DIWAN 1973). These agents also increase the passive permeability to ions, possibly by activating endogeneous ionophores (see Section C 4, below). Valinomycin and gramicidin increase active swelling (BRIERLEY et al. 1971 a) and have a similar effect on the passive swelling in the presence of KNO_3. In beef heart mitochondria removal of Mg^{2+} by chelators enhances Na and Li acetate accumulation with little effect on K^+ (SETTLEMIRE et al. 1968).

However, other findings are not in agreement with this transport model. Inducers of anion permeability (MEROLA and BRIERLEY 1970) or Cl^- and OH^- exchange (SELWYN et al. 1970) are without effect on transport. Tannic acid, which inhibits the transport of several anions (e.g., malate, succinate, malonate, glutamate, aspartate and phosphate), does not inhibit the energy dependent K^+ influx, but in fact stimulates it (DIWAN 1972). In addition, certain cations seem to be excluded from the mitochondrial interior in the absence of metabolism although they would be expected to penetrate even in the absence of the H^+ pump. Sodium acetate in isotonic concentration penetrates beef heart mitochondria in the absence of metabolism. Presumably, the acetate penetrates as the unionized acid and then Na^+ exchanges for H^+. However, the other cations (e.g., TMA^+ or choline$^+$) also present as acetate salts are unable to penetrate without metabolism although, presumably the same mechanism should be operative (BRIERLEY et al. 1970). These results suggest a more complex mechanism which may involve the cations directly in the pump mechanism.

ROTTENBERG (1973) analyzes data concerning the transport of K^+ and Na^+ in the presence or absence of valinomycin or nigericin. He rejects the alternative of a cation pump transferring cations inwardly. He considers the most likely alternative an outwardly directed proton pump which creates an electrical potential gradient responsible for the cation transport. The conclusions are based on the following considerations:

1. The final K^+ concentration gradient at steady state has been claimed not to be affected by the presence of valinomycin (ROTTENBERG and SOLOMON 1969).

2. The concentration of external K^+ at which there is no net uptake (i.e., the system is at steady state from the beginning) is the same in the presence or absence of valinomycin. This argues for the same electrochemical gradient for the two cases (with and without valinomycin).

3. The rate of uptake of K^+ shows saturation kinetics in relation to valinomycin concentration but not K^+ concentration.

4. Valinomycin stimulates both influx and efflux of K^+ so that the influx/outflux decreases until it approaches 1.

5. The presence of gramicidin leads to concentration ratios for inside/outside Na^+ or K^+ which are virtually identical for either ion.

These five points will be discussed in some detail below.

According to ROTTENBERG (1973) "the final potassium concentration gradient which is reached at steady state (*i.e.*, when potassium uptake vanishes) is not affected by valinomycin (ROTTENBERG and SOLOMON 1969)". The data presented by MITCHELL and MOYLE (1969 b) also suggests that this might be correct. This statement is not supported by the data of ROTTENBERG and SOLOMON 1969 (Table 1 and Fig. 2 of ref.). Other studies in which the valinomycin concentration is varied over a wide range make the opposite claim (MASSARI *et al.* 1972 a). Both MITCHELL and MOYLE, and MASSARI *et al.*, fail to correct for mitochondrial volume changes which are significant and for this reason this point remains questionable. The conclusion of ROTTENBERG is not justified by the data. In addition, the objection is not crucial. An inward K+ pump aided by valinomycin and a concomitant valinomycin induced backflow could well lead to the same steady state level.

The external concentration at which K+ is initially at steady state (*i.e.*, with no net uptake) in the presence or absence of valinomycin appears to be the same from the extrapolation of the lines shown in ROTTENBERG (1973, Fig. 5). However, the data presented are insufficient to support the conclusions. The lines could be drawn equally validly without intercepting at the same point. Since the scale on the abscissa (the external K+ concentration) is logarithmic, even a small displacement would correspond to a very large deviation. Without publication of the details of the additional experiments or the presentation of statistical data, this result cannot be evaluated critically. It could be argued, of course, that very large deviations in the predicted values are tolerated by the membrane potential model (since the calculation of the membrane potential using the Nernst equation involves the logarithm of the concentration ratios). However, this reasoning depends on a number of assumptions, including the validity of the model being tested. At best, the data show that the results are not inconsistent with the model.

The rate of uptake of K+ shows a measure of saturation in relation to both valinomycin *and* K+ despite the statement of ROTTENBERG (1973). This is shown in Fig. 5 of the paper by ROTTENBERG (1973). The relation is not apparent, in part, because the external concentration of K+ is plotted on a logarithmic scale, as already noted. In addition, rather than approaching a slope of zero, the slope decreases and eventually becomes constant. This is to be expected since at the upper concentration range, the concentration of external K+ is high (*i.e.*, the concentration outside is greater than inside). In this range, part of the penetration is likely to be the result of diffusion in the direction of the K+ concentration gradient (which would not be expected to be saturable). Saturation of K+ influx in relation to valinomycin (HARRIS *et al.* 1967, ROSSI and AZZONE 1969) or K+ (*e.g.*, see HARRIS *et al.* 1967, MASSARI *et al.* 1972 a) has been demonstrated previously. Ca²⁺ uptake also exhibits saturation kinetics (*e.g.*, CARAFOLI and AZZI 1972, VINOGRADOV and SCARPA 1973).

The results presented by ROTTENBERG (1973) show that both the initial influx and the efflux increase in the presence of valinomycin and the influx/ efflux approaches 1. ROTTENBERG (1973) considers this evidence that the system is practically at equilibrium. Nevertheless, the conditions could just as well be the result of a steady state. The results are equally consistent with the idea that an increased influx favored by the valinomycin is also accompanied by an increased backflow brought about by a valinomycin induced increase in permeability. An increase in efflux caused by valinomycin is shown by experiments measuring the influx under steady state conditions (at steady state, influx and outflux are equal). A more careful analysis of the results also permits estimates which are somewhat difficult to explain from the point of view of the presence of a membrane potential. The influx ratios brought about by diffusion in the presence of a membrane potential should follow the relationship shown below (*e.g.*, TEORELL 1953):

$$J_i / J_o = \frac{(K)_o}{(K)_i} \, e^{-\Delta EF/RT}$$

J_i and J_o represent the influx and the efflux, respectively. The subscripts i and o are used to indicate the concentration in the inside and the outside phase, respectively. R is the gas constant, T the temperature, ΔE the membrane potential and F the Faraday constant. When the system is at steady state or reasonably close to steady state, $J_i \cong J_o$ and the relationship reduces to the Nernst equation, *i.e.*, $\Delta E = RT/F \log_e (K)_o/(K)_i$. The equation shown should allow calculating the potential across the membrane from the flux ratios, provided the fluxes are passive (*i.e.*, caused by diffusion) as postulated by ROTTENBERG. In the presence of valinomycin the ΔE, calculated from the steady state concentrations at which there is no net flow, is approximately — 130 mv as reported by ROTTENBERG (1973). However, if the initial fluxes (Table 2, ROTTENBERG 1973) are used, the value calculated from the above equation (using the information provided in his Table 1 and his legend of Fig. 6) corresponds to — 57 mv. In the absence of valinomycin at 30 °C it corresponds to — 74 mv and at 4 °C, presumably at a much reduced metabolism, it becomes — 109 mv. These results are not consistent with the electrogenic pump model adopted by ROTTENBERG (1973).

Furthermore, the basic postulate of the chemiosmotic hypothesis used to calculate potentials (*e.g.*, ROTTENBERG 1970, MITCHELL and MOYLE 1969) assumes that valinomycin only redistributes the K^+ without affecting the system significantly, whereas in these experiments the chemiosmotic model would have to conclude that the membrane potential is changed by valinomycin.

In the presence of gramicidin, an ionophore which induces the passage of both Na^+ and K^+, the concentration ratios of these cations reach the same values at steady state (ROTTENBERG 1973). Similarly, in the presence of valinomycin (which increases the permeability to both K^+ and Rb^+), the Ca^{2+} and Rb^+ ratios approximately follow the relationship $[(Ca^{2+}_{in})/(Ca^{2+}_{out})]^{1/2} = (Rb^+_{in})/(Rb^+_{out})$ (ROTTENBERG and SCARPA 1974). These ion distributions are consistent with the interpretation that they are determined by the presence of a potential across the mitochondrial membrane and equally consistent to a Donnan distribution in the absence of a membrane potential (see p. 76). The presence of nigericin or valinomycin would increase the permeability to K^+ and hence create a diffusion potential not directly dependent on metabolism. Such an effect has been invoked to explain by the chemiosmotic hypothesis the phosphorylation resulting from valinomycin induced efflux in metabolically blocked mitochondria (GLYNN 1967).

PAPA *et al.* (1970, 1973 a, b) have presented arguments for the presence of an electrogenic H$^+$ pump coupled only secondarily to cation-H$^+$ counter exchange or anion coexchange. As already noted, the coupled exchange of ions to maintain electroneutrality need not result in a membrane potential. The results cannot be interpreted as the result of an electrogenic process. However the results argue for a primary role of the H$^+$ flux in the ion flux of submitochondrial particles under the conditions used. Whether this is related to normal transport of ions in mitochondria remains unresolved. The data has been obtained very indirectly (*e.g.*, by the use of inhibitors) and at times can be explained by alternative models. For example, divalent cations are not thought to be involved in the uptake of H$^+$ on the grounds that the chelators EDTA and EGTA are present in the medium. However, the presence of chelators in the medium is not likely to affect a counterflow of divalent cations to match the H$^+$ uptake.

PAPA *et al.* (1973) have observed a biphasic efflux of H$^+$ when previously aerobic submitochondrial particles are subject to anaerobiosis in the presence of substrate. The results can be interpreted on the basis of two independent processes; a fast process which depends on the nature of the cation in the medium and a slower process independent of the cations in the medium and considered an "electrogenic" flux. Other interpretations are also possible. For example, the slow process could be the result of the exit of H$^+$ and an anion from the internal phase.

b) Anion and Amino Acid Transport

The transport of anions, including adenine nucleotides has been recently reviewed (see KLINGENBERG 1970 b, MEIJER and VAN DAM 1974). MEIJER and VAN DAM discuss in particular the probable physiological significance of the various transport systems.

Mitochondria are thought to be permeable to monovalent anions such as hydroxybutyrate, acetoacetate, fatty acids, azide (PALMIERI and KLINGENBERG 1967), SCN$^-$ and NO$_3^-$ (MITCHELL and MOYLE 1969 a) by mechanisms which do not require a carrier. There are some indications that the anions of weak acids penetrate predominantly in their undissociated form (*e.g.*, CHAPPELL and CROFTS 1966, CHAPPELL and HAARHOFF 1967). It is not clear whether this mechanism is general since anions such as SCN$^-$, NO$_3^-$ and to some extent SO$_4^{2-}$ also penetrate (*e.g.*, MITCHELL and MOYLE 1969 a). [Note, however, that a special carrier has been proposed for SO$_4^{2-}$ (CROMPTON *et al.* 1974).] In addition, some of the undissociated divalent or trivalent acids are present in the medium at very low concentration indeed (10^{-5}–10^{-7} for some dicarboxylic acids) and as already discussed the correlation between pK and permeability is far from perfect. As already noted, in some cases the net uptake of citrate is not dependent on the pH of the suspending medium (GAMBLE 1973) and acetate cannot substitute for citrate in the uptake of cations.

Pyruvate is taken up by mitochondria by a process which exhibits saturation kinetics (PAPA *et al.* 1971, BROUWER *et al.* 1973, PAPA and PARADIES 1974) and the uptake is favored by a more acid pH. The uptake takes place either as an exchange for another anion (PAPA *et al.* 1971) or a net uptake when present as an isotonic NH_4 salt (BROUWER *et al.* 1973). The efflux of pyruvate increases when the pH of the suspending medium is increased (BROUWER *et al.* 1973). These results have been interpreted to mean that pyruvate enters by an exchange diffusion between this anion and OH^- and that this exchange requires a carrier. The uptake can be inhibited by mersalyl or NEM (PAPA and PARADIES 1974) as well as phenylpyruvate, α-oxo-4-methylpentonoate (HALESTRAP *et al.* 1974 a and b) and α-cyano-4-hydroxycinnamate (HALESTRAP and DENTON 1974).

The transfer of a number of other biologically significant anions is thought to occur by means of special transport mechanisms involving carriers or transporter molecules. Presumably, special mechanisms for the transport of substrates involved in oxidative phosphorylation are present in all mitochondria whereas amino acids are accumulated by these mechanisms only in the mitochondria from specialized organs such as liver (see KLINGENBERG 1970 a, b). The presence of special transport mechanisms is indicated by the following criteria, (a) the high specificity of the transport mechanisms in relation to the transported molecule, (b) saturability of the system in relation to the concentration of the anion transported, (c) the demonstration of blocks brought about by specific inhibitors and (d) a high dependence on temperature.

Inhibitors are not always specific. Tetraphenylboron, for example, has been found to block the entry of a variety of anions, presumably by increasing the negative charges on the mitochondrial surface (see MEISNER 1973). Conversely, cations added to mitochondria suspended in a low ionic strength medium increase the uptake of succinate, malonate and P_i. This effect has been interpreted to be the result of the increase in the positive charges of the mitochondrial surface (MEISNER *et al.* 1972), although alternate explanations are also possible (*e.g.*, a co-transport of the cations).

Inorganic phosphate (P_i) can be transported either in exchange for OH or in exchange for dicarboxylic acids (FONYÓ 1968, TYLER 1968, PAPA *et al.* 1969 b, MEIJER *et al.* 1970, JOHNSON and CHAPPELL 1974). The two systems can be distinguished by their differential sensitivity to inhibitors. A presumed phosphate translocator should be sensitive to mersalyl whereas the dicarboxylate translocator should be sensitive to *n*-butylmalonate (*e.g.*, see ROBINSON and CHAPPELL 1967). Dicarboxylic acids (malate, malonate, and succinate) are thought to exchange for other dicarboxylic acids such as ketoglutarate or P_i (DE HAAN and TAGER 1968, PAPA *et al.* 1969 a, b) in a carrier mediated process. Special mechanisms of transfer have also been proposed for glutamate, ketoglutarate and aspartate (AZZI *et al.* 1967, McGIVAN *et al.* 1969).

The reduction of nicotinamide nucleotides has been used to monitor the uptake of substrates. The swelling of mitochondria suspended in the appropriate isotonic concentration of ammonium salts has also been used as an indication of the permeability of a variety of anions. Results obtained with these approaches have suggested three carrier mediated transport systems (see CHAPPELL and HAARHOFF 1966, CHAPPELL and ROBINSON 1968). One appears specific for dicarboxylic acids such as L-malate, D-malate, malonate, and succinate but it appears inactive with others (e.g., fumarate and maleate). This dicarboxylic acid translocator system may also be involved in HCO_3^- transport (WÓZNIAK et al. 1973). Another system seems to be involved with tricarboxylic acids such as citrate, isocitrate and cis-aconitate (e.g., PALMIERI et al. 1972). Presumably the dicarboxylic acid carrier exchanges for P_i and the tricarboxylic acid carrier requires both P_i and dicarboxylates. Since a net transport of P_i can take place (e.g., see COTY and PEDERSEN 1974) the transport of the other anions could take place as a cascade mechanism where the transported phosphate exchanges for dicarboxylic acids (e.g., see JOHNSON and CHAPPELL 1973) and these in turn exchange for tricarboxylic acids.

A third carboxylic acid carrier is presumed to function for ketoglutarate, since the transport of ketoglutarate has distinct activation requirements (DE HAAN and TAGER 1968). One to one exchanges can take place between citrate and malate, malate and ketoglutarate, malate and phosphate (PAPA et al. 1969 a, b) and between citrate, malate and phosphate (GAMBLE 1965). The various exchanges could permit the functioning of the respiratory chain without net uptakes of anions by recycling the phosphate.

The transport of tricarboxylates is specifically inhibited by benzene 1, 2, 3 tricarboxylate (SHUG and SHRAGO 1973). It shares a sensitivity for atractyloside (SHUG and SHRAGO 1973) and carboxyatractyloside (MOREL et al. 1974) with the adenine nucleotide translocator. The binding sites for tricarboxylates also bind dicarboxylates (PALMIERI et al. 1972) and phosphoenolpyruvate (PALMIERI et al. 1972, ROBINSON 1971, KLEINEKE et al. 1973).

The phosphate transport is inhibited by sulfhydryl reagents such as mersalyl (FONYO 1968, TYLER 1968) and by phenylindoline (HOOPER et al. 1973). Specific inhibitors have been found for the dicarboxylic acid carrier, phenyl-succinate and butylmalonate (ROBINSON and CHAPPELL 1967) and probably phosphate esters and phosphonate compounds (JOHNSON and CHAPPELL 1974). Tannic acid has been shown also to inhibit the uptake of succinate, malonate, glutamate, aspartate and malate, and the exchange of P_i (DIWAN 1972, KING and DIWAN 1972, LUCIANI 1973). There is some disagreement on the effect of butylmalonate and the SH-reagents with respect to the di-carboxylate-phosphate exchange, the phosphate-phosphate exchange and the dicarboxylate-dicarboxylate exchange (see MEYER and TAGER 1969, CHAPPELL 1969).

Maleate, found to be a non-penetrant anion in at least some experiments with rat liver mitochondria (CHAPPELL et al. 1968) has been shown to be taken up in other studies (LÊ-QUÔC-BRUGUERA and GAUDEMER 1973). The transport is blocked by ethacrynic acid [2,3-dichloro-4 (2-methylenebutyril) phenoxyacetate] but not butylmalonate or N-ethylmaleimide. The ethacrynic block does not seem to depend on a reaction with sulhydryl groups since ethacrynate analogs incapable of reaction with sulfhydryl groups are also effective in inhibiting the transport. Maleate can substitute for P_i in inducing succinate and malate exchange. The biological role of this mechanism is not clear since maleate is not normally present.

A specific transport system for 2-oxoglutarate has been studied in some detail (DE HAAN and TAGER 1968, SLUSE et al. 1972, 1973). The results are consistent with the hypothesis that a mobile carrier is involved and that the movement of the carrier in the membrane is the rate limiting step in the transport.

Fatty acid acyl CoA has been found to have an inhibitory effect on the transport system for tricarboxylates, dicarboxylates and adenine nucleotides (HARRIS et al. 1972, HALPERIN et al. 1972, MOREL et al. 1974) but not on P_i translocation (HALPERIN et al. 1972). This effect is probably physiologically significant.

Accurate kinetic constants have been estimated for the transport of suc-cinate and malate (QUAGLIARIELLO et al. 1969) gluatamate (MEYER and VIGNAIS 1973), tricarboxylates (PALMIERI et al. 1972), P_i (COTY and PEDERSEN 1974) and pyruvate and acetoacetate (PAPA and PARADIES 1974).

The pattern of transport of a variety of anions may be rather complicated. For example, phosphoenol pyruvate (SHUG and SHRAGO 1973) is transported by a mechanism involving in part the tricarboxylate carrier and in part the adenine nucleotide carrier (discussed in the next section).

At least some amino acids are also transported by a carrier. This is the case with glutamate and aspartate (AZZI et al. 1967, MEIJER et al. 1972). The transport of aspartate may require the presence of glutamate (McGIVAN et al. 1969, LA NOUE et al. 1974). Glutamate is also thought to be translocated in exchange for OH^- (MEIJER et al. 1972), but it does not seem to exchange with aspartate. Glutamate translocation is blocked by certain SH reagents (e.g., N-ethylmaleimide), but not by others (e.g., mersalyl) (MEIJER et al. 1972). Apparently the inhibition depends on the lipid solubility of the reagents (e.g., see MEYER and VIGNAIS 1973). 1-difluoro-2,4-dinitrobenzene (FDNB) blocks glutamate transport but has no effect on aspartate transport (KING and DIWAN 1972). Uncouplers also facilitate the exit of glutamate in a mechanism which does not involve the translocator (BROUWER et al. 1973). The glutamate translocator-mediated uptake is energy dependent (BROUWER et al. 1973) and glutamate accumulation depends on energy and the presence of K^+ (HARRIS et al. 1973, BROUWER et al. 1973). The mechanism mediating glutamate uptake was found to be stereospecific (KING and DIWAN 1972). A proteolipid which has the properties excepted of a glutamate carrier has been isolated (JULLIARD and GAUTHERON 1973, see Section C 4 d, p. 108).

Rat liver mitochondria are readily permeable to L-leucine, D- and L-tyrosine, α-aminoisobutyric and L-lysine by a mechanism which does not require metabolism and which is unaffected by inhibitors of glutamate and aspartate transport (KING and DIWAN 1973). Uptake of the cation L-lysine is enhanced by conditions (e.g., nigericin addition) which cause efflux of endo-geneous K^+, and inhibited by conditions favoring energy-linked K^+ uptake (DIWAN and ARAM 1974). Ornithine (which also carries a net positive charge) does not penetrate in the absence of metabolism or in the presence of un-couplers or respiratory inhibitors. However, it does penetrate in the presence of metabolism when accompanied by anions of weak acids such as P_i, acetate or bicarbonate (GAMBLE and LEHNINGER 1973). Ornithine is presumed to be transported by a special mechanism since the system is highly specific for the L stereoisomer. Furthermore, the transport is tissue specific since the translocating mechanism is present in mitochondria of some tissues (e.g., rat liver) and not in others (e.g., rat heart).

Many of the translocator mediated transport mechanisms have been studied in the absence of metabolism, for example in the presence of rotenone and antimycin. However, there have been suggestions that several translocators may require metabolism for their functioning. For example, the uptake of glutamate (BROUWER et al. 1973) and the efflux of aspartate from rat heart mitochondria (LA NOUE and WILLIAMSON 1971, BROUWER et al. 1973) are thought to depend on metabolism. In addition, the adenine translocator is thought to favor the exit of ATP during metabolism (KLINGENBERG 1970 b).

Most transport functions seem to involve sulfhydryl components, although the sensitivity to the various reagents differs. For example fuscin, a quinonoid compound can block P_i, ADP as well as glutamate transport (VIGNAIS and VIGNAIS 1973). Glutamate transport is blocked by N-ethylmaleimide (MEYER and VIGNAIS 1973, DEBISE and DURAND 1974) and other liposoluble sulfhydryl reagents. Charged reagents such as mersalyl are ineffective in inhibiting glutamate transport.

The involvement of a mobile carrier in P_i transport has been suggested on the basis of experiments using various SH-reagents (GUÉRIN et al. 1970). Some of these [e.g., N-(N-Acetyl-4-sulfamyl-phenyl) maleinimide, (ASPM)] seem to block the inward passage of P_i but appear not to block its efflux, presumably because the inhibitors are unable to penetrate the mitochondrial membrane. The efflux can also be followed by generating internal phosphate with ATP and an uncoupler. In this case the efflux is also blocked. These results have been interpreted to mean that the ASPM blocks transport in both directions and that the carrier is mobile. The failure to block the exit of P_i in the absence of an internal generating system was thought to be caused by an unequal distribution of the carrier. This interpretation is questionable. If the carrier were truly mobile the inhibition of the carrier from a single interface should eventually block both influx and efflux. An inhibition of transport was seen only when the P_i was generated internally. It is entirely possible that the inhibitor blocks the mitochondrial ATPase (which also contains sulfhydryl groups) and hence inhibits the generation of internal P_i. It should also be noted that the osmotic method was used to monitor passage of P_i after adding P_i externally. Other more complex mechanisms could be responsible for the swelling (interpreted as an influx) or a shrinkage (interpreted as an efflux).

The functional significance of the various transport systems has been critically examined, particularly in relation to the transport of reducing equivalents (since NADH penetrates the mitochondria poorly) (see MEIJER and VAN DAM 1974).

There is general agreement that the anion translocases are preserved in yeast mitochondria which lack DNA or in the presence of an inhibitor of mitochondrial protein synthesis (KOLAROV et al. 1972, PERKINS et al. 1972, 1973). These results suggest that these components are synthesized on cytoplasmic ribosomes.

The equilibrium distribution of anions depends on the ΔpH between the inner mitochondrial compartment and the medium. The anion ratios are inversely related to the ΔpH. For monovalent anions the ratios are inversely proportional to the ΔpH. For divalent anions (e.g., malate) the square root of the concentration ratio is inversely proportional to ΔpH. This distribution has been considered evidence for a dependence of anion transport on a H^+ pump (e.g., PALMIERI et al. 1970, QUAGLIARIELLO et al. 1971). However, the distribution follows quantitatively the predictions of a Donnan distribution (see HARRIS and BERENT 1970, HARRIS and BANGHAM 1972, HARRIS 1973) and need not involve a H^+ pump. Non-penetrating anions such as Cl^- follow this distribution after anionic permeability is induced by alkyl tin salts (HARRIS et al. 1973 b).

The Donnan distribution predicts the following ratios:

$$r = \frac{(H^+)o}{(H^+)_i} = \frac{(A_i^{1-})}{(A_o^{1-})} = \left[\frac{(A_i^{2-})}{(A_o^{2-})}\right]^{\frac{1}{2}} = \left[\frac{(A_i^{n-})_i}{(A_o^{n-})}\right]^{1/n}$$

the charge balance would be as follows:

$$H^+ + K^+ + 2\,Ca^{2+} = (X^-) + r A_o^- + r^2 A_o^{2-} + r^3 A_o^{3-} + \Sigma n B_i^{n-}$$

B_i^{n-} express the internally generated anions which remain trapped and X^- represents the fixed charge. In this equation, (A) corresponds to the anion concentration, the subscript o indicates the outside phase and i the inside phase.

The equations show a dependence of anion content on the cation concentration. When cations are transported following the addition of valinomycin, permeant anions are found to enter in almost precise equivalence (HARRIS 1969). Similar findings are reported for P_i induced transport (ANAGNOSTI and TEDESCHI 1970) and the energy dependent uptake of citrate (GAMBLE 1973) or glutamate (HARRIS et al. 1973). Less extensive anion uptake has been described in Ca^{2+} transport (RASMUSSEN et al. 1965, ROSSI et al. 1967, HARRIS and BERENT 1970). However, at least in some cases the uptake of anions corresponds at least approximately to that of Ca^{2+} (TUPPER and TEDESCHI 1967).

The transient alkalinization of the mitochondrial interior accompanying Ca^{2+} uptake is also accounted for by the equation since the increase in internal cation concentration will reduce the H^+ (see above equation).

c) Adenine Nucleotide Transport

Adenine nucleotides seem to be transported by a carrier system (KLINGENBERG and PFAFF 1966). The kinetic parameters of the transport have been evaluated (PFAFF and KLINGENBERG 1968, PFAFF et al. 1969).

The translocation is highly specific for ADP and ATP and does not transfer AMP (CHAPPELL and HAARHOFF 1967, and KLINGENBERG 1968). The translocation takes place as a one to one exchange and is inhibited specifically by atractyloside (KLINGENBERG and PFAFF 1966, HELDT et al. 1969, WEIDMANN et al. 1969), atractyloside analogs (e.g., VIGNAIS et al. 1971, 1973 a, b) and bongkrekic acid (HENDERSON and LARDY 1970). The adenine nucleotide carrier has functional regulative significance since it is the endogenous adenine nucleotide which is phosphorylated (HELDT et al. 1965, HELDT 1966, DUÉÉ and VIGNAIS 1969).

The adenine nucleotide transport is also thought to involve a mobile carrier (KLINGENBERG and BUCHHOLTZ 1973). This conclusion is based on the interaction of bongkrekate and ADP binding. The binding of either ADP or bongkrekate is enhanced by the other component and the interaction of the two, results in irreversible binding. These results suggest that the ADP-carrier complex becomes trapped in the inner membrane interface by bongkrekate.

The interactions of the adenine nucleotide translocator system with inhibitors (e.g., carboxyatractyloside, VIGNAIS et al. 1971, 1972, 1973 a) suggest a cooperative behavior and hence the presence of the carrier in more than one conformation. A dependence of the conformation on energy state is indicated also by the affinities of the translocator for adenine nucleotides or for inhibitors which depend on the energy state of the mitochondria and the presence of ADP (see VIGNAIS and VIGNAIS 1972, 1973, SOUVERIJN et al. 1973, VERDOUX and BERTINA 1974). The presence of high affinity binding sites for inhibitors suggests a stoichiometry for the adenine nucleotide translocator of about 1 or 2 per respiratory chain assembly (VIGNAIS et al. 1971, 1973 a, b, KLINGENBERG et al. 1973). The stoichiometry opens the possibility for a close interaction between the translocator and F_1. Experiments with arsenate uncoupling (BERTAGNOLLI and HANSON 1973) and on dinitrophenol induced ATPase in the presence and absence of aurovertin (VERDOUX and BERTINA 1974) suggest a close interaction between the translocator and F_1 without a release of ADP into the mitochondrial matrix.

The adenine nucleotide translocator is inhibited by acyl CoA, an effect which is likely to have biological significance (PANDE and BLANCAER 1971, LERNER et al. 1972, VAARTJES et al. 1972, KLINGENBERG et al. 1973).

At least some components necessary for the adenine nucleotide translocase system are synthesized in the mitochondria, since the transport system is drastically altered in mitochondria isolated from yeast lacking mitochondrial DNA or where the mitochondrial protein synthesis has been inhibited (HASLAM et al. 1973 a).

d) Carriers and Ionophores

The study of the molecular mechanisms of the transport of ions has naturally involved searching for molecules which could act as carriers. In these studies, the search has been directed at protein molecules either capable of binding the ion under discussion or capable of acting in stimulating the transport of the ion in question. In this latter case the molecules have been referred to as ionophore molecules analogously to valinomycin and nigericin which have been used in mitochondria to induce the transport of ions.

The transport of Ca^{2+} into mitochondria was first observed by VASINGTON and MURPHY (1962). A similar accumulation of Mg^{2+} has been studied in beef heart mitochondria (BRIERLY et al. 1962). This rapidly advancing field has been recently reviewed (LEHNINGER et al. 1970, CARAFOLI 1973). The transport can be powered by either oxidative metabolism or ATP hydrolysis. When powered by oxidation, the process is sensitive to inhibitors of respiration and uncouplers but not oligomycin. On the other hand, the ATP powered process is sensitive to oligomycin and uncouplers but not respiratory inhibitors. The transport is inhibited by La^{3+} (MELA 1968, MELA and CHANCE 1969, LEHNINGER and CARAFOLI 1971), Ho^{3+} (holmium) and Pr^{3+} (praseodymium) (MELA and CHANCE 1969) or ruthenium red (MOORE 1971, VASINGTON et al. 1972). Ruthenium red is a dye which combines with glycoproteins and mucopolysaccharides. The Ca^{2+} transport shows saturation kinetics and the uptake is competitively inhibited by Sr^{2+}.

The K_m of the Ca^{2+} transport from a variety of studies ranges between 2–3 to 150 µM (CHANCE and SCHOENER 1966, BYGRAVE et al. 1972, CARAFOLI and AZZI 1972, VINOGRADOV and SCARPA 1973). The lack of agreement is probably produced in part by the indirect techniques used (e.g., CHANCE and SCHOENER 1966, CARAFOLI and AZZI 1972) or the lack of rapid kinetic measurements (BYGRAVE et al. 1972). In one study, the initial rate of Ca^{2+} uptake in rat liver mitochondria was estimated using a stop-flow technique and monitoring the Ca^{2+} with the indicator, murexide (VINOGRADOV and SCARPA 1973). The half saturation concentration of Ca^{2+} was found to be 55–70 µM. The rate of uptake as a function of Ca^{2+} concentrations is actually sigmoidal. The Hill plot suggests an involvement of 2 Ca^{2+} per molecule of transporter (BYGRAVE et al. 1972, VINOGRADOV and SCARPA 1973). The cooperativity of the interaction suggests that the presumed transporter molecule undergoes a conformational change.

In the absence of energy, mitochondria can bind Ca^{2+} at two different classes of binding sites, those of high affinity ($K_d = 0.1–1$ µM) and low affinity (K_d about 0.1 mM) (REYNAFARJE and LEHNINGER 1969, CHEN and LEHNINGER 1973). The low affinity groups can bind 50–70 nmoles Ca^{2+} per mg of mitochondrial protein. The high affinity sites bind 1 nmole per mg protein. The Ca^{2+} at the high affinity sites is blocked by La^{3+} or ruthenium red in the range of concentration at which transport is blocked. The high affinity sites also bind Sr^{2+} and Mn^{2+}. Mitochondria which lack a true Ca^{2+} transport system also lack the high affinity binding sites (e.g., yeast and blowfly mitochondria, CARAFOLI and LEHNINGER 1971).

The details of the results concerning high affinity binding have to be accepted with caution since La^{3+} sensitive sites can be detected in the apparent absence of Ca^{2+} binding sites (MELA and CHANCE 1969). In addition, some residual transport takes place despite the presence of metabolic inhibitors and may be responsible for some of the results (SOUTHARD and GREEN 1974 a).

The parallelisms in properties between Ca^{2+} transport and the high affinity binding sites suggests that the binding sites correspond to Ca^{2+} carrier molecules. Attempts to extract a protein molecule with a high affinity to Ca^{2+} has resulted in the isolation of an insoluble protein (GOMEZ-PUYOU *et al.* 1972) and a glycoprotein (SOTTOCASA *et al.* 1972, CARAFOLI *et al.* 1972, 1973, 1974). The glycoprotein is derived from the mitochondrial membrane and has a molecular weight of about 40,000 (CARAFOLI *et al.* 1973). It contains some phospholipid and carbohydrate, including 1 mole of sialic acid per mole of protein. The molecule binds with high affinity (K_d about 1 µM or less) 2 to 3 moles of Ca^{2+} per mole of glycoprotein and with low affinity (K_d between 10 µM and 1 mM) 10 moles of Ca^{2+} per mole of glycoprotein (CARAFOLI *et al.* 1972). The binding is inhibited by La^{3+} and ruthenium red (SOTTOCASA *et al.* 1972) at concentrations at which these inhibitors block transport. Blowfly and yeast mitochondria which do not carry out Ca^{2+} transport except very inefficiently, lack the glycoprotein (CARAFOLI *et al.* 1973).

The insoluble protein has a higher molecular weight (67,000). However, it resembles the glycoprotein in its affinity for Ca^{2+} and in some other properties (GOMEZ-PUYOU *et al.* 1972). Since the insoluble protein and the glycoprotein both contain lipid and other components, the difference in molecular weight may not be significant and the two may correspond to two different forms of the same molecule.

The glycoprotein decreases the Ca^{2+} conductance of lipid bilayers (CARAFOLI 1974, CARAFOLI *et al.* 1974, PRESTIPINO *et al.* 1974) and may correspond to the Ca^{2+} ionophore (BLONDIN 1974) discussed at the end of this section.

A component exhibiting an atractyloside-sensitive adenine nucleotide binding activity has been solubilized (EGAN and LEHNINGER 1974). In addition, it has been found possible to reconstitute vesicles capable of adenine nucleotide transport from lipids and a protein fraction extracted from mitochondria (SHERTZER and RACKER 1974).

A low molecular weight protein which binds P_i has been isolated from chloroform extracts of mitochondria and it contains SH groups (KADENBACH and HAVÁRY 1973, 1974). This protein may correspond to at least one of the postulated P_i carriers. However, the results should be regarded with caution since oxidative phosphorylation also involves SH groups (*e.g.*, FLUHARTY and SANADI 1960, FOUCHER and GAUDEMER 1971, SABADIE-PIALOUX and GAUTHERON 1971) and proteins involved in phosphorylation are likely to bind P_i. Some of the components of the rutamycin sensitive ATPase are soluble in organic solvent (TZAGOLOFF and MEAGHER 1972) and could correspond to the P_i binding site.

A number of attempts are now being made to isolated protein fractions capable of binding anions (*e.g.*, PALMIERI *et al.* 1974).

A proteolipid with a high affinity for glutamate has been isolated from pig heart mitochondria using a high affinity batch separation method (JUILLARD and GAUTHERON 1973). The proteolipid has a binding constant which approximately corresponds to the glutamate transport system and has no glutamate dehydrogenase activity. When added to liposomes it facilitated the entry of glutamate. For these reasons it is presumed to be involved in the glutamate transport system.

The transport of cations induced by ionophores such as valinomycin and nigericin has been studied for some time. The isolation of natural ionophores from mitochondria suggests that these may play a significant role in the natural active transport of ions. A Na^+ and K^+ ionophore has been isolated (BLONDIN et al. 1971). In mitochondria it seems to be activated by mercurials (SOUTHARD et al. 1973, 1974). More recently, a divalent cation ionophore has been isolated from beef heart mitochondria (BLONDIN 1974). These ionophores could function either in controlling the accessibility of the transport system to the ion or as carriers.

Oxidative phosphorylation is inversely related to the transport of either K^+ or Mg^{2+} induced by mercurials (SOUTHARD and GREEN 1974 b), suggesting that the coupling mechanism may be poised either to phosphorylate or transport ions. A similar reciprocal relationship between phosphorylation and transport was also observed in the case of P_i-induced transport (IZZARD and TEDESCHI 1970, 1973).

Bibliography

AAIJ, C., and P. BORST, 1972: The gel electrophoresis of DNA. Biochim. biophys. Acta **269**, 192.

— C. SACCONE, P. BORST, and M. N. GADALETA, 1970: Hybridization studies with RNA synthesized by isolated rat liver mitochondria. Biochim. biophys. Acta **199**, 373.

ABDELKADER, A. B., and P. MAZLIAK, 1970: Echange de lipides entre mitochondries, microsomes et surnageant cytoplasmique de cellules de pomme de terre ou de chou-fleur. Eur. J. Biochem. **15**, 250.

ADOUTTE, A., 1974: Mitochondria mutations in *Paramecium:* phenotypical characterization and recombination. In: The biogenesis of mitochondria. (KROON, A. M., and C. SACCONE, eds.), p. 263. New York-London: Academic Press.

AGSTERIBBE, E., A. M. KROON, and E. F. J. VAN BRUGGEN, 1972: Circular DNA from mitochondria of *Neurospora crassa*. Biochim. biophys. Acta **269**, 299.

— R. DATEMA, and A. M. KROON, 1974: Mitochondrial polysomes from *Neurospora crassa*. In: The biogenesis of mitochondria. (KROON, A. M., and C. SACCONE, eds.), p. 305. New York-London: Academic Press.

AINSWORTH, P. J., E. R. TUSTANOFF, and A. J. S. BALL, 1972: Membrane phase transitions as a diagnostic tool for studying mitochondriogenesis. Biochem. biophys. Res. Commun. **47**, 1299.

AKIMENKO, V. K., 1971: On the action of the uncouplers on soluble mitochondrial ATPase. Biokhimiya **36**, 655.

ALONI, Y., and G. ATTARDI, 1971 a: Expression of the mitochondrial genome in HeLa cells. II. Evidence for complete transcription of mitochondrial DNA. J. molec. Biol. **55**, 251.

— — 1971 b: Expression of the mitochondrial genome in HeLa cells. IV. Titration of mitochondrial genes for 16 s, 12 s and 4 s RNA. J. molec. Biol. **55**, 271.

— — 1971 c: Symmetrical *in vivo* transcription of mitochondrial DNA in HeLa cells. Proc. nat. Acad. Sci. (U.S.) **68**, 1757.

— — 1972: Expression of mitochondrial genome in HeLa cells. II. Isolation and characterization of transcription complexes of mitochondrial-DNA. J. molec. Biol. **70**, 363.

AMOORE, J. E., 1960: Exchange of potassium ions across a concentration difference by isolated rat-liver mitochondria. Biochem. J. **76**, 438.

— and W. BARTLEY, 1958: The permeability of isolated rat-liver mitochondria to sucrose, sodium chloride and potassium chloride at 0°. Biochem. J. **69**, 223.

ANAGNOSTI, E., and H. TEDESCHI, 1970: The mechanism of low-amplitude orthophosphate-induced swelling in isolated mitochondria. J. Cell Biol. **47**, 520.

ANDERSON, W. A., G. BARA, and A. M. SELIGMAN, 1975: The ultrastructural localization of cytochrome oxidase via cytochrome c. J. Histochem. and Cytochem. **23**, 13.

ANDRÉ, J., and V. MARINOZZI, 1965: Présence dans les mitochondrie, de particules ressemblant aux ribosomes. J. Micr. **4**, 615.

ARNBERG, A., E. F. J. VAN BRUGGEN, J. TER SCHEGGET, and P. BORST, 1971: The presence of DNA molecules with a displacement loop in standard mitochondrial DNA preparations. Biochim. biophys. Acta **246**, 353.

— — R. B. H. SCHUTGENS, R. A. FLAVELL, and P. BORST, 1972: Multiple D-loops in *Tetrahymena* mitochondrial DNA. Biochim. biophys. Acta **272**, 487.

ARNBERG, A., E. F. J. VAN BRUGGEN, R. A. CLEGG, W. B. UPHOLT, and P. BORST, 1974: An analysis by electron microscopy of intermediates in the replication of linear *Tetrahymena* mitochondrial DNA. Biochim. biophys. Acta **361**, 266.

ASAI, J., G. A. BLONDIN, W. J. VAIL, and D. E. GREEN, 1969: The mechanism of mitochondrial swelling. IV. Configurational changes during swelling of beef heart mitochondria. Arch. Biochem. Biophys. **132**, 524.

ASHHURST, D. E., 1965: Mitochondrial particles seen in sections. J. Cell Biol. **24**, 497.

ASHWELL, M., and T. S. WORK, 1970: Biogenesis of mitochondria. Ann. Rev. Biochem. **39**, 251.

ASHWORTH, C. T., J. S. LEONARD, E. H. EIGENBRODT, and F. J. WRIGHTSMAN, 1966: Hepatic intracellular osmiophilic droplets; effect of lipid solvents during tissue preparation. J. Cell Biol. **31**, 301.

ASTLE, L., and C. COOPER, 1974: Relationship of sidedness of mitochondrial inner membrane vesicles to their enzymic properties. Biochem. **13**, 154.

ATTARDI, B., and G. ATTARDI, 1967: A membrane-associated RNA of cytoplasmic origin in HeLa cells. Proc. nat. Acad. Sci. (U.S.) **58**, 1051.

— — 1971: Expression of the mitochondrial genome in HeLa cells. I. Properties of the discrete RNA components from the mitochondrial fraction. J. molec. Biol. **55**, 231.

ATTARDI, G., 1970: Transcription of mitochondrial DNA in HeLa cells. Cold Spring Harbor Symp. Quant. Biol. **35**, 599.

— Y. ALONI, B. ATTARDI, D. OJALA, L. PICA-MATTOCCIA, D. S. ROBBERSON, and G. STORRIE, 1970: Transcription of mitochondrial DNA in HeLa cells. Cold Spring Harbor Symp. Quant. Biol. **35**, 599.

AVADHANI, N. G., and D. E. BUETOW, 1972 a: Protein synthesis with isolated mitochondrial polysomes. Biochem. biophys. Res. Commun. **46**, 773.

— — 1972 b: Isolation of active polyribosomes from the cytoplasm, mitochondria and chloroplasts of *Euglena gracilis*. Biochem. J. **128**, 353.

— and R. J. RUTMAN, 1974: A sensitive *in vitro* protein synthesizing system from *Ehrlich ascites* mitochondria. Biochem. biophys. Res. Commun. **58**, 42.

— M. J. LYNCH, and D. E. BUETOW, 1971: Protein synthesis on polysomes in mitochondria isolated from *Euglena gracilis*. Exp. Cell Res. **69**, 226.

AZZI, A., J. B. CHAPPELL, and B. H. ROBINSON, 1967: Penetration of the mitochondrial membrane by glutamate and aspartate. Biochem. biophys. Res. Commun. **29**, 148.

AZZONE, G. F., 1972: Oxidative phosphorylation, a history of unsuccessful attempts: is it only an experimental problem? J. Bioenerg. **3**, 95.

— and S. MASSARI, 1971: Thermodynamic and kinetic aspects of interconversion of chemical and osmotic energies in mitochondria. Eur. J. Biochem. **19**, 97.

— — 1972: Osmotic properties of sonicated mitochondrial fragments. FEBS Lett. **28**, 61.

— — 1973: Active transport and binding in mitochondria. Biochim. biophys. Acta **301**, 195.

— — R. COLONNA, P. DELL'ANTONE, and L. FRIGERI, 1974: Two conceptions of active transport in mitochondria: principles and experimental tests. Ann. N.Y. Acad. Sci. **227**, 337.

BAILEY, E., C. B. TAYLOR, and W. BARTLEY, 1967: Turnover of mitochondrial components of normal and essential fatty acid-deficient rats. Biochem. J. **104**, 1026.

BAKEEVA, L. E., L. L. GRINIUS, A. A. JASAITIS, V. V. KULSENE, D. O. LEVITSKY, E. A. LIBERMAN, I. I. SEVERINA, and V. P. SKULACHEV, 1970: Conversion of biomembrane-produced energy into electric form. II. Intact mitochondria. Biochim. biophys. Acta **216**, 13.

BALTSCHEFFSKY, H., and M. BALTSCHEFFSKY, 1974: Electron transport phosphorylation. Ann. Rev. Biochem. **43**, 871.

BANK, H., 1974: Freezing injury in tissue cultured cells as visualized by freeze-etching. Exp. Cell Res. **85**, 367.

— and P. MAZUR, 1972: Relation between ultrastructure and viability of frozen-thawed chinese hamster tissue-culture cells. Exp. Cell Res. **71**, 441.

— — 1973: Visualization of freezing damage. J. Cell Biol. **57**, 729.

BARATH, Z., and H. KÜNTZEL, 1972 a: RNA polymerase-induction in mitochondria of *Neurospora crassa*. Nature, New Biol. **240**, 195.

BARATH, Z., and H. KÜNTZEL, 1972 b: Cooperation of mitochondria and nuclear genes specifying the mitochondrial genetic apparatus in *Neurospora crassa*. Proc. nat. Acad. Sci. (U.S.) **69**, 1371.

BARGOLIE, W., W. HASSELBACH, and M. MAKINOSE, 1971: Activation of calcium efflux by ADP and inorganic phosphate. FEBS Lett. **12**, 267.

BARNETT, W. E., and D. H. BROWN, 1967: Mitochondrial transfer ribonucleic acids. Proc. nat. Acad. Sci. (U.S.) **57**, 452.

— and J. L. EPLER, 1966: Fractionation and specificities of two aspartyl-ribonucleic acid and two phenylalanyl-ribonucleic acid synthetases. Proc. nat. Acad. Sci. (U.S.) **55**, 184.

— D. H. BROWN, and J. L. EPLER, 1967: Mitochondrial-specific aminoacyl-RNA synthetases. Proc. nat. Acad. Sci. (U.S.) **57**, 1775.

BARNHART, E. R., and C. E. TERRY, 1971: Cryobiology of *Neurospora crassa*. I. Freeze response of *Neurospora crassa* conidia. Cryobiol. **8**, 323.

BARTÓK, I., S. Z. VIRÁGH, and J. MENYHÁRT, 1973: Prompt divisions and peculiar transformation of cristae in liver-mitochondria of rats rehydrated after prolonged water deprivation. J. Ultrastruct. Res. **44**, 49.

BAUER, H., and K. TAMAKA, 1968: Ultrastructure of mitochondria and crystal containing bodies in mature ballsitospores of the fungus *Basidiobolus ranarum* as revealed by freeze-etching. J. Bact. **96**, 2132.

BAUER, W., and J. VINOGRAD, 1971: The use of intercalative dyes in the study of closed circular DNA. Progr. Mol. Subcell. Biol. **2**, 181.

BEALE, G. H., J. KNOWLES, and A. TAIT, 1972: Mitochondrial genetics in *Paramecium*. Nature **235**, 396.

BEATTIE, D., 1971: The synthesis of mitochondrial proteins. Subcell. Biochem. **1**, 1.

BEATTIE, D. S., R. E. BASFORD, and D. B. KORITZ, 1967 a: Bacterial contamination and amino acid incorporation by isolated mitochondria. J. biol. Chem. **342**, 336.

— — — 1967 b: The inner membrane as the site of the *in vitro* incorporation of L-[C^{14}] leucine into mitochondrial protein. Biochem. **6**, 3099.

— L.-R. H. LIN, and R. N. STUCHELL, 1974: Studies on the control of mitochondrial protein synthesis in yeast. In: The biogenesis of mitochondria. (KROON, A. M., and C. SACCONE, eds.), p. 465. New York-London: Academic Press.

BEAULATION, J. A., 1966: Modifications ultrastructurales des cellules sécrétrices de la gland prothoracique de vers à poie au cours des deux dernièrs âges larvaires. I. Le chondriome, et ses relations avec le reticulum agranulaire. J. Cell Biol. **39**, 501.

BEECHEY, R. B., and K. J. CATTELL, 1973: Mitochondrial coupling factors. Curr. Top. in Bioenerg. **5**, 306.

BEHNKE, O., 1965: Helical filaments in rat liver mitochondria. Exp. Cell Res. **37**, 687.

BEINERT, H., and R. H. SANDS, 1960: Studies in succinic and DPNH dehydrogenase preparations by paramagnetic resonance (EPR) spectroscopy. Biochem. biophys. Res. Commun. **3**, 41.

— B. A. C. ACKRELL, E. B. KEARNEY, and T. P. SINGER, 1974: EPR studies on the mechanism of action of succinate dehydrogenase in activated preparations. Biochem. biophys. Res. Commun. **58**, 564.

BEISSON, J., A. SAINSARD, A. ADOUTTE, G. H. BEALE, J. KNOWLES, and A. TAIT, 1974: Genetic control of mitochondria in *Paramecium*. Genetics **78**, 403.

BEMIS, J. A., G. M. BRYANT, J. C. ARCOS, and M. F. ARGUS, 1968: Swelling and contraction of mitochondrial particles: A re-examination of the existence of a contractile protein extractable with 0.6 M-potassium chloride. Journal of Molecular Biology **33**, 299.

BENDICH, A. J., and B. J. MCCARTHY, 1970: Ribosomal RNA homologies among distantly related organisms. Proc. nat. Acad. Sci. (U.S.) **65**, 349.

BERDEN, J. A., and E. C. SLATER, 1972: The allosteric binding of antimycin to cytochrome b in the mitochondrial membrane. Biochim. biophys. Acta **256**, 199.

BERGER, E. R., 1973: Two morphologically different mitochondrial populations in the rat hepatocyte as determined by quantitative three-dimensional electron microscopy. J. Ultrastruct. Res. **45**, 303.

BERNARDI, G., M. FAURES, G. PIPERNO, and P. P. SLONIMSKI, 1970: Mitochondrial DNA's from respiratory-sufficient and cytoplasmic respiratory-deficient mutant yeast. J. molec. Biol. **48**, 23.

BERNARDI, G., G. PIPERNO, and G. FONTY, 1972: The mitochondrial genome of wild-type yeast cells. I. Preparation and heterogeneity of mitochondrial DNA. J. molec. Biol. **65**, 173.

BERTAGNOLLI, B. L., and J. B. HANSON, 1973: Functioning of the adenine nucleotide transporter in the arsenate uncoupling of corn mitochondria. Plant Physiol. **52**, 431.

BERTINA, R. M., P. I. SHRIER, and E. C. SLATER, 1973: The binding of aurovertin to mitochondria and its effect on mitochondrial respiration. Biochim. biophys. Acta **305**, 503.

BIELAWSKY, J., T. E. THOMPSON, and A. L. LEHNINGER, 1966: The effect of 2,4—dinitrophenol on electrical resistance of phospholipid bilayer membranes. Biochem. biophys. Res. Commun. **24**, 948.

BIRT, L. M., and W. BARTLEY, 1960: The distribution and metabolism of intra- and extra-mitochondrial pyridine nucleotides in suspensions of liver mitochondria. Biochem. J. **75**, 303.

BLAMIRE, J., D. R. CRYER, D. B. FINKELSTEIN, and J. MARMUR, 1972 a: Sedimentation properties of yeast nuclear and mitochondrial DNA. J. molec. Biol. **67**, 11.

— D. B. FINKELSTEIN, and J. MARMUR, 1972 b: Isolation and fractionation of yeast nucleic acids. I. Characterization of poly(L-lysine) Kieselguhr chromatography using yeast nucleic acids. Biochem. **11**, 4848.

BLINZINGER, K., N. B. REWCASTLE, and H. HAGER, 1965: Observations on prismatic-type mitochondria within astrocytes of the Syrian hamster brain. J. Cell Biol. **25**, 293.

BLONDIN, G. A., 1974: Isolation of a divalent-cation ionophore from beef heart mitochondria. Biochem. biophys. Res. Commun. **56**, 97.

— and D. E. GREEN, 1969: Mechanism of mitochondrial swelling. III. Two forms of energized swelling. Arch. Biochem. Biophys. **132**, 509.

— W. J. VAIL, and D. E. GREEN, 1969: The mechanism of mitochondrial swelling. II. Pseudo-energized swelling in the presence of alkali metal salts. Arch. Biochem. Biophys. **129**, 158.

— A. F. DE CASTRO, and A. E. SENIOR, 1971: The isolation and properties of a peptide ionophore from beef heart mitochondria. Biochem. biophys. Res. Commun. **43**, 28.

BLOOMFIELD, D. K., and K. BLOCH, 1960: The formation of Δ^9-unsaturated fatty acids. J. Biol. Chem. **235**, 337.

BOLOTIN, M., D. COEN, J. DEUTSCH, B. DUJON, P. NETTER, E. PETROCHILO et P. SLONIMSKI, 1971: La recombination des mitochondries chez *Saccharomyces cerevisiae*. Bull Inst. Pasteur **69**, 215.

BONNER, W. D., JR., and E. C. SLATER, 1970: Effect of antimycin on the potato mitochondrial cytochrome b system. Biochim. biophys. Acta **223**, 349.

BORST, P., 1971: Size, structure and information content of mitochondrial DNA. In: Autonomy and biogenesis of mitochondria and chloroplasts. (BOARDMAN, N. K., A. W. LINNANE, and R. M. SMILLIE, eds.), p. 260. Amsterdam-London: North-Holland.

— 1972: Mitochondrial nucleic acids. Ann. Rev. Biochem. **41**, 333.

— 1974: Structure of petite mtDNA; prospects for mitochondrial gene isolation mapping and sequencing. In: The biogenesis of mitochondria. (KROON, A. M., and C. SACCONE, eds.), p. 147. New York-London: Academic Press.

— and C. AAIJ, 1969: Identification of the heavy strand of ratliver mitochondrial DNA as the messenger strand. Biochem. biophys. Res. Commun. **34**, 358.

— and R. A. FLAVELL, 1972: Mitochondrial DNA, genes, replication. In: Mitochondria: Biogenesis and bioenergetics. (VAN DEN BERGH, S. G., P. BORST, L. L. M. VAN DEENEN, J. C. RIEMERSMA, E. C. SLATER, and J. M. TAGER, eds.), p. 1. Amsterdam-London: North-Holland/American Elsevier.

— and L. A. GRIVELL, 1971: Mitochondrial ribosomes. FEBS Lett. **13**, 73.

— and A. M. KROON, 1969: Mitochondrial DNA: Physicochemical properties, replication and genetic function. Int. Rev. Cytol. **26**, 107.

— and G. J. C. M. RUTTENBERG, 1966: On the presence of DNA in mitochondria of animal tissues. In: Regulation of metabolic processes in mitochondria. (TAGER, J. M., S. PAPA, E. QUAGLIARIELLO, and E. C. SLATER, eds.), p. 454. Amsterdam-London-New York: Elsevier Publishing Co.

— — 1969: Mitochondrial DNA. IV. Interaction of ribopolynucleotides with the complementary strands of chick liver mitochondrial DNA. Biochim. biophys. Acta **190**, 391.

Bosmann, H. B., 1970: Camptothecin inhibits macromolecular synthesis in mammalian cells but not in isolated mitochondria or *E. coli*. Biochem. biophys. Res. Commun. **41**, 1412.

Boyer, P. D., 1965: Carboxyl activation as a possible common reaction in substrate level, muscle contraction and oxidative phosphorylation. In: Oxidases and related redox systems. (King, T. E., H. S. Mason, and M. Morrison, eds.), Vol. 2, p. 994. New York: J. Wiley.

— 1975: Energy transduction and proton translocation by adenosine triphosphatase. FEBS Lett. **50**, 91.

— R. L. Cross, and W. Momsen, 1973: A new concept for energy coupling in oxidative phosphorylation based on a molecular explanation of the oxygen exchange reaction. Proc. nat. Acad. Sci. (U.S.) **70**, 2837.

Bradford, N. M., and J. D. McGivan, 1973: Quantitative characteristics of glutamate transport in rat-liver mitochondria. Biochem. J. **134**, 1023.

Brandt, J. T., A. P. Martin, F. V. Lucas, and M. L. Vorbeck, 1974: The structure of rat liver mitochondria: a re-evaluation. Biochem. biophys. Res. Commun. **59**, 1097.

Branton, D., 1966: Fracture faces of frozen membranes. Proc. nat. Acad. Sci. (U.S.) **55**, 1048.

— 1967: Fracture faces of frozen myelin. Exp. Cell Res. **45**, 703.

— and D. W. Deamer, 1972: In: Membrane structure. (Alfert, M., H. Bauer, W. Sandwritter, and P. Sitte, eds.). Wien-New York: Springer-Verlag.

— and H. Moor, 1964: Fine structure in freeze-etched *Allium cepa*. L. Root tips. J. Ultrastruct. Res. **11**, 401.

— and R. B. Park, 1967: Subunits in chloroplast lamellae. J. Ultrastruct. Res. **19**, 283.

Brega, A., and C. Baglioni, 1971: A study of mitochondria protein synthesis in intact HeLa cells. Eur. J. Biochem. **22**, 415.

Brierley, G. P., 1974: Passive permeability and energy linked ion movements in isolated heart mitochondria. Ann. N.Y. Acad. Sci. **227**, 398.

— and C. T. Settlemire, 1967: Ion transport by heart mitochondria. IX. Induction of the energy-linked uptake of K^+ by zinc ions. J. Biol. Chem. **242**, 4324.

— E. Bachman, and D. E. Green, 1962: Active transport of inorganic phosphate and magnesium ions by beef heart mitochondria. Proc. nat. Acad. Sci. (U.S.) **48**, 1928.

— V. A. Knight, and C. T. Settlemire, 1968 a: Ion transport by heart mitochondria. XII. Activation of monovalent cation uptake by sulfhydril group reagent. J. biol. Chem. **243**, 5035.

— C. T. Settlemire, and V. A. Knight, 1968 b: Ion transport by heart mitochondria. XI. Spontaneous and induced permeability of heart mitochondria to cations. Arch. Biochem. **126**, 276.

— M. Jurkowitz, K. M. Scott, and A. J. Merola, 1970: Ion transport by heart mitochondria. XX. Factors affecting passive osmotic swelling of isolated mitochondria. J. biol. Chem. **245**, 5404.

— — — — 1971 a: Ion transport by heart mitochondria. XXII. Spontaneous energy-linked accumulation of acetate and phosphate salts of monovalent cations. Arch. Biochem. Biophys. **147**, 545.

— K. M. Scott, and M. Jurkowitz, 1971 b: Ion transport by heart mitochondria. XXI. Differential effects of mercurial reagents on adenosine triphosphatase activity and adenosine triphosphate-dependent swelling and contraction. J. biol. Chem. **246**, 2241.

— M. Jurkowitz, A. J. Merola, and K. M. Scott, 1972: Ion transport by heart mitochondria. XXV. Activation of energy-linked K^+ uptake by non-ionic detergents. Arch. Biochem. Biophys. **152**, 744.

— — K. H. Scott, 1973: Ion transport by heart mitochondria. XXVII. Relation of mercurial-dependent adenosine triphosphatase activity to ion movements. Arch. Biochem. Biophys. **159**, 742.

Brooks, J. C., and A. E. Senior, 1971: Studies on the mitochondrial oligomycin insensitive ATPase. II. The relationship of the specific protein inhibitor to the ATPase. Arch. Biochem. Biophys. **147**, 467.

Brouwer, A., G. G. Smits, J. Tas, A. J. Meijer, and J. M. Tager, 1973: Substrate anion transport in mitochondria. Biochimie **55**, 717.

Buck, C. A., and M. M. K. Nass, 1960: Chromatographic differences between cytoplasmic and mitochondrial transfer RNA. Fed. Proc. 27, 342.

— — 1969: Studies on mitochondrial tRNA from animal cells. I. A comparison of mitochondrial and cytoplasmic tRNA and amino-acyl-tRNA synthetases. J. molec. Biol. 41, 67.

Bullivant, S., 1973: Freeze-etching and freeze-fracturing. In: Advanced techniques in biological electron microscopy. (Koehler, J. K., ed.), p. 67. Berlin-New York: Springer-Verlag.

— and A. Ames, 1966: A simple freeze-fracture replication method for electron microscopy. J. Cell Biol. 29, 435.

Bulos, B., and E. Racker, 1968: Partial resolution of the enzyme catalyzing oxidative phosphorylation. XVII. Further resolution of rutamycin-sensitive adenosine triphosphatase. J. biol. Chem. 243, 3891.

Bunn, C. N., C. H. Mitchell, H. B. Lukins, and A. W. Linnane, 1970: Biogenesis of mitochondria. XVIII. A new class of cytoplasmically determined antibiotic resistant mutants in Saccharomyces cerevisiae. Proc. nat. Acad. Sci. (U.S.) 67, 1233.

Burke, J. P., and D. S. Beattie, 1974: Products of rat liver mitochondrial protein synthesis: electrophoretic analysis of the number and size of theseproteins and their solubility in chloroform: methanol. Arch. Biochem. Biophys. 164, 1.

Bygrave, F. L., K. C. Reed, and T. Spencer, 1971: Cooperative interactions in energy-dependent accumulation of Ca^{2+} by isolated rat liver mitochondria. Nature, New Biology 230, 89.

Cailloux, M., et L. Genevès, 1966: Variation des infrastructure mitochondriales dans le méristème radiculaire du Raphanus savitus (Crucifères) on fonction des conditions de culture. C. R. Acad. Sci. Série D, 263, 1699.

Callen, D. F., 1974 a: Recombination and segregation of mitochondrial genes in Saccharomyces cerevisiae. Mol. Gen. Genetics 134, 49.

— 1974 b: Segregation of mitochondrially inherited antibiotic resistance genes in zygote cell lineages of Saccharomyces cerevisiae. Mol. Gen. Genetics 134, 65.

Cantley, L. C., Jr., and G. G. Hammes, 1973: Activation of beef heart mitochondrial adenosine triphosphatase by 2,4-dinitrophenol. Biochem. 12, 4900.

Capaldi, R. A., 1974: Identification of the major enzymic activities of the mitochondrial inner member in terms of their migration in sodium dodecyl sulfate polyacrylamide gel electrophoresis. Arch. Biochem. Biophys. 163, 99.

Carafoli, E., 1973: Transport of calcium by mitochondria—problems and perspectives. Biochimie 55, 755.

— 1974: The interaction of Ca^{2+} with the mitochondrial membrane and with a soluble mitochondrial glycoprotein. In: Biomembranes: Architecture, Biogenesis, Bioenergetics and Differentiation. (Packer, L., ed.), p. 221. New York-London: Academic Press.

— and A. Azzi, 1972: The affinity of mitochondria for Ca^{++}. Experientia 28, 906.

— and A. L. Lehninger, 1971: A survey of the interaction of calcium ions with mitochondria from different tissues and species. Biochem. J. 122, 681.

— R. G. Hansford, B. Sacktor, and A. L. Lehninger, 1971: Interaction of Ca^{2+} with blowfly flight muscle mitochondria. J. biol. Chem. 246, 964.

— P. Gazzotti, F. D. Vasington, G. L. Sottocasa, G. Sandri, E. Panfili, and B. de Bernard, 1972: Soluble Ca^{2+} binding factors isolated from mitochondria. In: Biochemistry and biophysics of mitochondrial membranes. (Azzone, G. F., E. Carafoli, A. L. Lehninger, E. Quagliariello, and N. Siliprandi, eds.), p. 623. New York-London: Academic Press.

— — C. Saltini, C. S. Rossi, G. L. Sottocasa, G. Sandri, E. Panfili, and B. de Bernard, 1973: Further studies on the mitochondrial Ca^{2+}-binding glycoprotein. In: Mechanisms in bioenergetics. (Azzone, G. F., L. Ernster, S. Papa, E. Quagliariello, and N. Siliprandi, eds.), p. 293. New York-London: Academic Press.

CARAFOLI, E., G. F. PRESTIPINO, D. CECCARELLI, and F. CONTI, 1974: The interaction between Ca^{2+}, the mitochondrial Ca^{2+}-binding glycoprotein, and artificial lipid bilayer systems. In: Membrane Proteins in Transport and Phosphorylation. (AZZONE, G. F., M. E. KLINGEN-BERG, E. QUAGLIARIELLO, and N. SILIPRANDI, eds.), p. 85. North-Holland: Publishing Co. Amsterdam-London-New York: American Elsevier Publishing Co.

CARNEVALI, F., G. MORPURGO, and G. TECCE, 1969: Cytoplasmic DNA from petite colonies of *Saccharomyces cerevisiae:* A hypothesis on the nature of the mutation. Science **163**, 1331.

CASEY, J., M. COHEN, M. RABINOWITZ, H. FUKUHARA, and G. S. GETZ, 1972: Hybridization of mitochondrial transfer RNA's with mitochondrial and nuclear DNA of *grande* (wild type) yeast. J. molec. Biol. **63**, 431.

— P. GORDON, and M. RABINOWITZ, 1974: Characterization of mitochondrial deoxyribonucleic acid from *grande* and *petite* yeasts by renaturation and denaturation analysis and by transfer ribonucleic acid hybridization; evidence for internal repetition or heterogeneity in mitochondrial deoxyribonucleic acid populations. Biochem. **13**, 1059.

CASWELL, A. H., 1968: Potentiometric determination of inter-relationships of energy conservation and ion gradient in mitochondria. J. biol. Chem. **243**, 5827.

— 1971: The estimation of redox potential of cytochromes in mitochondria. Arch. Biochem. Biophys. **144**, 445.

CATTERALL, W. A., and P. L. PEDERSEN, 1971: Adenosine triphosphatase from rat liver mitochondria. I. Purification, homogeneity and physical properties. J. biol. Chem. **246**, 4987.

— W. A. COTY, and P. L. PEDERSEN, 1973: Adenosine triphosphatase III. Subunit composition. J. Biol. Chem. **248**, 7427.

CERVÓS-NAVARRO, J., E. TONUTTI, and J. M. BAYER, 1964: Endokrinologie (Leipzig) **47**, 23.

CHAKRABARTI, S., D. K. DUBE, and S. C. ROY, 1972: Effects of emetine and cycloheximide on mitochondria protein synthesis in different systems. Biochem. J. **128**, 461.

CHANCE, B., 1965: The energy-linked reaction of calcium with mitochondria. J. biol. Chem. **240**, 2729.

— and U. FUGMANN, 1961: ATP induced oxidation of exogenous cytochrome c in terminally inhibited phosphorylating particles. Biochem. biophys. Res. Commun. **4**, 317.

— and M. MONTAL, 1971: Ion translocation in energy-conserving membrane systems. Curr. Top. in Memb. Transport **2**, 100.

— and B. SCHOENER, 1966: High and low energy states of cytochromes in reactions with cations. J. Biol. Chem. **241**, 4577.

— and G. R. WILLIAMS, 1956: The respiratory chain and oxidative phosphorylation. Adv. Enz. **17**, 65.

— D. F. WILSON, P. L. DUTTON, and M. ERECIŃSKA, 1970: Energy coupling mechanisms in mitochondria: kinetic, spectroscopic and thermodynamic properties of an energy-transducing form of cytochrome b. Proc. nat. Acad. Sci. (U.S.) **66**, 1175.

CHANG, T. M., and H. S. PENEFSKY, 1973: Aurovertin, a fluorescent probe of conformational change in beef heart mitochondrial adenosine triphosphatase. J. Biol. Chem. **248**, 2746.

— 1974: Energy-dependent enhancement of aurovertin fluorescence, an indicator of conformational changes in beef heart mitochondrial adenosine triphosphatase. J. Biol. Chem. **249**, 1090.

CHAPPELL, J. B., 1969: Transport and exchange of anions in mitochondria. In: Inhibitors, tools in cell research. (BÜCHER, TH., and H. SIES, eds.), p. 335. New York-Berlin-Heidelberg: Springer-Verlag.

— and A. R. CROFTS, 1965 a: Gramicidin and ion transport in isolated inner mitochondria. Biochem. J. **95**, 393.

— — 1965 b: The effect of atractylate and oligomycin in the behavior of mitochondria towards adenine nucleotides. Biochem. J. **95**, 707.

— — 1966: Ion transport and reversible volume changes of isolated mitochondria. In: Regulation of metabolic processes in mitochondria. (TAGER, J. M., S. PAPA, E. QUAGLIA-RIELLO, and E. C. SLATER, eds.), p. 293. Amsterdam-London-New York: Elsevier Publishing Co.

CHAPPELL, J. B., and K. N. HAARHOFF, 1967: The penetration of the mitochondrial membrane by anions and cations. In: Biochemistry of mitochondria. (SLATER, E. C., Z. KANIUGA, and L. WOJTCZAK, eds.), p. 75. New York-London: Academic Press.

— and B. H. ROBINSON, 1968: Penetration of mitochondrial membrane by tricarboxylic acid anions. Biochem. Soc. Symp. 27, 123.

— M. COHN, and G. D. GREVILLE, 1963: The accumulation of divalent ions by isolated mitochondria. In: Energy-linked function of mitochondria. (CHANCE, B., ed.), p. 219. New York: Academic Press.

— P. J. F. HENDERSON, J. D. McGIVAN, and B. H. ROBINSON, 1968: The effect of drugs on mitochondrial function. In: The interaction of drugs and subcellular components in animal cells. (CAMPBELL, P. N., ed.), p. 71. London: J. and A. Churchill, Ltd.

CHEN, C. H., and A. L. LEHNINGER, 1973: Ca^{+2} transport activity in mitochondria from some plant tissues. Arch. Biochem. 157, 183.

CHEN, W. L., and CHARALAMPOUS, 1969: Mechanism of induction of cytochrome oxidase in yeast. I. Kinetics of induction and evidence for accumulation of cytoplasmic and mitochondrial precursors. J. biol. Chem. 244, 2767.

CHEN, W. U., B. EPHRUSSI, et H. HOTTINGUER, 1950: Nature génétique des mutants à deficience respiratoire de la souche B-11 de la levure de boulangerie. Heredity 4, 337.

CHI, J. C. H., and Y. SUYAMA, 1970: Comparative studies on mitochondrial and cytoplasmic ribosomes of Tetrahymena pyriformis. J. molec. Biol. 53, 531.

CHIU, N., A. O. S. CHIU, and Y. SUYAMA, 1974: Coding degeneracy in mitochondria. In: The biogenesis of mitochondria. (KROON, A. M., and C. SACCONE, eds.), p. 383. New York-London: Academic Press.

CHRISTENSEN, A. K., and D. W. FAWCETT, 1961: The normal fine structure of opossum testicular interstitial cells. J. Cell Biol. 9, 653.

CHRISTIANSEN, C., A. L. BAK, A. STENDERUP, and G. CHRISTIANSEN, 1971: Repetitive DNA in yeasts. Nature New Biol. 231, 176.

CHRISTIANSEN, R. O., A. LOYTER, J. STEENSLAND, and E. RACKER, 1969: Energy-linked ion translocation in submitochondrial particles. II. Properties of submitochondrial particles capable of Ca^{++} translocation. J. Biol. Chem. 244, 4428.

CLARK, W. M., 1960: Oxidation-reduction potential of organic systems. Baltimore: Williams and Wilkins Co.

CLARK-WALKER, G. D., and A. W. LINNANE, 1966: In vivo differentiation of yeast cytoplasmic and mitochondrial protein synthesis with antibiotics. Biochem. biophys. Res. Commun. 25, 8.

— — 1967: The biogenesis of mitochondria in Saccharomyces cerevisiae. A comparison between cytoplasmic respiratory-deficient mutant yeast and chloramphenicol-inhibited wild-type cells. J. Cell. Biol. 34, 1.

CLAYTON, D. A., and R. M. BRAMBL, 1972: Detection of circular DNA from mitochondria of Neurospora crassa. Biochem. biophys. Res. Commun. 6, 1477.

— R. W. DAVIS, and J. VINOGRAD, 1970: Homology and structural relationships between the dimeric and monomeric circular forms of mitochondrial DNA from human leukemic leukocytes. J. molec. Biol. 47, 137.

CLEGG, R. A., P. BORST, and P. J. WEIJERS, 1974: Intermediates in the replication of the mitochondrial DNA of Tetrahymena pyriformis. Biochim. biophys. Acta 361, 277.

COBLEY, J. G., S. GROSSMAN, H. BEINERT, and T. P. SINGER, 1973: Catalytic activity and EPR signals of DPNH dehydrogenase in relation to the acquisition and loss of piericidin sensitivity and of coupling site I. Biochem. biophys. Res. Commun. 53, 1273.

COBON, G. S., P. D. CROWFOOT, and A. W. LINNANE, 1974: Biogenesis of Mitochondria: Phospholipid synthesis in vitro by yeast. Biochem. J. 144, 265.

COCKRELL, R. S., and E. RACKER, 1969: Respiratory control and K^+ transport in submitochondrial particles. Biochem. biophys. Res. Commun. 35, 414.

— E. J. HARRIS, and B. C. PRESSMAN, 1966: Energetics of potassium transport in mitochondria induced by valinomycin. Biochem. 5, 2326.

— — — 1967: Synthesis of ATP driven by a potassium gradient in mitochondria. Nature 215, 1487.

COEN, D., J. DEUTSCH, P. NETTER, E. PETROCHILO, and P. SLONIMSKI, 1970: Mitochondrial Genetics. Symp. Soc. Exp. Bio. **24**, 449.

COHEN, L. B., B. M. SALZBERG, H. V. DAVILA, W. N. ROSS, D. LANDOWNE, A. S. WAGGONER, and C.-H. WANG, 1974: Changes in axon fluorescence during activity; molecular probes of membrane potential. J. Memb. Biol. **19**, 1.

COHEN, L. H., C. P. HOLLENBERG, and P. BORST, 1970: An analysis of a possible base sequence complementarity of mitochondria and nuclear DNA in yeast. Biochim. biophys. Acta **224**, 610.

COHEN, M., and M. RABINOWITZ, 1972: Analysis of *grande* and *petite* yeast mitochondrial DNA by tRNA hybridization. Biochim. biophys. Acta **281**, 192.

— J. CASEY, M. RABINOWITZ, and G. S. GETZ, 1972: Hybridization of mitochondrial transfer RNA and mitochondrial DNA in *petite* mutants of yeast. J. molec. Biol. **63**, 441.

COLE, J. S., III, and H. ALEEM, 1973: Electron transport-linked compared with proton-induced ATP generation in *Thiobacillus novellus*. Proc. nat. Acad. Sci. (U.S.) **70**, 3571.

COLE, K. S., and J. W. MOORE, 1960: Potassium ion current in the squid giant axon: dynamic characteristics. Biophys. J. **1**, 1.

CONNELLY, J. L., and H. A. LARDY, 1964: Antibiotics as tools for metabolic studies. III. Effects of oligomycin and aurovertin on the swelling and contraction processes of mitochondria. Biochem. **3**, 1969.

CONOVER, T. E., and M. BÁRÁNY, 1966: The absence of a myosin-like protein in liver mitochondria. Biochim. biophys. Acta **127**, 235.

COOPER, C. S., and C. J. AVERS, 1974: Evidence of involvement of mitochondrial polysomes and messenger RNA in synthesis of organelle proteins. In: The biogenesis of mitochondria. (KROON, A. M., and C. SACCONE, eds.), p. 289. New York-London: Academic Press.

COOTE, J. L., and T. S. WORK, 1971: Proteins coded by mitochondrial DNA of mammalian cells. Eur. J. Biochem. **23**, 564.

COPELAND, L., C. J. DEUTSCH, S.-I. TU, and J. H. WANG, 1974: Chemical modification of mitochondria. II. Effect of labelling on oxidative phosphorylation. Arch. Biochem. Biophys. **160**, 451.

CORNEO, G., C. MOORE, D. R. SANADI, L. I. GROSSMAN, and J. MARMUR, 1966: Mitochondrial DNA in yeast and some mammalian species. Science **151**, 687.

— E. GINELLI, and E. POLLI, 1968 a: Isolation of the complementary strands of a human satellite DNA. J. molec. Biol. **33**, 331.

— L. ZARDI, and E. POLLI, 1968 b: Human mitochondrial DNA. J. molec. Biol. **36**, 419.

COSTER, H. G. L., 1965: A quantitative analysis of the voltage-current relationships of fixed charge membranes and the associated property of "punch-through". Biophys. J. **5**, 669.

COTTER, D. A., L. Y. MIURA-SANTO, and H. R. HOYL, 1969: Ultrastructural changes during germination of *Dictostelium discoideum* spores. J. Bact. **100**, 1020.

COTY, A., and P. L. PEDERSEN, 1974: Phosphate transport in rat liver mitochondria. Kinetics and energy requirement. J. biol. Chem. **249**, 2593.

CRANE, F. L., J. L. GLENN, and D. E. GREEN, 1956: Studies on the electron transfer system IV. The electron transfer particle. Biochim. biophys. Acta **22**, 475.

CROFTS, A. R., 1969: see Addendum, Ann. N.Y. Acad. Sci. **147**, 801.

CROMPTON, M., F. PAMIERI, M. CAPANO, and E. QUAGLIARIELLO, 1974: Mitochondrial sulphate and sulphite transport. In: Biomembranes: Architecture, Biogenesis, Bioenergetics and Differentiation. (PACKER, L., ed.), p. 213. New York-London: Academic Press.

CURGY, J.-J., G. LEDOIGT, B. J. STEVENS, and J. ANDRÉ, 1974: Mitochondrial and cytoplasmic ribosomes from *Tetrahymena pyriformis*. Correlative analysis by gel electrophoresis and electron microscopy. J. Cell Biol. **60**, 628.

D'AGOSTINO, M. A., K. M. LOWRY, and G. G. KALF, 1975: DNA biosynthesis in rat liver mitochondria. Inhibition by sulfhydryl compounds and stimulation by cytoplasmic proteins. Arch. Biochem. Biophys. **166**, 400.

DANIELSON, L., and L. ERNSTER, 1963: Energy-dependent reduction of triphosphopyridine nucleotide by reduced diphosphopyridine nucleotide, coupled to the energy-transfer system of the respiratory chain. Biochem. Z. **338**, 188.

DARGEL, R., 1967: ATPase-Aktivität und Kontraktion von Mitochondrien. Acta biol. med. german. **19**, 345

DAS, H. K., S. K. CHATERJEE, and J. C. ROY, 1964: Protein synthesis in plant mitochondria. I. Incorporation of amino acid in peptide linkage. J. biol. Chem. **239**, 1126.

DAVEY, P. J., R. YU, and A. W. LINNANE, 1969: Intracellular site of formation of mitochondrial protein synthetic system. Biochem. biophys. Res. Commun. **36**, 30.

DAVIDIAN, N., and R. PENNIALL, 1971: Origin of mitochondrial enzymes. IV. On the character of the product of cytochrome c synthesis by the endoplasmic reticulum. Biochem. biophys. Res. Commun. **44**, 15.

DAVIS, K. A., and Y. HATEFI, 1969: Kinetics of the resolution of complex I (reduced diphosphopyridine nucleotide reductase) of the mitochondrial electron transport chain by chaotropic agents. Biochem. **8**, 3355.

— — 1972: Resolution and reconstitution of complex II (succinate-ubiquinone reductase) by salts. Arch. Biochem. Biophys. **148**, 505.

— — K. C. POFF, and W. L. BUTLER, 1972: The b-type cytochromes of beef heart mitochondria. Biochem. biophys. Res. Commun. **46**, 1984.

— — — — 1973: The b-type cytochromes of bovine heart mitochondria: absorption spectra, enzymatic properties and distribution in the electron transfer complexes. Biochim. biophys. Acta **325**, 341.

DAVIS, L. E., 1967: Intramitochondrial crystals in *Hydra*. J. Ultrastruct. Res. **21**, 125.

DAVIDSON, J. B., and N. Z. STANACEV, 1974: Evidence for the biosynthetic difference between isolated mitochondria and microsomes from guinea-pig and rat liver regarding lysophosphatidic acid, phosphatidic acid, CDP-diglyceride, phosphatidyl glycerol, and cardiolipin. Can. J. Biochem. **52**, 936.

DAWID, I. B., 1970: The nature of mitochondrial RNA in oocytes of *Xenopus laevis* and its relation to mitochondrial DNA. In: Control of organelle development. (MILLER, P. L., ed.), p. 227. Cambridge: Cambridge Univ. Press/Academic Press, Int'l.

— 1972 a: Mitochondrial RNA in *Xenopus laevis*. I. The expression of the mitochondrial genome. J. molec. Biol. **63**, 201.

— 1972 b: Evolution of mitochondrial DNA sequences in *Xenopus*. Develop. Biol. **29**, 139.

— and A. W. BLACKLER, 1972: Maternal and cytoplasmic inheritance of mitochondrial DNA in *Xenopus*. Develop. Biol. **29**, 152.

— and J. W. CHASE, 1972: Mitochondrial RNA in *Xenopus laevis*. II. Molecular weights and other physical properties of mitochondrial ribosomal and 4s RNA. J. molec. Biol. **63**, 217.

— and D. R. WOLSTENHOME, 1967: Ultracentrifuge and electron microscope studies on the structure of mitochondrial DNA. J. molec. Biol. **28**, 233.

— I. HORAK, and H. G. COON, 1974: Propagation and recombination of parental mtDNAs in hybrid cells. In: The biogenesis of mitochondria (KROON, A. M., and C. SACCONE, eds.), p. 255. New York-London: Academic Press.

DEAMER, D. W., and R. J. BASKIN, 1972: ATP synthesis in sarcoplasmic reticulum. Arch. Biochem. Biophys. **153**, 47.

— and D. BRANTON, 1967: Fracture planes in an ice-bilayer model membrane system. Science **158**, 655.

DEBISE, R., and F. DURAND, 1974: Inhibitory effect of N-ethylmaleimide on glutamate and phosphate transport in mitochondria. Biochimie **56**, 161.

DE HAAN, E. J., and J. M. TAGER, 1968: Evidence for a permeability barrier for α-oxoglutarate in rat liver mitochondria. Biochim. biophys. Acta **153**, 98.

DEMEL, R. A., K. W. A. WIRTZ, H. H. KAMP, W. S. M. GEURTS VAN KESSEL, and L. L. M. VAN DEENEN, 1973: Phosphatidylcholine exchange protein from beef liver. Nature, N. B. **246**, 102.

DENNIS, E. A., and E. P. KENNEDY, 1972: Intracellular sites of lipid synthesis and the biogenesis of mitochondria. J. Lipid Res. **13**, 263.

DEUTSCH, J., B. DUJON, P. NETTER, E. PETROCHILD, P. P. SLONIMSKI, M. BOLOTIN-FUKUHARA, and D. COEN, 1974: Mitochondrial genetics. VI. The *petite* mutation in *Saccharomyces cerevisiae*: interrelations between the loss of the ϱ + factor and the loss of the drug resistance mitochondrial genetic markers. Genetics **76**, 195.

De Vault, D., 1971: Energy transduction in electron transport. Biochim. biophys. Acta 226, 193.

De Vries, H., and A. M. Kroon, 1974: Physicochemical and functional characterization of the 55 S ribosomes from rat-liver mitochondria. In: The biogenesis of mitochondria. (Kroon, A. M., and C. Saccone, eds.), p. 357. New York-London: Academic Press.

— and R. van der Koogh-Schuuring, 1973: Physicochemical characteristics of isolated 55 S mitochondrial ribosomes from rat liver. Biochem. biophys. Res. Commun. 54, 308.

Diacumakos, E. G., L. Garnjobst, and E. L. Tatum, 1965: A cytoplasmic character in Neurospora crassa, the role of nuclei and mitochondria. J. Cell Biol. 26, 413.

Di Jeso, F., R. O. Christensen, H. Steensland, and A. Loyter, 1969: Localization of inner mitochondrial membrane component. Fed. Proc. 28, 663 (abst.).

Dimitriadis, G. J., and J. G. Georgatsos, 1974: Induction of protein synthesis of mitochondria by exogenous RNA. Synthesis of rabbit globin by isolated mitochondria of Tetrahymena pyriformis. FEBS Lett. 46, 96.

Diwan, J. J., 1972: Effects of tannic acid on ion transport in rat-liver mitochondria. Arch. Biochem. Biophys. 151, 316.

— 1973: Mitochondrial K+ transport; effect of N-ethylmaleimide on 42K flux. Biochem. biophys. Res. Commun. 50, 384.

— and J. P. Aram, 1974: L-lysine uptake by rat liver mitochondria; dependence on L-lysine concentration, pH and induced K+flux. Biophys. J. 14, 805.

Dixon, H., G. M. Kellerman, C. H. Mitchell, N. H. Towers, and A. W. Linnane, 1971: Mikamycin and inhibitor of both mitochondrial protein synthesis and respiration. Biochem. biophys. Res. Commun. 43, 780.

Dubin, D. T., 1972: Mitochondrial ribonucleic-acid from cultured animal cells—comparison of pulse-labelled with steady state-labelled ribonucleic acid. J. biol. Chem. 247, 2662.

Du Buy, H. G., and F. L. Riley, 1967: Hybridization between the nuclear and kinetoplast DNA's of Leishmani enrietti and between nuclear and mitochondrial DNA's of mouse liver. Proc. nat. Acad. Sci. (U.S.) 57, 790.

Dueé, E. D., and P. V. Vignais, 1969: Kinetics of phosphorylation of intramitochondrial and extramitochondrial adenine nucleotide as related to nucleotide translocation. J. biol. Chem. 244, 3932.

Duncan, D., and R. Morales, 1973: Fine structure of astrocyte mitochondria in the spinal cord of the dog, cat and monkey. Anat. Rec. 175, 519.

Dutton, P. L., 1971: Oxidation-reduction potential dependence of the interaction of cytochromes, bacteriochlorophyll and carotenoids at 77 °K in chromatophores of Chromatium and Rhodopseudomonas gelatinosa. Biochim. biophys. Acta 226, 63.

— and B. Storey, 1971: The respiratory chain of plant mitochondria. IX. Oxidation-reduction potentials of the cytochromes of mung bean mitochondria. Plant Phys. 47, 282.

— and D. F. Wilson, 1974: Redox potentiometry in mitochondrial and photosynthetic bioenergetics. Biochim. biophys. Acta 346, 165.

— — and C. P. Lee, 1971: Energy dependence of oxidation-reduction potential of the b and c cytochromes in beef heart submitochondrial particles. Biochem. biophys. Res. Commun. 43, 1186.

— M. Erecińska, Y. Mukai, N. Sato, M. Pring, and D. F. Wilson, 1972: Reactions of b-cytochrome with ATP and antimycin A in pigeon heart mitochondria. Biochim. biophys. Acta 267, 15.

Ebner, E., and T. Mason, 1972: Effect of nuclear mutations on mitochondrial protein synthesis. Fed. Proc. 31, 464.

— and G. Schatz, 1973: Mitochondrial assembly in respiration-deficient mutants of Saccharomyces cerevisiae. III. A nuclear mutant lacking mitochondrial adenosine triphosphatase. J. biol. Chem. 248, 5379.

— L. Menucci, and G. Schatz, 1973 a: Mitochondrial assembly in respiration-deficient mutants of Saccharomyces cerevisiae. I. Effect of nuclear mutations on mitochondrial protein synthesis. J. biol. Chem. 248, 5360.

EBNER, E., T. MASON, and G. SCHATZ, 1973 b: Mitochondrial assembly in respiration-deficient mutants of *Saccharomyces cerevisiae*. II. Effect of nuclear and extrachromosomal mutations on the formation of cytochrome-c-oxidase. J. biol. Chem. **248**, 5369.

EDELMAN, M., I. M. VERMAN, and U. Z. LITTAUER, 1970: Mitochondrial ribosomal RNA from *Aspergillus nidulans:* characterization of a novel molecular species. J. molec. Biol. **49**, 67.

EDWARDS, D. L., F. KWIECINSKI, and J. HORSTMANN, 1973: Selection of respiratory mutants of *Neurospora crassa*. J. Bact. **116**, 164.

— E. ROSENBERG, and P. E. MARONEY, 1974: Induction of cyanide-insensitive respiration in *Neurospora crassa*. J. biol. Chem. **247**, 3551.

EGAN, R. W., and A. L. LEHNINGER, 1974: Solubilization of atractyloside-sensitive ADP (ATP) binding activity of rat liver mitochondria. Biochem. biophys. Res. Commun. **59**, 195.

EHNOLM, C., and D. B. ZILVERSMIT, 1973: Exchange of various phospholipids and of cholesterol between liposomes in the presence of highly purified phospholipid exchange proteins. J. Biol. Chem. **248**, 1719.

ELLIOTT, A. M., and I. J. BAK, 1964: The fate of mitochondria during aging in *Tetrahymena pyriformis*. J. Cell Biol. **20**, 113.

EPHRUSSI, B., 1950: The interplay of heredity and environment in the synthesis of respiratory enzymes in yeast. The Harvey Lectures **46**, 45.

— 1953: In: Nuclear cytoplasmic relations in microorganisms. Their bearing on cell heredity and differentiation. Oxford: Clarendon Press.

— 1956: Die Bestandteile des Cytochrombildenden Systems der Hefe. Naturwissenschaften **43**, 505.

— P. L'HERITIER et H. HOTTINGUER, 1949 a: Action de l'acriflavine sur les levures. VI. Analyse quantitative de la transformation des populations. Ann. Inst. Pasteur. **77**, 64.

— H. HOTTINGUER et A. M. CHIMENES, 1949 b: Action de l'acriflavine sur les lévures. I. La mutation "petite colonie". Ann. Inst. Pasteur **76**, 351.

EPLER, J. L., and W. E. BARNETT, 1967: Coding properties of *Neurospora* mitochondrial and cytoplasmic leucine transfer RNA's. Biochem. biophys. Res. Commun. **28**, 328.

— 1969: The mitochondrial and cytoplasmic transfer ribonucleic acids of *Neurospora crassa*. Biochem. **8**, 2285.

— L. R. SHUGART, and W. E. BARNETT, 1970: N-formylmethionyl transfer ribonucleic acid in mitochondria from *Neurospora*. Biochem. **9**, 3575.

ERECIŃSKA, M., D. F. WILSON, Y. MUKAI, and B. CHANCE, 1970: Oxidation-reduction midpoint potentials of mitochondrial flavoproteins. Biochem. biophys. Res. Commun. **41**, 386.

— B. CHANCE, and D. F. WILSON, 1971: The oxidation-reduction potential of the copper signal in pigeon heart mitochondria. FEBS Lett. **16**, 284.

— D. F. WILSON, N. SATO, and P. NICHOLLS, 1972: The energy dependence of the chemical properties of cytochrome c oxidase. Arch. Biochem. Biophys. **151**, 188.

— R. L. VEECH, and D. F. WILSON, 1974: Thermodynamic relationships between the oxidation-reduction reactions and the ATP synthesis in suspensions of isolated pigeon heart mitochondria. Arch. Biochem. Biophys. **160**, 412.

ERLICH, D. S., J.-P. THIERY, and G. BERNARDI, 1972: The mitochondrial genome of wild-type ycast cells. III. The pyrimidine tracts of mitochondrial DNA. J. molec. Biol. **65**, 207.

ERNSTER, L., and B. KUYLENSTIERNA, 1970: Outer membrane of mitochondria. In: Membranes of Mitochondria and Chloroplasts. (RACKER, E., ed.), p. 172. New York: Van Nostrand, Reinhold Co.

— and C. P. LEE, 1964: Biological oxidoreductions. Ann. Rev. Biochem. **33**, 729.

— K. JUNTTI, and K. ASAMI, 1973: Mechanisms of energy conservation in mitochondrial membranes. J. Bioenerg. **4**, 149.

EVANS, D. A., and D. LLOYD, 1967: Effect of chloramphenicol on mitochondria of *Polytomella caeca*. Biochem. J. **103**, 22.

EYTAN, G. D., and G. SCHATZ, 1975: Cytochrome c oxidase from bakers yeast. V. Arrangement of subunits in isolated and membrane bound enzyme. J. Biol. Chem. **250**, 767.

FAUMAN, M., and M. RABINOWITZ, 1972: Analysis of *grande* and *petite* mitochondrial DNA by DNA-DNA hybridization. FEBS Lett. **28**, 317.

FAYE, G., H. FUKUHARA, C. GRANDCHAMP, J. LAZOWSKA, F. MICHEL, J. CASEY, G. S. GETZ, J. LOCKER, M. RABINOWITZ, M. BOLOTIN-FUKUHARA, D. COEN, J. DEUTSCH, B. DUJON, P. NETTER, and P. P. SLONIMSKI, 1973: Mitochondrial nucleic acids in *petite* colony mutants: deletion and repetition of genes. Biochimie **55**, 779.

KUJAWA, C., and H. FUKUHARA, 1974: Physical and genetic organization of *petite* and *grande* yeast mitochondrial DNA IV. *In vivo* transcription products of mitochondrial DNA and localization of 23 S ribosomal RNA in *petite* mutants of *Saccharomyces cerevisiae*, 1974. J. Mol. Biol. **88**, 185.

FELDMAN, F., and H. R. MAHLER, 1974: Mitochondrial biogenesis. Retention of terminal formylmethionine in membrane proteins and regulation of their synthesis. J. biol. Chem. **249**, 3702.

FESSENDEN, J. M., and E. RACKER, 1966: Partial resolution of the enzymes catalyzing oxidative phosphorylation. XI. Stimulation of oxidative phosphorylation by coupling factors and oligomycin; inhibition by an antibody against coupling factor 1. J. biol. Chem. **241**, 2483.

FESSENDEN-RADEN, J. M., and E. RACKER, 1971: Structural and functional organization of mitochondrial membranes. In: Structure and Function of Biological Membranes. (ROTHFIELD, L. I., ed.), p. 401. New York-London: Academic Press.

FIRKIN, F. C., and A. W. LINNANE, 1968: Differential effects of chloramphenicol on the growth and respiration of mammalian cells. Biochem. biophys. Res. Commun. **32**, 398.

FISHBEIN, W. N., and R. E. STOWELL, 1969: Studies on the mechanism of freezing damage to mouse liver using a mitochondrial enzyme assay. II. Comparison of slow and rapid cooling rate. Cryobiol. **6**, 234.

FISHER, R. J., J. C. CHEN, B. P. SANI, S. S. KAPLAY, and D. R. SANADI, 1971: A soluble mitochondrial ATP synthetase complex catalyzing ATP-phosphate and ATP-ADP exchange. Proc. nat. Acad. Sci. (U.S.) **68**, 2181.

— E. N. MONDRIANAKIS, and D. R. SANADI, 1972: ATP synthetase from beef heart mitochondria. Fed. Proc. **31**, Abstract 1115.

FLAVELL, R. A., and E. A. C. FOLLET, 1970: Size and configuration of *Tetrahymena* mitochondrial deoxyribonucleic acid. Biochem. J. **119**, 61 P.

— and I. G. JONES, 1970: Mitochondrial deoxyribonucleic acid from *Tetrahymena pyriformis* and its kinetic complexity. Biochem. J. **116**, 811.

FLEISCHER, S., and G. ROUSER, 1965: Lipids of subcellular particles. J. Amer. Oil Chem. Soc. **42**, 588.

— B. FLEISCHER, and W. STOECKENIUS, 1967: Fine structure of lipid-depleted mitochondria. J. Cell Biol. **32**, 193.

— W. L. ZAHLER, and H. OZAWA, 1972: Membrane associated proteins. In: Biomembranes. (MANSON, L. A., ed.), Vol. 2, p. 105. New York-London: Pelnum Press.

FLETCHER, M. J., and D. R. SANADI, 1966: Turnover of rat-liver mitochondria. Biochim. biophys. Acta **51**, 356.

FLUHARTY, A., and D. R. SANADI, 1960: Evidence for a vicinal dithiol in oxidative phosphorylation. Proc. nat. Acad. Sci. (U.S.) **46**, 609.

FONYO, A., 1968: Phosphate carrier of rat liver mitochondria: its role in phosphate outflow. Biochem. biophys. Res. Commun. **32**, 624.

FORTE, G., L. ROSA, and F. GARLASCHII, 1972: Synthesis of ADP by isolated "coupling factor" from chloroplasts. FEBS Lett. **27**, 23.

FOUCHER, B., and Y. GAUDEMER, 1971: Implication of SH-groups in mitochondria energy-coupling system revealed by measurements of C^{14}-ethacrynate incorporation in rat liver mitochondria. FEBS Lett. **13**, 95.

FOWLER, C. F., and B. KOK, 1974: Direct observation of a light induced electric field in chloroplasts. Biochim. biophys. Acta **357**, 308.

FOWLER, C. R., S. H. RICHARDSON, and Y. HATEFI, 1962: A rapid method for the preparation of highly purified cytochrome oxidase. Biochim. biophys. Acta **64**, 168.

FRANK, H. S., and M. W. EVANS, 1965: Free volume and entropy in condensed systems. III. Entropy in binary liquid mixture; partial molar entropy in dilute solutions; structure and thermodynamics in aqueous electrolytes. J. Chem. Phys. **13**, 507.

FREEMAN, K. B., 1967: The morphological site of synthesis of cytochrome *c* in mammalian cells (Krebs cells). Biochem. J. **105**, 947.

FREI, J. V., and H. SHELDON, 1961: Corpus intra cristam: a dense body within mitochondria of cells in hyperplastic mouse epidermis. J. Cell Biol. **11**, 724.

FUJITA, A., and M. MACHINO, 1964: Fine structure of intramitochondrial crystals in rat thyroid follicular cell. J. Cell Biol. **23**, 383.

FUKAMACHI, S., B. BARTOOV, and K. B. FREEMAN, 1972: Synthesis of ribonucleic acid by isolated rat liver mitochondria. Biochem. J. **128**, 299.

FUKUHARA, H., 1967: Informational role of mitochondrial DNA studied by hybridization with different classes of RNA in yeast. Proc. nat. Acad. Sci. (U.S.) **58**, 1065.

— 1970: Transcriptional origin of RNA in a mitochondrial fraction of yeast and its bearing on the problem of sequence homology between mitochondrial and nuclear DNA. Mol. Gen. Genet. **107**, 58.

— M. FAURES, and C. GENIN, 1969: Comparison of RNA's transcribed *in vivo* from mitochondrial DNA of cytoplasmic and chromosomal respiratory deficient mutants. Mol. Gen. Genet. **104**, 264.

GAITSKHOKI, V. S., O. I. KISSELEV, N. A. KLIMOV, N. K. MLNAKHOV, G. V. MUKHA, A. L. SCHWARTZMAN, and S. A. NEIFAKH, 1974: On the intracellular distribution of polyribosomes synthesizing mitochondrial proteins. FEBS Lett. **43**, 151.

GALPER, J. B., and J. E. DARNELL, 1971: Mitochondrial protein synthesis in HeLa cells. J. molec. Biol. **57**, 363.

GAMBLE, J. L., 1965: Accumulation of citrate and malate by mitochondria. J. biol. Chem. **240**, 2668.

— 1973: Transport of potassium and sodium with citrate across mitochondrial membrane. Biochim. biophys. Acta **323**, 240.

— and A. L. LEHNINGER, 1973: Transport of ornithine and citrulline across the mitochondrial membrane. J. biol. Chem. **248**, 610.

GARLAND, P. B., 1970: Biochemical applications of continuous culture; energy-conservation mechanisms in *Torulopsis utilis*. Biochem. J. **118**, 329.

— R. A. CLEGG, P. A. LIGHT, and C. I. RAGAN, 1969: Mechanisms and inhibitors acting on electron transport and energy conservation between NADH and the cytochrome chain. In: Inhibitors, Tools in Cell Research. (BÜCHER, TH., and H. SIES), p. 217. Berlin-Heidelberg-New York: Springer-Verlag.

GAUSE, G. G., JR., and S. M. DOLGILEVISH, 1975: Replication of mitochondrial DNA. Selective inhibition of the H-strand synthesis in isolated mitochondria by sibiromycin. Biochim. biophys. Acta **383**, 9.

GAUTHERON, D. C., J. H. JULLIARD, and C. GODINOT, 1974: Protein-lipid associations in glutamate transport across mitochondrial membranes. In: Membrane Proteins in Transport and Phosphorylation. (AZZONE, G. F., M. E. KLINGENBERG, E. QUAGLIARIELLO, N. SILIPRANDI, eds.), p. 91. Amsterdam-London: North-Holland Publishing Co. New York: American Elsevier Publishing Co.

GILLHAM, N. G., 1974: Genetic analysis of the chloroplast and mitochondrial genomes. Ann. Rev. Gen. **8**, 347.

GINGOLD, E. B., G. W. SAUNDERS, H. B. LUKINS, and A. W. LINNANE, 1969: Biogenesis of mitochondria. X. Reassortment of cytoplasmic genetic determinants for respiratory competence and erythromycin resistance in *Saccharomyces cerevisiae*. Genetics **62**, 735.

GLOVER, A. J., and Z. S. GARVITCH, 1974: The freezing rate of freeze-etch specimens for electron microscopy. Cryobiol. **11**, 248.

GLYNN, I. M., 1967: Involvement of a membrane potential in the synthesis of ATP by mitochondria. Nature **216**, 1318.

— and V. L. LEW, 1970: Synthesis of adenosine triphosphate at the expense of downhill cation movements in intact red cell. J. Physiol. **207**, 393.

GOFFEAU, A., A. M. COLSON, Y. LANDRY, and F. FOURY, 1972: Modifications of mitochondrial ATPase in chromosomal respiratory-deficient mutants of a "petite-negative" yeast, *Schizosaccharomyces pombe*. Biochem. biophys. Res. Commun. **48**, 1448.

— Y. LANDRY, F. FOURY, M. BRIQUET, and A. M. COLSON, 1973: Oligomycin resistance of mitochondrial adenosine triphosphatase in a pleiotropic chromosomal mutant of a "petite-negative" yeast, *Schizosaccharomyces pombe*. J. Biol. Chem. **248**, 7097.

— A. M. COLSON, Y. LANDRY, F. FOURY, and M. BRIQUET, 1974: Stable pleiotropic chromosomal mutations with modified mitochondrial ATPase and cytochromes in *Schizosaccharomyces pombe*. In: Biomembranes: Architecture, Biogenesis, Bioenergetics, and Differentiation. (PACKER, L., ed.), p. 35. New York-London: Academic Press.

GOLDBERGER, R., A. M. PUMPHREY, and A. SMITH, 1962: Studies on the electron transport system. XLVI. On the modification of the properties of cytochrome *b*. Biochim. biophys. Acta. **58**, 307.

GOLDRING, J. M., and M. P. BLAUSTEIN, 1973: Synaptosome membrane potential changes monitored with a fluorescent probe. Soc. Neurosci. (Abst.) **15**.

GOMEZ-PUYOU, A., M. T. GOMEZ-PUYOU, G. BECKER, and A. L. LEHNINGER, 1972: An insoluble Ca^{2+} binding factor from rat liver mitochondria. Biochem. biophys. Res. Commun. **47**, 814.

GOMPEL, C., 1964: Structure fine des mitochondries de la cellule glandulaire endométriale humaine au cours du cycle menstruel. J. Microscopie (Paris) **3**, 427.

GONZÁLEZ-CADAVID, N. F., and P. N. CAMPBELL, 1967: The biosynthesis of cytochrome *c*. Sequence of incorporation *in vivo* of [^{14}C] lysine into cytochrome *c* and total proteins of rat-liver subcellular fractions. Biochem. J. **105**, 443.

— and C. S. DE CORDOVA, 1974: Role of membrane-bound and free polyribosomes in the synthesis of cytochrome *c* in rat liver. Biochem. J. **140**, 157.

GORDON, P., and M. RABINOWITZ, 1973: Evidence for deletion and changed sequence in the mitochondrial *petite* mutant of *Saccharomyces cerevisiae*. Biochem. **12**, 116.

— J. CASEY, and M. RABINOWITZ, 1974: Characterization of mitochondrial deoxyribonucleic acid from a series of *petite* yeast strains by deoxyribonucleic acid-deoxyribonucleic acid hybridization. Biochem. **13**, 1067.

GRAY, E. G., 1960: Regular organization of material in certain mitochondria of neuroglia of lizard brain. J. Cell Biol. **8**, 282.

GRECO, M., P. CANTATORE, G. PEPE, and C. SACCONE, 1973: Isolation and characterization of rat-liver mitochondrial ribosomes highly active in poly (U)-directed polyphenylalanine synthesis. Eur. J. Biochem. **37**, 171.

— G. PEPE, and C. SACCONE, 1974: Characterization of the monomer form of rat-liver mitochondrial ribosomes and its activity in poly (U)-directed polyphenylalanine synthesis. In: The biogenesis of mitochondria. (KROON, A. M., and C. SACCONE, eds.), p. 367. New York-London: Academic Press.

GREEN, D. E., 1974: The electromechanochemical model for energy coupling in mitochondria. Biochim. biophys. Acta. **346**, 27.

— and S. JI, 1972 a: The electromechanochemical model of mitochondrial structure and function. J. Bioenerg. **3**, 159.

— — 1972 b: The electromechanochemical model of mitochondrial structure and function. Proc. nat. Acad. Sci. (U.S.) **29**, 726.

— — 1973: Transductional principle and structural principles of the mitochondrial transducing unit. Proc. nat. Acad. Sci. (U.S.) **70**, 904.

— and S. REIBLE, 1974: Paired moving charges in mitochondrial energy coupling. Proc. nat. Acad. Sci. (U.S.) **71**, 4850.

— — 1975: Paired moving charges in mitochondria energy coupling II. Universality of the principles of energy coupling in biological systems. Proc. nat. Acad. Sci. (U.S.) **72**, 253.

— J. ASAI, R. A. HARRIS, and J. T. PENNINSTON, 1968: Conformational basis of energy transformations in membrane systems. III. Configurational changes in the mitochondrial inner membrane induced by changes in functional states. Arch. Biochem. Biophys. **125**, 684.

GREENAWALT, J. W., and E. CARAFOLI, 1966: Electron microscope studies on the active accumulation of Sr^{++} by rat-liver mitochondria. J. Cell Biol. **29**, 37.

GREENAWALT, J. W., C. S. ROSSI, and A. L. LEHNINGER, 1964: Effect of the active accumulation of calcium and phosphate ions on the structure of rat liver mitochondria. J. Cell Biol. **23**, 21.

GREENGARD, O., and P. N. CAMPBELL, 1959: Factors influencing the incorporation of amino acid into the protein of microsome and mitochondria preparations of rat liver and liver tumour. Biochem. J. **72**, 305.

GREVILLE, G. D., 1969: A scrutiny of Mitchell's chemiosmotic hypothesis of respiratory chain and photosynthetic phosphorylation. Curr. Top. Bioenerg. **3**, 1.

GRIFFITHS, D. E., and D. C. WHARTON, 1961 a: Studies of the electron transport system. XXXV. Purification and properties of cytochrome oxidase. J. biol. Chem. **236**, 1850.

— — 1961 b: Studies of the electron transport system. XXXVI. Properties of copper in cytochrome oxidase. J. biol. Chem. **236**, 1857.

— and R. L. HOUGHTON, 1974: Studies on energy-linked reactions: modified mitochondrial ATPase of oligomycin-resistant mutants of *Saccharomyces cerevisiae*. Eur. J. Biochem. **46**, 157.

— — and W. E. LANCASHIRE, 1974: Mitochondrial genes and ATP-synthetase. In: The biogenesis of mitochondria. (KROON, A. M., and C. SACCONE, eds.), p. 215. New York-London: Academic Press.

— P. R. AVNER, W. E. LANCASHIRE, and J. R. TURNER, 1972: Studies of energy-linked reactions: isolation and properties of mitochondrial oligomycin-resistant, trialkyl tin-resistant and uncoupler-resistant mutants of yeast. In: Biochemistry and Biophysics of Mitochondrial Membranes. (AZZONE, G. F., E. CARAFOLI, A. L. LEHININGER, E. QUAGLIA-RIELLO, and N. SILIPRANDI, eds.), p. 505. New York-London: Academic Press.

GRIMES, G. W., H. R. MAHLER, and P. S. PERLMAN, 1974: Nuclear gene dosage effects in mitochondrial mass and DNA. J. Cell Biol. **61**, 565.

GRINIUS, L. L., A. A. JASAITIS, Y. P. KADZIAUSKAS, E. A. LIBERMAN, V. P. SKULACHEV, V. P. TOPALI, L. M. TSOFINA, and M. A. VLADIMIROVA, 1970: Conversion of biomembrane-produced energy into electric form. Biochim. biophys. Acta **216**, 1.

— T. I. GUDS, and V. P. SKULACHEV, 1971: Arrangement of the electric potential-generating redox chain in the mitochondrial membrane. J. bioenerg. **2**, 101.

GRIVELL, L. A., L. REIJNDERS, and P. BORST, 1971: Isolation of yeast mitochondrial ribosomes highly active in protein synthesis. Biochim. biophys. Acta **247**, 91.

GROOT, G. S. P., 1974: The biosynthesis of mitochondrial ribosomes in *Saccharomyces cerevisiae*. In: The biogenesis of mitochondria. (KROON, A. M., and C. SACCONE, eds.), p. 443. New York-London: Academic Press.

— L. KOVÁČ, and G. SCHATZ, 1971: Promitochondria of anaerobically grown yeast. V. Energy transfer in the absence of an electron transfer chain. Proc. nat. Acad. Sci. (U.S.) **68**, 308.

— W. ROUSLIN, and G. SCHATZ, 1972: Promitochondria of anaerobically grown yeast. VI. Effects of oxygen on promitochondrial protein synthesis. J. biol. Chem. **247**, 1735.

— R. A. FLAVELL, G. J. B. VAN OMMEN, and L. A. GRIVELL, 1974: Yeast mitochondrial RNA does not contain poly (A). Nature **252**, 167.

GROSS, N. J., and M. RABINOWITZ, 1969: Synthesis of new strands of mitochondrial and nuclear deoxyribonucleic acid by semiconservative replication. J. biol. Chem. **244**, 1563.

— M. T. McCoy, and E. G. GILMORE, 1968: Evidence for the involvement of a nuclear gene in the production of the mitochondrial leucyl-tRNA synthesis of *Neurospora*. Proc. nat. Acad. Sci. (U.S.) **61**, 253.

GROSSMAN, L. I., R. WATSON, and J. VINOGRAD, 1973: The presence of ribonucleotides in mature closed-circular mitochondrial DNA. Proc. nat. Acad. Sci. (U.S.) **70**, 3339.

GUÉRIN, B., M. GUÉRIN, and M. KLINGENBERG, 1970: Differential inhibition of phosphate efflux and influx and a possible discrimination between an inner and outer location of the phosphate carrier in mitochondria. FEBS Lett. **10**, 265.

GULIK-KRZYWICKI, T., E. RIVAS, and V. LUZZATI, 1967: Structure et polymorphisme des Lipides: Étude par diffraction des rayon X du système formé de lipides de mitochondries de coeur de boeuf et d'eau. J. Mol. Biol. **27**, 303.

GURR, M. I., C. PROTTEY, and J. N. HAWTHORNE, 1965: The phospholipids of liver-cell fractions. II. Incorporation of [^{32}P] orthophosphate *in vivo* in normal and regeneration rat liver. Biochim. biophys. Acta **106**, 357.

HACKENBROCK, C. R., 1966: Ultrastructural bases for metabolically linked mechanical activity in mitochondria. I. Reversible ultrastructural changes with change in metabolic steady state in isolated liver mitochondria. J. Cell Biol. **30**, 269.

— 1968: Chemical and physical fixation of isolated mitochondria in low-energy and high-energy states. Proc. nat. Acad. Sci. (U.S.) **61**, 598.

— 1972 a: Energy linked ultrastructural transformations in isolated mitochondria and mitoplasts. Preservation of configurations by freeze-cleaving compared to chemical fixation. J. Cell Biol. **53**, 450.

— 1972 b: States of activity and structure in mitochondrial membranes. Ann. N.Y. Acad. Sci. **195**, 492.

— 1973: Structural transformations in the molecular core of mitochondrial membranes during change in energy state. In: Mechanisms in bioenergetics. (AZZONE, G. F., L. ERNSTER, S. PAPA, E. QUAGLIARIELLO, and N. SILIPRANDI, eds.), p. 77. New York-London: Academic Press.

— T. G. REHN, E. C. WEINBACH, and J. L. LEMASTERS, 1971 a: Oxidative phosphorylation and ultrastructural transformation in mitochondria in the intact ascites tumor cell. J. Cell Biol. **51**, 123.

— — J. L. GAMBLE, JR., E. C. WEINBACH, and J. L. LEMASTERS, 1971 b: Ultrastructural transformation in the mitochondrion: its relationship to the energy state of the mitochondrion and the energy state of the cell. In: Energy transduction in respiration and photosynthesis. (QUAGLIARIELLO, E., S. PAPA, and C. S. ROSSI, eds.), p. 285. Bari: Adriatica Editrice.

HADDOCK, B. A., and P. B. GARLAND, 1971: Effect of sulphate-limited growth on mitochondrial electron transfer and energy conservation between reduced nicotinamide-adenine dinucleotides and the cytochromes in *Torulopsis utilis*. Biochem. J. **124**, 155.

HALBREICH, A., and M. RABINOWITZ, 1971: Isolation of *Saccharomyces cerevisiae* mitochondrial formyltetrahydrofolic acid: methionyl-tRNA transformylase and the hybridization of mitochondrial DNA. Proc. nat. Acad. Sci. (U.S.) **68**, 294.

HALESTRAP, A. P., and R. M. DENTON, 1974: Specific inhibition of pyruvate transport in rat liver mitochondria and human erythrocytes by α-cyano-4-hydroxycinnamate. Biochem. J. **138**, 313.

— M. D. BRAND, and R. M. DENTON, 1974 a: Inhibition of mitochondrial pyruvate transport by phenylpyruvate and α-oxo-4-methylpentanoate. Biochem. Soc. Trans. **2**, 980.

— — — 1974 b: Inhibition of mitochondrial pyruvate transport by phenylpyruvate and α-ketoisocaproate. Biochim. biophys. Acta **367**, 102.

HALL, J. D., and F. L. CRANE, 1970: An intracristal structure in beef heart mitochondria. Exp. Cell Res. **62**, 480.

HALLBERG, R. L., 1974: Mitochondrial DNA in *Xenopus laevis* oocytes. I. Displacement loop occurrence. Develop. Biol. **38**, 346.

HALLERMAYER, G., and W. NEUPERT, 1974 a: Lipid composition of mitochondrial outer and inner membranes of *Neurospora crassa*. Hoppe-Seyler's Z. für Physiol. Chem. **355**, 279.

— — 1974 b: Immunological difference of mitochondrial and cytoplasmic ribosomes of *Neurospora crassa*. FEBS Letter **41**, 264.

HALPERIN, M. L., B. H. ROBINSON, and I. B. FRITZ, 1972: Effects of palmitoyl CoA on citrate and malate transport in rat liver mitochondria. Proc. Nat. Acad. Sci. (U.S.) **69**, 1003.

HANSTEIN, W. G., and Y. HATEFI, 1974 a: Characterization and localization of mitochondrial uncoupler binding-sites with an uncoupler capable of photoaffinity labelling. J. biol. Chem. **249**, 1356.

— 1974 b: Trinitrophenol: a membrane-impermeable uncoupler of oxidative phosphorylation. Proc. nat. Acad. Sci. (U.S.) **71**, 288.

— K. A. DAVIS, M. A. GHALAMBOR, and Y. HATEFI, 1971: Succinate dehydrogenase II enzymatic properties. Biochem. **10**, 2517.

HANZELY, L., and O. A. SCHJEIDE, 1971: Fine structural observations of mitochondria undergoing division in *Allium savitum* root tip cells. Cytobiol. **4**, 207.

HARMON, H. J., J. D. HALL, and F. L. CRANE, 1974: Structure of the mitochondrial cristae membranes. Biochim. biophys. Acta **344**, 119.

HARRIS, D. A., J. ROSING, R. J. VAN DE STADT, and E. C. SLATER, 1973: Tight binding of adenine nucleotides to beef heart mitochondrial ATPase. Biochim. biophys. Acta 314, 338.

HARRIS, E. J., 1969: Mitochondrial anion uptake. In: Energy level and metabolic control in mitochondria. (PAPA, S., J. M. TAGER, E. QUAGLIARIELLO, and E. C. SLATER, eds.), p. 31. Bari: Adriatica Editrice.

— 1973: Physicochemical basis for anion, cation and proton distributions between rat-liver mitochondria and suspending medium. J. Bioenerg. 4, 179.

— and J. A. BANGHAM, 1972: Titration of mitochondrial buffer by accumulated anions. J. Membr. Biol. 9, 141.

— and D. J. BASSETT, 1972: Distribution of ammonia and methylamine between mitochondria and suspension medium. FEBS Lett. 19, 214.

— and C. BERENT, 1970: The applicability of the Donnan relation to the distribution of certain anions between mitochondria and medium. FEBS Lett. 10, 6.

— and B. C. PRESSMAN, 1969: The direction of polarity of the mitochondrial transmembrane potential. Biochim. biophys. Acta 172, 66.

— and K. VAN DAM, 1968: Changes of total water and sucrose space accompanying induced low uptake or phosphate swelling of rat liver mitochondria. Biochem. J. 106, 759.

— G. CATLIN, and B. C. PRESSMAN, 1967: Effect of transport-inducing antibiotics and other agents on potassium flux in mitochondria. Biochem. 6, 1360.

— J. A. BANGHAM, and J. M. WIMHURST, 1973 a: Dependence on energy and K⁻ ions of accumulation of glutamate by rat-liver mitochondria. Arch. Biochem. 158, 236.

— — and B. ZUKOVIC, 1973 b: Equilibration of chloride and pyruvate distribution between liver mitochondria and medium mediated by organo-tin salts. FEBS Lett. 29, 339.

— J. T. PENNINSTON, J. ASAI, and D. E. GREEN, 1968: The conformational basis of energy conservation in membrane systems. II. Correlation between conformational change and functional states. Proc. nat. Acad. Sci. (U.S.) 59, 830.

HARRIS, R. A., B. FARMER, and T. OZAWA, 1972: Inhibition of the mitochondrial adenine nucleotide transport system by oleyl CoA. Arch. Biochem. Biophys. 150, 199.

HARTROFT, W. S., 1964: Electron microscopy of liver and kidney cells in dietary deficiencies. In: CIBA foundation symposium on cellular injury. (DE REUCK, A. V. S., and J. KNIGHT, eds.), p. 248. Boston: Little, Brown & Co.

HARTWELL, L. H., 1967: Macromolecular synthesis in temperature-sensitive mutants of yeast. J. Bact. 93, 1662.

HARVEY, M. S., K. W. A. WIRTZ, H. H. KAMP, B. J. M. ZEGER, and L. L. M. VAN DEENEN, 1973: A study on phospholipid exchange proteins present in the soluble fraction of beef liver and brain. Biochim. biophys. Acta 323, 234.

HASLAM, J. M., M. PERKINS, and A. W. LINNANE, 1973 a: Biogenesis of mitochondria, 32. Requirement for mitochondrial protein synthesis for formation of normal adenine-nucleotide transporter in mitochondria. Biochem. J. 134, 935.

— T. W. SPITHILL, A. W. LINNANE, and J. B. CHAPELL, 1973 b: Biogenesis of mitochondria. 33. Effects of altered membrane lipids on cation transport of mitochondria of Saccharomyces cerevisiae. Biochem. J. 134, 949.

HASSELBACH, W., M. MAKINOSE, and A. MIGALA, 1973: Calcium transport and ATP turnover in the sarcoplasmic membrane. In: Mechanisms in bioenergetics. (AZZONE, G. F., L. ERNSTER, S. PAPA, E. QUAGLIARIELLO, and N. SILIPRANDI, eds.), p. 219. New York-London: Academic Press.

HATEFI, Y. A., 1966: The functional complexes of the mitochondrial electron-transfer system. Comprehensive Biochem. 14, 199.

— 1973: Oxidation of reduced triphosphopyridine nucleotide by submitochondrial particles from beef heart. Biochem. biophys. Res. Commun. 50, 978.

— and W. C. HANSTEIN, 1973: Interactions of reduced and oxidized triphosphopyridine nucleotides with the electron-transport system of bovine heart mitochondria. Biochem. 12, 3515.

— and K. E. STEMPEL, 1967: Resolution of complex I (DPNH-coenzyme A reductase) of the mitochondrial electron transfer chain. Biochem. biophys. Res. Commun. 26, 301.

— — 1969: Isolation and enzymatic properties of the mitochondrial reduced diphosphopyridine nucleotide dehydrogenase. J. biol. Chem. 244, 2350.

HATEFI, Y. A., A. G. HAAVIK, and D. E. GRIFFITHS, 1961 a: Reconstitution of the electron transport system. I. Preparation and properties of the interacting enzyme complexes. Biochem. biophys. Res. Commun. **4**, 441.

— — — 1961 b: Reconstitution of the electron transport system. II. Reconstitution of DPNH-cytochrome reductase, succinic-cytochrome *c* reductase and DPNH, succinic-cytochrome *c* reductase. Biochem. biophys. Res. Commun. **4**, 447.

— — — 1962 a: Studies on the electron transfer system. XL. Preparation and properties of mitochondrial DPNH-coenzyme Q reductase. J. biol. Chem. **237**, 1676.

— — — 1962 b: Studies on the electron transfer system. XLI. Reduced coenzyme Q (QH_2)-cytochrome *c* reductase. J. biol. Chem. **237**, 1681.

— K. E. STEMPEL, and W. HANSTEIN, 1969: Inhibitors and activators of mitochondrial reduced diphosphopyridine nucleotide dehydrogenase. J. biol. Chem. **244**, 2358.

— W. HANSTEIN, K. A. DAVIS, and K. S. YOU, 1974: Structure of the mitochondrial electron transport system. Ann. N.Y. Acad. Sci. **227**, 504.

— D. L. STIGGAL, Y. GALANTE, and W. G. HANSTEIN, 1974 b: Mitochondrial ATP-P_i exchange complex. Biochem. biophys. Res. Commun. **61**, 313.

HAWLEY, E. S., and J. W. GREENAWALT, 1970: An assessment of *in vivo* mitochondrial protein synthesis in *Neurospora crassa*. J. biol. Chem. **245**, 3574.

HELDT, H. W., 1966: The participation of endogenous nucleotides in mitochondrial phosphate-transfer reactions. In: Regulation of metabolic processes in mitochondria. (TAGER, J. M., S. PAPA, E. QUAGLIARIELLO, and E. C. SLATER, eds.), p. 51. Amsterdam-London-New York: Elsevier Publishing Co.

— 1969: The inhibition of adenine nucleotide translocation by atractyloside. In: Inhibitors, tools in cell research. (BUCHER, T. H., and H. SIES, eds.), p. 201. Heidelberg-New York-Berlin: Springer-Verlag.

— H. JACOBS, and M. KLINGENBERG, 1965: Endogenous ADP of mitochondria, and early phosphate acceptor of oxidative phosphorylation as disclosed by kinetic studies with C^{14} labelled ADP and ATP and with atractyloside. Biochem. biophys. Res. Commun. **18**, 174.

HELINSKI, D. R., and D. B. CLEWELL, 1971: Circular DNA. Ann. Rev. Biochem. **40**, 899.

HELMKAMP, G. M., JR., M. S. HARVEY, K. W. A. WIRTZ, and L. L. M. VAN DEENEN, 1974: Phospholipid exchange between membranes. Purification of bovine brain proteins that preferentially catalyze the transfer of phosphatidylinositol. J. Biol. Chem. **249**, 6382.

HENDERSON, P. J. F., and H. A. LARDY, 1970: Bongkrekic acid. An inhibitor of the adenine nucleotide translocase of mitochondria. J. biol. Chem. **245**, 1319.

— J. D. McGIVAN, and J. B. CHAPPELL, 1969: The action of certain antibiotics on mitochondrial erythrocyte and artificial phopholipid membranes. The role of induced proton permeability. Biochem. J. **111**, 521.

HENRY, M. L., and E. J. NYNS, 1975: Cyanide-insensitive respiration. An alternative mitochondrial pathway. Sub. Cell. Biochem. **4**, 1.

HENSON, C. P., P. PERLMAN, C. N. WEBER, and H. R. MAHLER, 1968: Formation of yeast mitochondria. II. Effects of antibiotics on enzyme activity during derepression. Biochem. **7**, 4445.

HERMAN, H. B., and C. A. RECHNITZ, 1974: Carbonate ion-selective membrane electrode. Science **184**, 1074.

HERNANDEZ, A., I. BURDETT, and T. S. WORK, 1971: Protein synthesis by brain cortex mitochondria. Characterization of a 55 S mitochondrial ribosome as the functional unit in protein synthesis by cortex mitochondria and its distinction from a contaminant cytoplasmic protein-synthesizing system. Biochem. J. **124**, 327.

HINKLE, P. C., and L. L. HORSTMAN, 1971: Respiration-driven proton transport in submitochondrial particles. J. biol. Chem. **246**, 6024.

— and P. MITCHELL, 1970: Effect of membrane potential on equilibrium poise between cytochrome *a* and cytochrome *c* in rat-liver mitochondria. J. Bioenerg. **1**, 45.

— H. S. PENEFSKY, and E. RACKER, 1967: Partial resolution of the enzymes catalyzing oxidative phosphorylation. XII. The $H_2^{18}O$ inorganic phosphate and $H_2^{18}O$-adenosine triphosphate exchange reactions in submitochondrial particles from beef heart. J. biol. Chem. **242**, 1788.

HIRSCH, M., and S. PENMAN, 1973: Mitochondrial polyadenylic acid-containing RNA: localization and characterization. J. molec. Biol. **80**, 379.
— — 1974 a: Post-transcriptional addition of polyadenylic acid to mitochondrial RNA by
a cordycepin-insensitive process. J. Mol. Biol. **83**, 131.
— — 1974 b: The messenger-like properties of poly(A)-RNA in mammalian mitochondria.
Cell **3**, 335.
— A. SPRADLING, and S. PENMAN, 1974: The messenger-like poly(A)-containing RNA species
from the mitochondria of mammals and insects. Cell **1**, 31.
HOFFMAN, H.-P., and C. J. AVERS, 1973: Mitochondrion of yeast: ultrastructural evidence
for one giant, branched organelle per cell. Science **181**, 749.
HOFFMAN, J. F., and P. C. LARIS, 1974: Determination of membrane potentials in human
and *Amphiuma* red blood cells by means of a fluorescent probe. J. Physiol. **239**, 519.
HOLLENBERG, C. P., P. BORST, and E. F. J. VAN BRUGGEN, 1970: Mitochondrial DNA.
V. A 25 μ closed circular duplex DNA molecule in wild-type yeast mitochondria. Structure
and genetic complexity. Biochim. biophys. Acta **209**, 1.
— — R. A. FLAVELL, G. F. VAN KREIJL, E. F. J. VAN BRUGGEN, and A. C. ARNBERG, 1972:
The unusual properties of mtDNA from a low density *petite* mutant. Biochim. biophys.
Acta **277**, 44.
HOMMES, F. A., 1964: The kinetics of cytochrome *b* and *c* during oxidative phosphorylation
in rat liver mitochondria. Arch. Biochem. **197**, 78.
HOOPER, M., A. P. GREEN, and A. J. SWEETMAN, 1973: Effect of 2-phenylindolenone on
phosphate transport in liver mitochondria. FEBS Lett. **33**, 297.
HOPFER, U., A. L. LEHNINGER, and T. E. THOMPSON, 1968: Protonic conductions across
phospholipid bilayer membrane induced by uncoupling agents for oxidative phosphoryla-
tion. Proc. nat. Acad. Sci. (U.S.) **49**, 486.
HORNE, R. W., 1965: Negative staining methods. In: Techniques for electron microscopy.
(KAY, D. H., ed.), p. 328. Philadelphia: FA Davis Co.
HORSTMAN, L. L., and E. RACKER, 1970: Partial resolution of the enzymes catalyzing
oxidative phosphorylation. XXII. Interaction between adenosine triphosphatase inhibitor
and mitochondrial adenosine triphosphatase. J. biol. Chem. **245**, 1336.
HRUBAN, Z., and H. SWIFT, 1964: Uricase: localization in hepatic microbodies.
Science **146**, 1316.
HUANG, C., L. WHEELDON, and T. E. THOMPSON, 1964: The properties of bilayer mem-
branes separating two aqueous phases: formation of a membrane of simple composition.
J. molec. Biol. **8**, 148.
HUDSON, B., W. B. UPHOLT, J. DEVINNY, and J. VINOGRAD, 1969: The use of an ethidium
analogue in the dye-buoyant density procedure for the isolation of closed circular DNA:
the variation of the superhelix density of mitochondrial DNA. Proc. nat. Acad. Sci.
(U.S.) **62**, 813.
HUNTER, G. R., Y. KAMISHIMA, and G. P. BRIERLEY, 1969: Ion transport by heart mitochondria. XV. Morphological changes associated with pentration of solutes into isolated heart
mitochondria. Biochim. biophys. Acta **180**, 81.
HUNTER, D. R., H. KOMAI, and R. A. HAWORTH, 1974: Oxidative phosphorylation and
respiratory control in lysolecithin treated electron transport particles. Biochem. biophys.
Res. Commun. **56**, 647.
HWANG, K. M., K. M. SCOTT, and G. P. BRIERLEY, 1972: Ion transport by heart mitochondria. The effects of Cu^{2+} on membrane permeability. Arch. Biochem. Biophys. **150**, 746.

IBRAHIM, N. G., J. P. BURKE, and D. S. BEATTIE, 1974: The sensitivity of rat liver and yeast
mitochondrial ribosomes to inhibitors of protein synthesis. J. Biol. Chem. **249**, 6806.
INESI, G., S. BLANCHET, and D. WILLIAMS, 1973: ATPase and ATP binding sites in the
sarcoplasmic reticulum membrane. In: Organization of energy-transducing membranes.
(NAKAO, M., and L. PACKER, eds.). Baltimore-London-Tokyo: University Park Press.
ISHIHARA, T., C. TSUKAYAMA, F. UCHINO, and N. MATSUMOTO, 1973: Intramitochondrial
filamentous structures in human reticulum cells in the bone marrow. J. Electr. Micr. **22**, 39.
ITOH, N., T. KAWASAKI, and I. YAMASHINA, 1974 a: The carbohydrate composition of submitochondrial fractions from rat liver. FEBS Lett. **47**, 225.

ITOH, N., T. KAWASAKI, and I. YAMASHINA, 1974 b: Isolation and characterization of glyco-
    peptides from rat liver mitochondria. J. Biochem. **76**, 459.
IZZARD, S., and H. TEDESCHI, 1970: Ion transport underlying metabolically controlled
    volume changes of isolated mitochondria. Proc. nat. Acad. Sci. (U.S.) **67**, 702.
— — 1973: Characterization of orthophosphate-induced active transport in isolated
    mitochondria. Arch. Biochem. Biophys. **154**, 527.

JACKSON, J. B., and A. R. CROFTS, 1969: The high energy state in chromatophores from
    Rhodopseudomonas spheroides. FEBS Lett. **4**, 185.
JACKSON, K. L., and N. PACE, 1956: Some permeability properties of isolated rat liver cell
    mitochondria. J. gen. Physiol. **40**, 47.
JACOB, S. T., and D. G. SCHINDLER, 1972: Polyriboadenylate polymerase solubilized from
    rat liver mitochondria. Biochem. biophys. Res. Commun. **48**, 126.
— — and H. P. MORRIS, 1972: Mitochondrial polyadenylate polymerase: relative lack of
    activity in hepatomas. Science **178**, 639.
JACOVCIC, S., G. S. GETZ, M. RABINOWITZ, H. JAKOB, and H. SWIFT, 1971: Cardiolipin
    content of wild type and mutant yeasts in relation to mitochondrial function and develop-
    ment. J. Cell Biol. **48**, 490.
JAGENDORF, A. T., and E. URIBE, 1966: ATP formation caused by acid-base transitions of
    spinach chloroplasts. Proc. nat. Acad. Sci. (U.S.) **55**, 170.
JANKI, R. M., H. N. AITHAL, W. C. MCMURRAY, and E. R. TUSTANOFF, 1974 a: The effect
    of altered membrane-lipid composition on enzyme activities of outer and inner mito-
    chondrial membranes. Biophys. biochem. Res. Commun. **56**, 1078.
— — E. R. TUSTANOFF, and A. J. S. BALL, 1974 b: Mechanism for the biogenesis of mito-
    chondrial membranes in yeast. In: Biomembranes, Architecture, Biogenesis, Bioenergetics
    and Differentiation. (PACKER, L., ed.). New York-London: Academic Press.
— — — — 1975: The biogenesis of mitochondrial membranes in the yeast *Saccharomyces
    cerevisiae*. Biochim. biophys. Acta **375**, 446.
JOHNSON, R. N., and J. B. CHAPPELL, 1973: Transport of inorganic-phosphate by mito-
    chondrial dicarboxylate carrier. Biochem. J. **134**, 769.
— — 1974: The inhibition of mitochondrial dicarboxylate transport by inorganic phosphate,
    some phosphate esters and some phosphate compounds. Biochem. J. **138**, 171.
JONAH, M., and J. A. ERWIN, 1971: The lipids of the membraneous cell organelles isolated
    from the ciliate, *Tetrahymena pyriformis*. Biochim. biophys. Acta **231**, 80.
JONES, D. H., and P. D. BOYER, 1969: The apparent absolute requirement of adenosine
    diphosphate for the inorganic phosphate water exchange in oxidative phosphorylation.
    J. biol. Chem. **244**, 5767.
JUILLIARD, J. H., and D. C. GAUTHERON, 1973: High glutamate affinity proteolipid from
    pig heart mitochondria. Is it a component of a glutamate translocator? FEBS Lett. **37**, 10.
JULIAN, F. J., J. W. MOORE, and D. E. GOLDMAN, 1962: Current-voltage relations in the
    lobster giant axon membrane under voltage clamp conditions. J. gen. Physiol. **45**, 1217.
JUNGAWALA, F. B., W. FRENKEL, and R. M. C. DAWSON, 1971: The metabolism of phos-
    phatidylinositol in the thyroid gland of the pig. Biochem. J. **123**, 19.

KADENBACH, B., 1966: Synthesis of mitochondrial proteins; demonstration of a transfer of
    proteins from microsomes into mitochondria. Biochim. biophys. Acta **134**, 430.
— and P. HADVARY, 1973: Specific binding of phosphate by a chloroform-soluble protein
    from rat-liver mitochondria. Eur. J. Biochem. **39**, 21.
— — 1974: Specific binding of phosphate to chloroform-soluble proteins from rat liver
    mitochondrial membranes. In: Membrane Proteins in Transport and Phosphorylation.
    (AZZONE, G. F., M. E. KLINGENBERG, E. QUAGLIARIELLO, and N. SILIPRANDI, eds.), p. 275.
    Amsterdam-London: North-Holland Publishing Co. New York: American Elsevier
    Publishing Co.
KADER, J. C., 1975: Proteins and the intracellular exchange of lipids. I. Stimulation of
    phospholipid exchange between mitochondria and microsomal fractions by proteins
    isolated from potato tuber. Biochim. biophys. Acta **380**, 31.
KAGAWA, Y., 1972: Reconstitution of oxidative phosphorylation. Biochim. biophys.
    Acta **265**, 297.

KAGAWA, Y., and E. RACKER, 1966: Partial resolution of the enzymes catalyzing oxidative phosphorylation IX. Reconstruction of oligomycin-sensitive adenosine triphosphatase. J. biol. Chem. 241, 2467.

— — 1971: Partial resolution of the enzymes catalyzing oxidative phosphorylation. XXV. Reconstitution of vesicles catalyzing $^{32}P_i$-adenosine triphosphate exchange. J. biol. Chem. 246, 5477.

— A. KANDRACH, and E. RACKER, 1973: Partial resolution of the enzymes catalyzing oxidative phosphorylation. XXVI. Specificity of phospholipids required for energy transfer reactions. J. biol. Chem. 248, 676.

KALF, G. F., 1963: The incorporation of leucine-1-C^{14} into the protein of rat heart sarcosomes; an investigation of optimal conditions. Arch. Biochem. Biophys. 101, 350.

— 1964: Deoxyribonucleic acid in mitochondria and its role in protein synthesis. Biochem. 3, 1702.

— and A. S. FAUST, 1969: The inner membranes of the rat liver mitochondrion as the site of incorporation of radioactively labelled precursors into nucleic acid and protein in vitro. Arch. Biochem. Biophys. 134, 103.

— and M. V. SIMPSON, 1959: The incorporation of valine-1-C^{14} into the protein of submitochondrial fractions. J. biol. Chem. 234, 2943.

KAMP, H. H., K. W. A. WIRTZ, and L. L. M. VAN DEENEN, 1973: Some properties of the phosphatidylcholine exchange protein purified from beef liver. Biochim. biophys. Acta 318, 313.

KANAZAWA, T., S. YAMADA, and Y. TONOMURA, 1970: ATP formation from ADP and a phosphorylated intermediate of Ca^{2+}-dependent ATPase in fragmented sarcoplasmic reticulum. J. Biochem. 68, 593.

— — T. YAMAMOTO, and Y. TONOMURA, 1971: Reaction mechanism of Ca^{2+}-dependent ATPase. V. Vectorial requirement for calcium and magnesium ions of three partial reactions of ATPase: formation and decomposition of a phosphorylated intermediate from ADP and the intermediate. J. Biochem. 70, 95.

KAROL, M. H., and M. V. SIMPSON, 1968: DNA biosynthesis by isolated mitochondria: a replicative rather than a repair process. Science 162, 470.

KASAMATSU, H., D. L. ROBBERSON, and J. VINOGRAD, 1971 a: Replication of mitochondrial DNA. I. The occurrence and composition of D-loops in MDNA from exponentially-growing mouse L cells. Fed. Proc. 30, 1177.

— — — 1971 b: A novel closed-circular mitochondrial DNA with properties of a replicating intermediate. Proc. nat. Acad. Sci. (U.S.) 68, 2252.

— L. I. GROSSMAN, D. L. ROBBERSON, R. WATSON, and J. VINOGRAD, 1973: The replication and structure of mitochondrial DNA in animal cells. Cold Spring Harbor Symp. Quant. Biol. 38, 289.

KATYARE, S. S., P. FATTERPAKER, and A. SREENIVASAN, 1971: Effect of 2,4-dinitrophenol (DNP) on oxidative phosphorylation in rat liver mitochondria. Arch. Biochem. Biophys. 144, 209.

KAUZMANN, W. L, 1969: Some factors in the interpretation of protein denaturation. Adv. Prot. Chem. 14, 1.

KEILIN, D., and E. T. HARTREE, 1939: Cytochrome and cytochrome oxidase. Proc. Roy. Soc. Series B. 127, 167.

KELLEMS, R. E., and R. A. BUTOW, 1972: Cytoplasmic-type 80 S ribosomes associated with yeast mitochondria. I. Evidence for ribosomes binding sites on yeast mitochondria. J. biol. Chem. 24, 8043.

— — 1974: Cytoplasmic-type 80 S ribosomes associated with yeast mitochondria. III. Changes in the amount of bound ribosomes in response to changes in metabolic state. J. biol. Chem. 249, 3304.

— V. F. ALLISON, and R. A. BUTOW, 1974 a: Cytoplasmic type 80 S ribosomes associated with yeast mitochondria. II. Evidence for the association of cytoplasmic ribosomes with the outer mitochondrial membrane in situ. J. biol. Chem. 249, 3297.

— — — 1974 b: Cytoplasmic ribosomes associated with yeast mitochondria. In: The biogenesis of mitochondria. (KROON, A. M., and C. SACCONE, eds.), p. 511. New York-London: Academic Press.

KENNEDY, K. E., and G. A. THOMPSON, JR., 1970: Phosphonolipids localization in surface membranes of *Tetrahymena*. Science **168**, 989.

KEYHANI, E., 1973: Ribosomal granules associated with outer mitochondrial membrane in aerobic yeast cells. J. Cell Biol. **58**, 480.

— et J. J. KRIZ, 1969: Biologie cellulaire. Ultrastructure de la membrane mitochondriale. Etude par coloration négative et cryodécapage. C. R. Acad. Sci. (Paris) **268**, 1643.

KING, M. J., and J. J. DIWAN, 1972: Transport of glutamate and aspartate across the membranes of rat liver mitochondria. Arch. Biochem. Biophys. **152**, 670.

— — 1973: Permeability of rat-liver mitochondria to leucine, tyrosine, alpha-amino-isobutyric acid and lysine. Arch. Biochem. Biophys. **159**, 166.

KIRSCHNER, R. H., D. R. WOLSTENHOLME, and N. J. GROSS, 1968: Replicating molecules of circular mitochondrial DNA. Proc. nat. Acad. Sci. (U.S.) **60**, 1466.

KJAERHEIM, A., 1967: Crystallized tubules in the mitochondrial matrix of adrenal cortical cells. Exp. Cell Res. **45**, 236.

KLEINEKE, J., H. SAUER, and H. D. SÖLING, 1973: On the specificity of the tricarboxylic acid carrier system in rat liver mitochondria. FEBS Lett. **29**, 82.

KLEINOW, W., W. NEUPERT, and F. MILLER, 1974: Fine structure of mitochondrial ribosomes of locust flight muscle. In: The biogenesis of mitochondria. (KROON, A. M., and C. SACCONE, eds.), p. 337. New York-London: Academic Press.

KLINGENBERG, M., 1967: Kinetics of adenine nucleotide exchange. In: Mitochondrial structure and compartmentation. (QUAGLIARIELLO, E., S. PAPA, E. C. SLATER, and J. M. TAGER, eds.), p. 271. Bari: Adriatica Editrice.

— 1968: The respiratory chain. In: Biological oxidation. (SINGER, T. P., ed.), p. 3. New York: Wiley (Interscience).

— 1970 a: Mitochondria metabolite transport. FEBS Lett. **6**, 145.

— 1970 b: Metabolite transport in mitochondria: An example for intracellular membrane function. Essays in Biochem. **6**, 119.

— 1972: Abstr. 8th Congress Biochem., p. 154.

— and M. BUCHOLZ, 1970: Localization of the glycerol-phosphate dehydrogenase in the outer phase of the mitochondrial inner membrane. Eur. J. Biochem. **13**, 247.

— — 1973: On the mechanism of bongkrekate effect on the mitochondrial adenine-nucleotide carrier as studied through the binding of ADP. Eur. J. Biochem. **38**, 346.

— and E. PFAFF, 1966: Structural and functional compartmentation in mitochondria. In: Regulation of metabolic processes in mitochondria. (TAGER, J. M., S. PAPA, E. QUAGLIA-RIELLO, and E. C. SLATER, eds.), p. 180. Amsterdam-London-New York: Elsevier Publishing Co.

— — 1967: Means of terminating reactions. Methods in Enzymol. **10**, 680.

— and G. VON JAGOW, 1970: Topochemistry of the respiratory chain in the mitochondrial (cristae) membrane. In: Electron transport and energy conservation. (TAGER, J. M., S. PAPA, E. QUAGLIARIELLO, and E. C. SLATER, eds.), p. 281. Bari: Adriatica Editrice.

— B. SCHERER, L. STENGEL-RUTKOWSKI, M. BUCHHOLZ, and K. GREBE, 1973: Experimental demonstration of the reorienting (mobile) carrier mechanism exemplified by the mito-chondrial adenine nucleotide translocator. In: Mechanisms in Bioenergetics. (AZZONE, G. F., L. ERNSTER, S. PAPA, E. QUAGLIARIELLO, and N. SILIPRANDI, eds.), p. 257. New York-London: Academic Press.

— P. RICCIO, H. AQUILA, B. SCHMIEDT, K. GREBE, and P. TOPITSCH, 1974: Characterization of the ADP/ATP carrier in mitochondria. In: Membrane Proteins in Transport and Phosphorylation. (AZZONE, G. F., M. E. KLINGENBERG, E. QUAGLIARIELLO, and N. SILI-PRANDI, eds.), p. 229. Amsterdam-London: North-Holland Publishing Co. New York: American Elsevier Publishing Co.

KNOWLES, A. F., and H. S. PENEFSKY, 1972: The subunit structure of beef heart mito-chondrial adenosine triphosphatase, physical and chemical properties of isolated subunits. J. biol. Chem. **247**, 6624.

— and E. RACKER, 1975: Formation of adenosine triphosphate from P_i and adenosine diphosphate by purified Ca^{2+}-adenosine triphosphatase. J. Biol. Chem. **250**, 1949.

KOIKE, K., and M. KOBAYASHI, 1973: Synthesis of mitochondrial DNA *in vitro:* two classes of nascent DNAs. Biochim. biophys. Acta **324**, 452.

— and D. R. WOLSTENHOLME, 1974: Evidence for discontinuous replication of circular mitochondrial DNA molecules from Novikoff rat ascites hepatoma cells. J. Cell Biol. **61**, 14.

KOLAROV, J., J. SUBIK, and L. KOVAC, 1972: Oxidative phosphorylation in yeast. VIII. Osmotic and permeability properties of mitochondria isolated from wild-type yeast and from a respiratory deficient mutant. Biochim. biophys. Acta **267**, 457.

KOLODNER, R., and K. K. TEWARI, 1972: Circular mitochondrial DNA (70 × 10⁶ dalton) from pea leaves. Fed. Proc. **31**, 876, abstr.

KOMAI, H., D. R. HUNTER, and Y. TAKAHASHI, 1973: Effect of lysolecithin treatment on the structure and functions of the mitochondrial inner membrane. Biochem. biophys. Res. Commun. **53**, 82.

KOVÁC, Á. Č., and K. WEISSOVÁ, 1968: Oxidative phosphorylation in yeast. III. ATPase activity of the mitochondrial fraction from a cytoplasmic respiratory-deficient mutant. Biochim. biophys. Acta **153**, 55.

KRAML, J., and H. R. MAHLER, 1967: Biochemical correlates of respiratory deficiency. VIII. A precipitating antiserum against cytochrome oxidase of yeast and its use in the study of respiratory deficiency. Immunoch. **4**, 213.

KRAUSE, W., 1967: Elektronenmikroskopische Darstellung von elektronendichten globulären Teilchen an isolierten Mitochondrienmembranen der Rattenleber im Ultradünnschnittpräparat. Acta Biol. Med. German. **19**, 791.

— 1968: Elektronenmikroskopische Beobachtung von fibrillären Elementen und isolierten Mitochondrienmembranen der Rattenleber. Acta Biol. Med. German. **21**, 241.

KREBS, W., D. SCHWAB, and H. SCHWAB-STEY, 1972: Some observations on the fine structure of the mitochondrial inner membrane of *Tetrahymena pyriformis.* J. Ultrastruct. Res. **38**, 605.

KROON, A. M., 1963 a: Protein synthesis in heart mitochondria. I. Amino acid incorporation into the proteins of isolated beef-heart mitochondria and fractions derived from them by sonic oscillation. Biochim. biophys. Acta **72**, 391.

— 1963 b: Inhibitors of mitochondrial protein synthesis. Biochim. biophys. Acta **76**, 165.

— and R. J. JANSEN, 1968: The effect of low concentrations of chloramphenicol on beating rat-heart cells in tissue culture. Biochim. biophys. Acta **155**, 629.

— C. SACCONE, and M. J. BOTMAN, 1967: RNA and protein synthesis by sterile rat-liver mitochondria. Biochim. biophys. Acta **142**, 552.

— E. AGSTERIBBE, and H. DE VRIES, 1972: Protein synthesis in mitochondria and chloroplasts. In: The mechanism of protein synthesis and its regulation. (BOSCH, L., ed.), p. 539. Amsterdam: North Holland.

KUNER, J. M., and R. E. BEYER, 1970: An ultrastructural study of isolated rat skeletal muscle mitochondria in various metabolic states. J. Membr. Biol. **2**, 71.

KÜNTZEL, H., 1969: Proteins of mitochondrial and cytoplasmic ribosomes from *Neurospora crassa.* Nature **222**, 142.

— 1971: The genetic apparatus of mitochondria from *Neurospora* and yeast. Curr. Top. Microb. Imm. **54**, 94.

— und Z. BARATH, 1972: Kerngesteuerte Biosynthese des mitochondrialen genetischen Apparates in *Neurospora crassa.* Hoppe-Seyler's Z. physiol. Chem. **353**, 690.

— and H. C. BLOSSEY, 1974: Translation products *in vitro* of mitochondrial messenger RNA from *Neurospora crassa.* Eur. J. Biochem. **47**, 165.

— and H. NOLL, 1967: Mitochondrial and cytoplasmic polysomes from *Neurospora crassa.* Nature **214**, 1340.

KURIYAMA, Y., and D. J. L. LUCK, 1973 a: Ribosomal RNA synthesis in mitochondria of *Neurospora crassa.* J. molec. Biol. **73**, 425.

— — 1973 b: Membrane-associated ribosomes in mitochondria of *Neurospora crassa.* J. Cell Biol. **59**, 776.

KUROSOMI, K., T. MATSUZAWA, N. WATARI, 1966: Mitochondrial inclusions in the snake renal tubules. J. Ultrastruct. Res. **16**, 269.

LAMB, A. J., G. D. CLARK-WALKER, and A. W. LINNANE, 1968: The biogenesis of mito-
    chondria. 4. The differentiation of mitochondrial and cytoplasmic protein synthesis systems
    in vitro by antibiotics. Biochim. biophys. Acta **161**, 415.
LAMBETH, D. O., and H. A. LARDY, 1971: Purification and properties of rat-liver mito-
    chondrial adenosine triphosphatase. Eur. J. Biochem. **22**, 355.
— — A. E. SENIOR, and J. C. BROOKS, 1971: Reassessment of the molecular weight of
    mitochondrial ATPase from beef heart. FEBS Lett. **17**, 330.
LAMBOWITZ, A. M., and W. D. BONNER, JR., 1974: The b-cytochromes of plant mitochondria.
    A spectrophotometric and potentiometric study. J. biol. Chem. **249**, 2428.
— and C. W. SLAYMAN, 1971: Cyanide-resistant respiration in *Neurospora crassa.* J.
    Bact. **108**, 1087.
— — C. C. SLAYMAN, and W. D. BONNER, JR., 1972 a: The electron transport components
    of wild type and *poky* strains of *Neurospora crassa.* J. biol. Chem. **247**, 1536.
— E. W. SMITH, and C. W. SLAYMAN, 1972 b: Oxidative phosphorylation in *Neurospora*
    mitochondria. J. biol. Chem. **247**, 4859.
— W. D. BONNER, JR., and N. K. E. WIKSTRÖM, 1974: On the lack of ATP-induced
    midpoint potential shift for cytochrome-b-566 in plant mitochondria. Proc. nat. Acad. Sci.
    (U.S.) **71**, 1183.
LA NOUE, K., and J. R. WILLIAMSON, 1971: Interrelationships between malate-aspartate
    shuttle and citric acid cycle in rat heart mitochondria. Metabolism **20**, 119.
— E. I. WALAJTYS, and J. R. WILLAMSON, 1973: Regulation of glutamate metabolism and
    interactions with citric acid cycle in rat heart mitochondria. J. Biol. Chem. **248**, 717.
— A. J. MEIJER, and A. BROUWER, 1974: Evidence for electrogenic aspartate transport in
    rat liver mitochondria. Arch. Biochem. Biophys. **161**, 544.
LANSMAN, R. A., M. J. ROWE, and D. O. WOODWARD, 1974: Pulse-recovery studies on
    cycloheximide-insensitive protein synthesis in *Neurospora.* Association of products with
    cytochrome oxidase. Eur. J. Biochem. **41**, 15.
LARDY, H. A., and C. H. LIN, 1969: Inhibition of mitochondrial oxidative phosphorylation
    by aurovertin. In: Inhibitors, tools in cell research. (BUCHER, T. H., and H. SIES, eds.),
    p. 279. New York-Heidelberg-Berlin: Springer-Verlag.
— J. L. CONNELLY, and D. JOHNSON, 1964: Antibiotics as tools for metabolic studies.
    II. Inhibition of phosphoryl transfer in mitochondria by oligomycin and aurovertin.
    Biochem. **3**, 1961.
— P. WITONSKY, and D. JOHNSON, 1965: Antibiotics as tools of metabolic studies:
    IV. Comparative effectiveness of oligomycin A, B, C and rutamycin as inhibitors of phos-
    phoryl transfer reactions in mitochondria. Biochem. **4**, 552.
LARIS, P. C., D. P. BAHR, and R. R. J. CHAFFEE, 1975: Membrane potentials in mitochondrial
    preparations as measured by means of cyanine dyes. Biochim. biophys. Acta **376**, 415.
LASSEN, U. V., A. M. T. NIELSEN, L. PAPE, and L. O. SIMONSEN, 1971: The membrane
    potential of Ehrlich ascites tumor cells. Microelectrode measurements and their critical
    evaluation. J. Membr. Biol. **6**, 269.
LAZOWSKA, J., F. MICHEL, G. FAYE, H. FUKUHARA, and P. P. SLONIMSKI, 1974: Physical
    and genetic organization of *petite* and *grande* yeast mitochondrial DNA. II. DNA-DNA
    hybridization studies and buoyant density determination. J. molec. Biol. **85**, 393.
LEDERMAN, M., and G. ATTARDI, 1970: *In vitro* protein synthesis in a mitochondrial fraction
    from HeLa cells: sensitivity to antibiotics and ethidium bromide. Biochem. biophys.
    Res. Commun. **40**, 1492.
— — 1973: Expression of the mitochondrial genome in HeLa cells. XV. Electrophoretic
    properties of the products *in vivo* and *in vitro* mitochondrial protein synthesis. J. molec.
    Biol. **78**, 275.
LEE, C. P., 1970: Orientation of the respiratory chain in the mitochondrial inner mem-
    brane. In: Electron transport and energy conservation. (TAGER, J. M., S. PAPA, E. QUA-
    GLIARIELLO, and E. C. SLATER, eds.), p. 291. Bari: Adriatica Editrice.
— 1971: In: Probes of structure and function of macromolecules and membranes. (CHANCE, B.,
    ed.), p. 417. New York-London: Academic Press.
— and L. ERNSTER, 1968: Studies of the energy-transfer system of submitochondrial particles,
    effects of oligomycin and aurovertin. Eur. J. Biochem. **3**, 391.

LEFFLER, A. T., II, E. CRESKOFF, S. W. LUBORSKY, V. McFARLAND, and P. T. MORA, 1970: Isolation and characterization of rat liver mitochondrial DNA. J. molec. Biol. **48**, 455.

LEHNINGER, A. L., 1962: A heat-labile factor required for the extrusion of water from mitochondria. J. Biol. Chem. **237**, 946.

— 1965: The mitochondrion, molecular basis of structure and function. Amsterdam-New York: Benjamin, Inc.

— 1970: Mitochondria and calcium transport. Biochem. J. **119**, 129.

— 1974: Role of phosphate and other proton-donating anions in respiration-coupled ion transport of Ca^{2+} by mitochondria. Proc. nat. Acad. Sci. (U.S.) **71**, 1520.

— and E. CARAFOLI, 1971: The interaction of La^{3+} with mitochondria in relation to respiration-coupled Ca^{2+} transport. J. biol. Chem. **143**, 506.

— — and C. S. ROSSI, 1967: Energy-linked ion movements in mitochondrial systems. Advanc. Enzymol. **29**, 259.

LEIGH, JR., J. S., D. F. WILSON, C. S. OWEN, and T. E. KING, 1974: Heme-heme interaction in cytochrome oxidase: the cooperativity of the hemes of cytochrome c oxidase, its existence in the reaction with CO. Arch. Biochem. **160**, 476.

LENARD, J., and S. J. SINGER, 1968: Alteration of the conformation of proteins in red blood cell membranes and in solution by fixatives used in electron microscopy. J Cell Biol. **37**, 117.

LENAZ, G., 1965: Effect of aurovertin on energy linked processes related to oxidative phosphorylation. Biochem. biophys. Res. Commun. **21**, 170.

LÊ-QUÔC-BRUGUERA, D., and Y. GAUDEMER, 1973: Evidence for maleate penetration into rat liver mitochondria. Biochimie **55**, 1511.

LERNER, E., A. L. SHUG, C. ELSON, and E. SHRAGO, 1972: Reversible inhibition of adenine nucleotide translocation by long chain fatty acyl coenzyme A esters in liver mitochondria of diabetic and hibernating animals. J. Biol. Chem. **247**, 1513.

LEVY, M., and M.-T. SAUNER, 1967: Compositin en phospholipides des membranes interne et externe des mitochondries. Compt. Rend., Societé Biol. **161**, 277.

LIBERMAN, E. A., and V. P. SKULACHEV, 1970: Conversion of biomembrane-produced energy into electric form. IV. General discussion. Biochim. biophys. Acta **216**, 30.

— and V. P. TOPALY, 1968: Selective transport of ions through bimolecular phospholipid membranes. Biochim. biophys. Acta **163**, 125.

LIGHT, P. A., C. I. RAGAN, R. A. CLEGG, and P. B. GARLAND, 1968: Iron-limited growth of *Torulopsis utilis* and the reversible loss of mitochondrial energy conservation at site 1 and of sensitivity to rotenone and piericidin A. FEBS Lett. **1**, 4.

LIN, H. S., 1965: Microcylinders within mitochondrial cristae in the rat pinealocyte. J. Cell Biol. **25**, 435.

LINDSAY, J. G., 1974: ATP-induced oxidation of a^{3+}-CO compound in pigeon heart mitochondria. Arch. Biochem. Biophys. **163**, 705.

— and D. F. WILSON, 1972: Apparent adenosine triphosphate induced ligand change in cytochrome a_3 of pigeon heart mitochondria. Biochem. **11**, 4613.

— P. L. DUTTON, and D. F. WILSON, 1972: Energy-dependent effects on the oxidation-reduction midpoint potentials of the b and c cytochromes in phosphorylating submitochondrial particles from pigeon heart. Biochem. **11**, 1937.

LINNANE, A. W., and J. M. HASLAM, 1970: The biogenesis of mitochondria. Curr. Top. Cell. Reg. **2**, 101.

— G. W. SAUNDER, E. B. GINGOLD, and H. B. LUKINS, 1968: The biogenesis of mitochondria. V. Cytoplasmic inheritance of erythromycin resistance in *Saccharomyces cerevisiae* Proc. nat. Acad. Sci (U.S.), **59**, 903.

LIZARDI, P. M., and D. J. L. LUCK, 1972: The intracellular site of synthesis of mitochondrial ribosomal proteins in *Neurospora crassa*. J. Cell Biol. **54**, 56.

LOCKER, J., M. RABINOWITZ, and G. L. GETZ, 1974: Tandem inverted repeats in mitochondrial DNA of petite mutants of *Saccharomyces cerevisiae*. Proc. nat. Acad. Sci. (U.S.) **71**, 1366.

LORENZ, B., W. KLEINOW, and H. WEISS, 1974: Mitochondrial translation of cytochrome b in *Neurospora crassa* and *Locusta migratoria*. Hoppe-Seyler's Z. physiol. Chem. **355**, 300.

LOUD, A. V., 1968: A quantitative sterological description of the ultrastructure of normal rat liver parenchymal cells. J. Cell Biol. **37**, 27.

LOW, H., and I. VALLIN, 1963: Succinate-linked diphosphopyridine nucleotide reduction in submitochondrial particles. Biochim. biophys. Acta **69**, 361.

LUCIANI, S., 1973: Inhibition by tannic acid of succinate and malate translocation across mitochondrial membrane. Biochem. Pharmacol. **22**, 1821.

LUCK, D. J. L., 1963 a: Formation of mitochondria in *Neurospora crassa:* a quantitative radioautographic study. J. Cell Biol. **16**, 483.

— 1963 b: Genesis of mitochondria in *Neurospora crassa.* Proc. nat. Acad. Sci. (U.S.) **49**, 233.

— 1965 a: The influence of precursor pool size on mitochondrial composition in *Neurospora crassa.* J. Cell Biol. **24**, 445.

— 1965 b: Formation of mitochondria in *Neurospora crassa.* A study based on mitochondrial density changes. J. Cell Biol. **24**, 461.

— 1966: Probleme der biologischen Reduplikation (SITTE, P., ed.). Berlin-Heidelberg-New York: Springer-Verlag.

— and E. REICH, 1964: DNA in mitochondria of *Neurospora crassa.* Proc. nat. Acad. Sci. (U.S.) **52**, 931.

LUCY, J. A., and A. M. GLAUERT, 1964: Structure and assembly of macromolecular lipid complexes composed of globular micelles. J. molec. Biol. **8**, 727.

LUFT, R., D. IKKOS, G. PALMIERI, L. ERNSTER, and B. AFZELIUS, 1962: A case of severe hypermetabolism of non-thyroid origin with a defect in the maintenance of mitochondrial respiratory control: a correlated clinical, biochemical and morphological study. J. clin. Invest. **41**, 1776.

LUSENA, C. V., and F. DEPOCAS, 1966: Heterogeneity and differential fragility of rat liver mitochondria. Canad. J. Biochem. **44**, 497.

MACLENNAN, D. H., 1970 a: Molecular architecture of the mitochondrion. Curr. Top. Membr. Transp. **1**, 177.

— 1970 b: Purification and properties of an adenosine triphosphatase from sarcoplasmic reticulum. J. biol. Chem. **245**, 4508.

— and J. ASAI, 1968: Studies on the mitochondrial adenosine triphosphatase system. V. Localization of oligomycin-sensitivity conferring protein. Biochem. biophys. Res. Commun. **33**, 441.

— and A. TZAGOLOFF, 1968: Studies on the mitochondrial adenosine triphosphatase system. IV. Purification and characterization of the oligomycin-sensitivity conferring protein. Biochem. **7**, 1603.

— P. SEEMAN, G. H. ILES, and C. C. YIP, 1971: Membrane formation by the adenosine triphosphatase of sarcoplasmic reticulum. J. Biol. Chem. **246**, 2702.

MAGER, J., 1960: Chloramphenicol and chlortetracycline inhibition of amino acid incorporation into proteins in a cell-free system from *Tetrahymena pyriformis.* Biochim. biophys. Acta, **38**, 150.

MAHLER, H. R., 1973: Biogenetic autonomy of mitochondria. Crit. Rev. Biochem. **1**, 381.

— and K. DAWIDOWICZ, 1973: Autonomy of mitochondria in *Saccharomyces cerevisiae* in their production of messenger RNA. Proc. nat. Acad. Sci. (U.S.) **70**, 111.

— P. S. PERLMAN, P. SLONIMSKI, M. J. DEUTSCH, H. FUKUHARA, and C. FAYE, 1971 a: Information content of mitochondrial DNA. Fed. Proc. **30**, 1149.

— — and B. D. MEHROTRA, 1971 a: Mitochondrial specification of the respiratory chain. In: Autonomy and biogenesis of mitochondria and chloroplasts. (BOARDMAN, N. K., A. W. LINNANE, and R. M. SMILLIE, eds.), p. 492. Amsterdam-New York: Elsevier.

— L. R. JONES, and W. J. MOORE, 1971 b: Mitochondrial contribution to protein synthesis in cerebral cortex. Biochem. biophys. Res. Commun. **42**, 384.

— K. DAWIDOWICZ, and F. FELDMAN, 1972: Formate as a specific label for mitochondrial translational products. J. biol. Chem. **247**, 7439.

— F. FELDMAN, S. H. PHAN, P. HAMILL, and K. DAWIDOWICZ, 1974: Initiation, identification and integration of mitochondrial proteins. In: The biogenesis of mitochondria. (KROON, A. M., and C. SACCONE, eds.), p. 423. New York-London: Academic Press.

MAHLER, H. R., P. S. PERLMAN, F. FELDMAN, and R. BASTOS, 1974 b: Regulation of the mitochondrial genetic system and its expression. In: Biomembranes. Architecture, Biogenesis, Bioenergetics and Differentiation. (PACKER, L., ed.), p. 3. New York-London: Academic Press.

MAIO, J. J., 1971: DNA strand reassociation and polyribonucleotide binding in the African green monkey *Cercopithecus aethiops.* J. molec. Biol. **56**, 579.

MAKINOSE, M., 1971: Calcium efflux-dependent formation of ATP from ADP and othophosphate by the membranes of the sarcoplasmic vesicles. FEBS Lett. **12**, 269.

— 1972 a: The conversion of osmotic into chemical energy coupled with calcium translocation across the sarcoplasmic membrane. Cold Spring Harbor Symposia on Quantit. Biol. **37**, 681.

— 1972 b: Phosphoprotein formed during osmo-chemical energy conversion in the membrane of the sarcoplasmic reticulum. FEBS Lett. **25**, 113.

— and W. HASSELBACH, 1971: ATP synthesis by the reverse of the sarcoplasmic calcium pump. FEBS Lett. **12**, 271.

MALHOTRA, S. K., 1966: A study of structure of the mitochondrial membrane system. J. Ultrastruct. Res. **15**, 14.

MARTIN, S. S., and H. B. BOSMANN, 1971: Glycoprotein nature of mitochondrial structural proteins and neutral sugar content of mitochondrial proteins and structural proteins. Exp. Cell Res. **66**, 59.

MARTONOSI, A., 1968: Sarcoplasmic reticulum. IV. Solubilization of microsomal adenosine triphosphatase. J. biol. Chem. **243**, 71.

— and R. A. HALPIN, 1971: Sarcoplasmic reticulum. X. The preotein composition of sarcoplasmic reticulum membranes. Arch. Biochem. Biophys. **144**, 66.

MASON, T. L., and R. O. POYTON, 1972: The biosynthesis of cytochrome oxidase in *Saccharomyces cerevisiae.* Fed. Proc. **31**, 1401.

— and G. SCHATZ, 1973: Cytochrome *c* oxidase from bakers' yeast. II. Site of translation of the protein components. J. biol. Chem. **248**, 1355.

— E. EBNER, R. O. POYTON, J. SALTZGABER, D. C. WHARTON, L. MENUCCI, and G. SCHATZ, 1972: The participation of mitochondrial and cytoplasmic protein synthesis on mitochondrial formation. Fed. Eur. Biochem. Soc. Eighth Meeting **28**, 53.

— R. O. POYTON, D. C. WHARTON, and G. SCHATZ, 1973: Cytochrome *c* oxidase from bakers yeast. I. Isolation and properties. J. biol. Chem. **248**, 1346.

MASSARI, S., and G. F. AZZONE, 1970 a: The mechanism of ion translocation in mitochondria. I. Coupling of K$^+$ and H$^+$ fluxes. Eur. J. Biochem. **12**, 301.

— — 1970 b: The mechanism of ion translocation in mitochondria. 2. Active transport and proton pump. Eur. J. Biochem. **12**, 310.

— — 1972 a: A thermodynamic analysis of the interconversion of osmotic and chemical energies. In: Biochemistry and biophysics of mitochondrial membranes. (AZZONE, G. F., E. CARAFOLI, A. L. LEHNINGER, E. QUAGLIARIELLO, and N. SILIPRANDI, eds.), p. 603. New York-London: Academic Press.

— — 1972 b: The equivalent pore radius of intact and damaged mitochondria and the mechanism of active shrinkage. Biochim. biophys. Acta, **283**, 23.

— E. BALBONI, and G. F. AZZONE, 1972 a: Distribution of permeant cations in rat liver mitochondria under steady state conditions. Biochim. biophys. Acta **283**, 16.

— L. FRIGERI, and G. F. AZZONE, 1972 b: The permeability to water, dimension of surface and structural changes during swelling in rat liver mitochondria. J. Memb. Biol. **9**, 57.

— — — 1972 c: A quantitative correlation between the kinetics of solutes and water translocation in liver mitochondria. J. Memb. Biol. **9**, 71.

MAY, R., 1974 a: Licht- und elektronenoptische Untersuchungen an Proteinkristaller und Mikrotubuli in Hefeprotoplasten. Z. allg. Mikrobiol. **14**, 409.

— 1974 b: Microfilaments in yeast mitochondria. Protoplasma **82**, 395.

MAZUR, P., 1970: Cryobiology: the freezing of biological systems. Science **168**, 939.

— and J. J. SCHMIDT, 1968: Interactions of cooling velocity temperature and warming velocity on survival of frozen and thawed yeast. Cryobiol. **5**, 1.

MAZUR, P., J. FARRANT, S. P. LEIBO, and E. H. Y. CHU, 1969: Survival of hamster tissue culture cells after freezing and thawing—interactions between protective solutes and cooling and warming rates. Cryobiol. 6, 1.

McFARLAND, B. H., and G. INESI, 1971: Solubilization of sarcoplasmic reticulum with Triton X-100. Arch. Biochem. Biophys. 145, 456.

McGIVAN, J. D., N. M. BRADFORD, and J. B. CHAPPELL, 1969: The inhibition of α-oxoglutarate entry into rat liver mitochondria by L-aspartate. FEBS Lett. 4, 247.

McINTYRE, J. A., M. J. KARNOVSKY, and N. B. GILULA, 1973: Intramembranous particle aggregation in lymphoid cells. Nature (N.B.) 245, 147.

McLEAN, J. R., G. L. COHN, I. K. BRANDT, and M. U. SIMPSON, 1958: Incorporation of labelled amino acids into the protein of muscle and liver mitochondria. J. biol. Chem. 233, 657.

McMURRAY, W. C., and R. M. C. DAWSON, 1969: Phospholipid exchange reactions within the liver cell. Bioch. J. 112, 91.

MEEK, G. A., and M. J. MOSES, 1963: Localization of tritiated thymidine in HeLa cells by electron autoradiography. J. roy. micr. Soc. 81, 187.

MEHROTRA, B. D., and H. R. MAHLER, 1968: Characterization of some unusual DNAs from the mitochondria from certain "petite" strains of Saccharomyces cerevisiae. Arch. Biochem. Biophys. 128, 685.

MEIJER, A. J., and K. VAN DAM, 1974: The metabolic significance of anion transport in mitochondria. Biochim. biophys. Acta 346, 213.

— G. S. P. GROOT, and J. M. TAGER, 1970: Effect of sulfhydril-blocking reagents on mitochondrial anion-exchange reactions involving phosphate. FEBS Lett. 8, 41.

— D. J. REINGOUD, A. BROUWER, J. B. HOEK, and J. M. TAGER, 1972: Transport of glutamate in rat liver mitochondria. Biochim. biophys. Acta 283, 421.

MEISNER, H., 1973: Inhibition of metabolite anion uptake in mitochondria by tetraphenylboron. Biochim. biophys. Acta 318, 383.

— F. PALMIERI, and E. QUAGLIARIELLO, 1972: Effect of cations and protons on the kinetics of substrate uptake in rat liver mitochondria. Biochem. 11, 949.

MEISSNER, G., and S. FLEISCHER, 1971: Characterization of sarcoplasmic reticulum from skeletal muscle. Biochim. biophys. Acta 241, 356.

— — 1973: Ca^{2+} uptake in reconstituted sarcoplasmic reticulum vesicles. Biochem. biophys. Res. Commun. 52, 22.

— — 1974: Dissociation and reconstitution of functional sarcoplasmic reticulum vesicles. J. biol. Chem. 249, 302.

MELA, L., 1968: Interactions of La^{3+} and local anesthetic drugs with mitochondrial Ca^{++} and Mn^{++} uptake. Arch. Biochem. Biophys. 123, 286.

— and B. CHANCE, 1969: Calcium carrier and the "high affinity" calcium binding site in mitochondria. Biochem. biophys. Res. Commun. 35, 556.

MELNICK, R. L., and L. PACKER, 1971: Freeze-fracture faces of inner and outer membranes of mitochondria. Biochim. biophys. Acta 253, 503.

MEROLA, A. J., and G. P. BRIERLEY, 1970: Respiratory control associated with cyclic pH transitions induced by N', N'-bis(dichloroacetyl)-12-diaminodecane. Biochem. biophys. Res. Commun. 41, 628.

MEYER, A. J., and J. M. TAGER, 1969: Effect of butyl malonate and mersalyl on anion-exchange reactions in rat liver mitochondria. Biochim. biophys. Acta 189, 136.

— and P. M. VIGNAIS, 1973: Kinetic study of glutamate transport in rat liver mitochondria. Biochim. biophys. Acta, 325, 375.

MEYER, H. W., and H. WINKELMANN, 1967: Freeze-etching and the structure of biological membranes. Protoplasma 68, 253.

MICHAELIS, G., S. DOUGLASS, M.-J. TSAI, and R. S. CRIDDLE, 1971: Mitochondrial DNA and suppressiveness of petite mutants in Saccharomyces cerevisiae. Biochem. Gen. 5, 487.

— — — K. BUZCHIEL, and R. S. CRIDDLE, 1972: In vitro transcription of mitochondrial deoxyribonucleic acid from yeast. Biochem. 12, 2026.

MICHEL, F., J. LAZOWSKA, G. FAYE, H. FUKUHARA, and P. P. SLONIMSKI, 1974: Physical and genetic organization of petite and grande yeast mitochondrial DNA. III. High resolution melting and reassociation studies. J. molec. Biol. 85, 411.

MICHEL, R., and W. NEUPERT, 1973: Mitochondrial translation products before and after integration into mitochondrial membrane in *Neurospora crassa*. Eur. J. Biochem. **36**, 53.

MILLER, E. K., and R. M. C. DAWSON, 1972: Exchange of phospholipids between brain membranes in vitro. Biochem. J. **126**, 823.

MITCHELL, C. H., C. L. BUAN, H. B. LUKINS, and A. W. LINNANE, 1973: Biogenesis of mitochondria. 23. The biochemical and genetic characteristics of two different oligomycin resistant mutant of *Saccharomyces cerevisiae* under the influence of cytoplasmic genetic modification. J. Bioenerg. **4**, 161.

MITCHELL, M. B., and H. K. MITCHELL, 1952: A case of "maternal" inheritance in *Neurospora crassa*. Proc. nat. Acad. Sci. (U.S.) **38**, 442.

— — and J. TISSIÈRES, 1953: Mendelian and non-mendelian factor affecting the cytochrome system in *Neurospora crassa*. Proc. nat. Acad. Sci. (U.S.) **39**, 606.

MITCHELL, P., 1961: Coupling of phosphorylation to electron and hydrogen transfer by a chemiosmotic type of mechanism. Nature **191**, 144.

— 1966 a: Chemiosmotic coupling in oxidative and photosynthetic phosphorylation. Biol. Rev. **41**, 445.

— 1966 b: Chemiosmotic coupling in oxidative and photosynthetic phosphorylation". Glynn Research Ltd., Bodmin, Cornwall, England.

— 1966 c: Metabolic flow in the mitochondrial multiphase system: an appraisal of the chemiosmotic theory of oxidative phosphorylation. In: Regulation of metabolic processes in mitochondria (TAGER, J. M., S. PAPA, E. QUAGLIARIELLO, and E. C. SLATER, eds.), p. 65. Amsterdam-London-New York: Elsevier Publishing Co.

— 1967: Proton-translocation phosphorylation in mitochondria, chloroplasts and bacteria: natural fuel cells and solar cells. Fed. Proc. **26**, 1370.

— 1968: "Chemiosmotic coupling and energy transduction". Glynn Research Ltd., Bodmin, Cornwall, England.

— 1969 a: In: "Mitochondria, structure and function". Symposium 5th Meeting Fed. Eur. Biochem. Soc., Prague.

— 1969 b: Orientated chemical reactions and ion movements in membranes. In: The molecular basis of membrane function. (TOSTESON, D. C., ed.), p. 483. Englewood Cliffs, N.J.: Prentice-Hall, Inc.

— 1974: A chemiosmotic molecular mechanism for proton translocating adenosine triphosphatases. FEBS Lett. **43**, 189.

— 1975: Proton translocation mechanisms and energy transduction by adenosine triphosphatase; an answer to criticisms. FEBS Lett. **50**, 95.

— and J. MOYLE, 1965: Stoichiometry of proton translocation through the respiratory chain and adenosine triphosphatase systems of rat liver mitochondria. Nature **208**, 147.

— — 1967 a: Acid-base titration across a membrane system of rat liver mitochondria. Catalysis by uncouplers. Biochem. J. **104**, 588.

— — 1967 b: Respiration-driven proton translocation in rat liver mitochondria. Biochem. J. **105**, 1147.

— — 1967 c: Proton-transport phosphorylation: some experimental tests. In: Biochemistry of mitochondria. (SLATER, E. C., Z. KANUIGA, and L. WOJTCZAK, eds.), p. 53. London-New York: Academic Press.

— — 1968: Proton translocation coupled to ATP hydrolysis in rat liver mitochondria. Eur. J. Biochem. **4**, 530.

— — 1969 a: Translocation of some anions, cations and acids in rat liver mitochondria. Eur. J. Biochem. **9**, 149.

— — 1969 b: Estimation of membrane potential and pH difference across the cristae membrane of rat liver mitochondria. Eur. J. Biochem. **7**, 471.

MITRA, R. S., and I. A. BERSTEIN, 1970: Thymidine incorporation into deoxyribonucleic acid by isolated rat liver mitochondria. J. biol. Chem. **245**, 1255.

— B. BARTOOU, J. MONAHAN, and K. B. FREEMAN, 1972: Comparison of mammalian mitochondrial ribonucleic acid from different species. Biochem. J. **128**, 1033.

MIYAMOTO, V. K., and T. E. THOMPSON, 1967: Some electrical properties of lipid bilayer membranes. J. Colloid Interface Sci. **25**, 16.

MOCHAN, B. S., R. W. LANG, and W. B. ELLIOTT, 1970: Studies on a cytochrome oxidase antibody. II. Inhibition kinetics. Biochim. biophys. Acta **216**, 106.

MONTAL, M., B. CHANCE, and C.-P. LEE, 1970: Ion transport and energy conservation in submitochondrial particles. J. Memb. Biol. **2**, 201.

MOOR, H., 1964: Die Gefrierfixation lebender Zellen und ihre Anwendung in der Elektronenmikroskopie. Z. Zellforsch. **62**, 546.

— and K. MUHLETHALER, 1963: Fine structure in frozen-etched yeast cells. J. Cell Biol. **17**, 609.

MOORE, C. L., 1971: Specific inhibition of mitochondrial Ca^{++} transport by ruthenium red. Biochem. biophys. Res. Commun. **42**, 298.

MORA, P. T., A. T. LEFELER, II and S. W. LUBORSKY, 1970: Properties of the complementary strands of a mitochondrial DNA. Hoppe-Seyler's Z. physiol. Chem. **351**, 955.

MORALES, R., and D. DUNCAN, 1971: Prismatic and other unusual arrays of mitochondrial cristae in astrocytes of cats and hamsters. Anat. Rec. **171**, 545.

MOREL, F., G. LANQUIN, J. LUNARDI, J. DUSZYNSKI, and P. V. VIGNAIS, 1974: An appraisal of the functional significance of the inhibitory effect of long chain acyl CoAs in mitochondrial transport. FEBS Lett. **39**, 133.

MORELIS, R., P. BROQUET, and P. LOUISOT, 1974: Glycoprotein biosynthesis in liver mitochondria. II. Mitochondrial localization of mannosyltransferase. Biochim. biophys. Acta **373**, 10.

MORRIS, G. J., and J. FARRANT, 1972: Interactions of cooling rate and protective additive on survival of washed human erythrocytes frozen to — 196 degrees C. Cryobiol. **9**, 173.

MORTON, D. J., R. W. D. ROWE, and J. J. MACFARLANE, 1973: The formation of intracristal structures induced in skeletal muscle mitochondria by high pressure. J. Bioenerg. **4**, 445.

MOUNOLOU, J. C., H. JAKOB, and P. P. SLONIMSKI, 1966: Mitochondrial DNA from yeast "petite" mutants: specific changes of buoyant density corresponding to different cytoplasmic mutations. Biochem. biophys. Res. Commun. **24**, 218.

MOUSTACCHI, E., and D. H. WILLIAMSON, 1966: Physiological variations in satellite components of yeast DNA detected by density gradient centrifugation. Biochem. biophys. Res. Commun. **23**, 56.

MUGNAINI, E., 1964 a: Filamentous inclusions in the matrix of mitochondria from human livers. J. Ultrastruct. Res. **11**, 525.

— 1964 b: Helical filaments in astrocytic mitochondria of the *corpus striatum* in the rat. J. Cell Biol. **23**, 176.

MUSCATELLO, U., V. GUARRIERA-BOBYLEVA, and P. BUFFA, 1972: Configurational changes in isolated rat liver mitochondria as revealed by negative staining. I. Modification caused by osmotic and other factors. J. Ultrastruct. Res. **40**, 215.

NAGLEY, P., and A. W. LINNANE, 1972: Biogenesis of mitochondria. XXI. Studies on the nature of the mitochondrial genome in yeast: the degenerative effects of ethidium bromide on mitochondrial genetic information in a respiratory competent strain. J. molec. Biol. **66**, 181.

— E. B. GINGOLD, H. B. LUKINS, and A. W. LINNANE, 1973: Biogenesis of mitochondria. XXV. Studies on the mitochondrial genomes of petite mutants of yeast using ethidium bromide as a probe. J. molec. Biol. **78**, 335.

— P. L. MOLLOY, H. B. LUKINS, and A. W. LINNANE, 1974 a: Studies on mitochondrial gene purification using petite mutants of yeast. Characterization of mutants enriched in ribosomal RNA cistrons. Biochem. biophys. Res. Commun. **57**, 232.

— E. B. GINGOLD, and A. W. LINNANE, 1974 b: The purification of mitochondrial genes using petite mutants of yeast. In: biogenesis of mitochondria. (KROON, A. M., and C. SACCONE, eds.), p. 157. New York-London: Academic Press.

NASS, M. M. K., 1966: The circularity of mitochondrial DNA. Proc. nat. Acad. Sci. (U.S.) **56**, 1215.

— and C. A. BUCK, 1970: Studies on mitochondrial tRNA from animal cells. II. Hybridization of aminoacyl-tRNA from rat liver mitochondria with heavy and light complementary strands of mitochondrial DNA. J. molec. Biol. **54**, 187.

NASS, M. M. K., and S. NASS, 1962: Fibrous structures within the matrix of developing chick embryo mitochondria. Exp. Cell Res. **26**, 424.

NASS, M. M. K., and C. A. BUCK, 1963 a: Intramitochondrial fibers with DNA characteristics. I. Fixation and electron staining reactions. J. Cell Biol. **19**, 593.

— — and AFZELIUS, 1965: The general occurrence of mitochondrial DNA. Exp. Cell Res. **37**, 516.

NASS, S., and M. M. K. NASS, 1963 b: Intramitochondrial fibers with DNA characteristics. II. Enzymatic and other hydrolytic treatments. J. Cell. Biol., **19**, 613.

NEIFAKH, S. A., and T. B. KAZAKOVA, 1963: Actomyosin-like protein in mitochondria of the mouse liver. Nature **197**, 1106.

NELSON, N., H. NELSON, and E. RACKER, 1972: Partial resolution of the enzymes catalyzing photophosphorylation. XII. Purification and properties of an inhibitor isolated from chloroplast coupling factor 1. J. biol. Chem. **247**, 7657.

NEUBERT, D., and H. HELGE, 1965: Studies on nucleotide incorporation into mitochondrial RNA. Biochem. biophys. Res. Commun. **18**, 600.

— und H. P. MORRIS, 1966: RNS- und Proteinsynthese in Zellkernen und Mitochondrien aus Rattenleber mit Hepatozellularen Tumoren. Arch. Exp. Path. Pharm. **255**, 51.

— H. P. HELGE und S. TESKE, 1966 a: Einige Eigenschaften der RNS-Polymerase-Reaktion in Warmblüter-Mitochondrion. Arch. Exp. Path. Pharm. **252**, 452.

— R. BASS und H. HELGE, 1966 b: Umsatzgeschwindigkeit der DNS in Mitochondrien von Warmblutzellen. Naturwissenschaften **53**, 23.

NEUPERT, W., and G. D. LUDWIG, 1971: Sites of biosynthesis of outer and inner membrane proteins of *Neurospora crassa* mitochondria. Eur. J. Biochem. **19**, 523.

— D. BRDICZKA, and TH. BÜCHER, 1967: Incorporation of amino acids into the outer and inner membrane of isolated rat liver mitochondria. Biochem. biophys. Res. Commun. **27**, 488.

— W. SEBALD, A. J. SCHWAB, P. MASSINGER, and TH. BÜCHER, 1969: Incorporation *in vivo* of ^{14}C-labelled amino acids into the proteins of mitochondrial ribosomes from *Neurospora crassa* sensitive to cycloheximide and insensitive to chloramphenicol. Eur. J. Biochem. **10**, 589.

NEWCOMB, E. H., W. STEER, P. K. HEPLER, and W. P. WERGIN, 1968: An atypical crista resembling a "tight junction" in bean root mitochondria. J. Cell Biol. **39**, 35.

NICHOLLS, D. G., 1974: The influence of respiration and ATP hydrolysis on the proton-electrochemical gradient across the inner membrane of rat-liver mitochondria as determined by ion distribution. Eur. J. Biochem. **50**, 305.

NICHOLLS, P., and L. C. PETERSEN, 1974: Haem-haem interactions in cytochrome aa$_3$ during the anaerobic-aerobic transition. Biochim. biophys. Acta **357**, 462.

NILSSON, O., 1958: Ultrastructure of mouse uterine surface epithelium under different estrogenic influences. J. Ultrastruct. Res. **1**, 375.

NIRENBERG, M., T. CASKEY, R. MARSHALL, R. BRIMACOMBE, D. KELLOG, B. DOCTOR, D. HATFIELD, J. LEVIN, F. ROTTMAN, S. PESTKA, M. WILCOX, and F. ANDERSON, 1966: The RNA code and protein synthesis. Cold Spring Harbor Symp. Quant. Biol. **31**, 11.

O'BRIEN, T. W., D. N. DENSLOW, and G. R. MARTIN, 1974: The structure, composition and function of 55 S ribosomes. In: The biogenesis of mitochondria. (KROON, A. M., and C. SACCONE, eds.), p. 347. New York-London: Academic Press.

OESTERHELT, D., and W. STOECKENIUS, 1971: Rhodopsin-like protein from the purple membrane of *Halobacterium halobium*. Nature (N.B.) **233**, 149.

OGAWA, K., and H. MAYAHARA, 1969: Intramitochondrial localization of adenosine triphosphatase activity. J. Histochem. Cytochem. **17**, 487.

OHNISHI, T., 1970: Induction of the site. I. Phosphorylation *in vivo* in *Saccharomyces carlbergensis*. Biochem. biophys. Res. Commun. **41**, 344.

— 1973: Mechanism of electron transport and energy conservation in the site I region of the respiratory chain. Biochim. biophys. Acta **301**, 105.

— and T. OHNISHI, 1962: A contractile protein of mitochondria. J. Biochem. (Tokyo) **51**, 380.

— H. SCHLEYER, and B. CHANCE, 1969: Studies on non-heme iron proteins and the piericidin A binding sites of mitochondrial particles from *Candida utilis* cells grown in media of varying iron concentrations. Biochem. biophys. Res. Commun. **36**, 487.

OHNISHI, T., T. ASAKURA, H. WOHLRAB, T. YONETANI, and B. CHANCE, 1970: Electron paramagnetic resonance studies on iron-sulfur proteins of submitochondrial particles from *Candida utilis* cells. J. biol. Chem. **245**, 900.

— — T. YONETANI, and B. CHANCE, 1971: Electron paramagnetic resonance studies at temperature below 77 °K on iron-sulfur proteins of yeast and bovine heart submitochondrial particles. J. biol. Chem. **246**, 5960.

— D. F. WILSON, T. ASAKURA, and B. CHANCE, 1972 a: Studies on ironsulfur proteins in the site I region of the respiratory chain in pigeon heart mitochondria and submitochondrial particles. Biochem. biophys. Res. Commun. **46**, 1631.

— — and B. CHANCE, 1972 b: Energy dependence of the half-reduction potentials of iron-sulfur center 1 in the site 1 region of the respiratory chain in pigeon heart mitochondria. Biochem. biophys. Res. Commun. **49**, 1087.

— T. ASAKURA, D. F. WILSON, and B. CHANCE, 1972 b: Oxidation-reduction potentials of iron-sulfur centers in the site 1 region of respiratory chain of *C. utilis* mitochondrial particles. FEBS Lett. **21**, 59.

— D. B. WINTER, J. LIM, and T. E. KING, 1973: Low temperature electron paramagnetic resonance studies on two iron-sulfur centers in cardiac succinic dehydrogenase. Biochem. biophys. Res. Commun. **53**, 231.

— J. S. LEIGH, D. B. WINTER, J. LIM, and T. E. KING, 1974 a: EPR studies on two ferredoxin-type iron sulfur centers in reconstituted active, inactive and reactivated soluble succinate dehydrogenase. Biochem. biophys. Res. Commun. **61**, 1026.

— D. B. WINTER, J. LIM, and T. E. KING, 1974 b: EPR studies on a Hipip type iron-sulfur center in the succinate dehydrogenase segment of the respiratory chain. Biochem. biophys. Res. Commun. **61**, 1017.

OJALA, D., and G. ATTARDI, 1972: Expression of the mitochondrial genome in HeLa cells. X. Properties of mitochondrial polysomes. J. molec. Biol. **65**, 273.

— and G. ATTARDI, 1974: Identification and partial characterization of multiple discrete polyadenylic acid-containing RNA components coded for by HeLa cell mitochondrial DNA. J. Mol. Biol. **88**, 205.

ONO, B., G. FINK, and G. SCHATZ, 1975: Mitochondrial assembly in respiration-deficient mutants of *Saccharomyces cerevisiae*. IV. Effects of nuclear amber suppressors on the accumulation of a mitochondrially made subunit of cytochrome c oxidase. J. Biol. Chem. **250**, 775.

ORME-JOHNSON, N. R., W. H. ORME-JOHNSON, R. E. HANSEN, H. BEINERT, and Y. HATEFI, 1971: EPR detectable electron acceptors in submitochondrial particles from beef heart with special reference to iron-sulfur components of DPN H-ubiquinone reductase. Biochem. biophys. Res. Commun. **44**, 446.

— — — — 1973: EPR detectable electron acceptors in submitochondrial particles from beef heart. In: Oxidases and related redox systems. (KING, T. E., H. S. MASON, and M. MORRISON, eds.). Baltimore-London-Tokyo: Univ. Park Press.

OSAFUNE, T., 1973: Three-dimensional structures of giant mitochondria, dictyosomes and "concentric lamellar bodies" formed during the cell cycle of *Euglena gracilis* (Z) in synchronous culture. J. Elect. Micr. **22**, 51.

OSHINO, N., T. SUGANO, R. OSHINO, and B. CHANCE, 1974: Mitochondrial function under hypoxic conditions: the steady states of cytochromes a + a₃ and their relationship to mitochondrial energy states. Biochim. biophys. Acta **368**, 298.

PACKER, L., 1960: Metabolic and structural states of mitochondria. I. Regulation by adenosine diphosphate. J. biol. Chem. **235**, 242.

— 1961: Metabolic and structural states of mitochondria. II. Regulation by phosphate. J. biol. Chem. **236**, 214.

— 1972: Functional organization of intramembrane particles of mitochondrial inner membranes. J. Bioenerg. **3**, 115.

— 1973: Membrane particles of mitochondria. In: Mechanisms in bioenergetics. (AZZONE, G. F., L. ERNSTER, S. PAPA, E. QUAGLIARIELLO, N. SILIPRANDI, eds.), p. 33. New York-London: Academic Press.

— K. UTSUMI, and M. G. MUSTAFA, 1966: Oscillatory states of mitochondria. I. Electron and energy transfer pathways. Arch. Biochem. Biophys. **117**, 381.

PACKER, L., J. M. WRIGGLESWORTH, P. A. G. FORTES, and B. C. PRESSMAN, 1968: Expansion of inner membrane compartment and its relation to mitochondrial volume and ion transport. J. Cell Biol. **39**, 382.

— J. A. WILLIAMS, and R. S. CRIDDLE, 1973: Freeze-fracture studies on mitochondria from wild-type and respiratory-deficient yeast. Biochim. biophys. Acta **292**, 92.

PADAN, E., and H. ROTTENBERG, 1973: Respiratory control and the proton electrochemical gradient in mitochondria. Eur. J. Biochem. **40**, 431.

PALADE, G. E., 1953: The fine structure of mitochondria. An electron microscope study. J. Hist. Cytochem. **1**, 188.

PALMIERI, F., and M. KLINGENBERG, 1967: Inhibiton of respiration under control of azide uptake by mitochondria. Eur. J. Biochem. **1**, 439.

— E. QUAGLIARIELLO, and M. KLINGENBERG, 1970: Quantitative correlation between the distribution of anions and the pH difference across the mitochondrial membrane. Eur. J. Biochem. **17**, 230.

— I. STIPANI, E. QUAGLIARIELLO, and M. KLINGENBERG, 1972: Kinetic study of the tricarboxylate carrier in rat liver mitochondria. Eur. J. Biochem. **26**, 587.

— S. PASSARELLA, I. STIPANI, and E. QUAGLIARIELLO, 1974 a: Mechanism of inhibition of the dicarboxylate carrier of mitochondria by thiol reagents. Biochim. biophys. Acta **333**, 195.

— G. GENCHI, I. STIPANI, F. FRANCIA, and E. QUAGLIARIELLO, 1974 b: The isolation of metabolite-binding proteins from submitochondrial particles. In: Membrane Proteins in Transport and Phosphorylation. (AZZONE, G. F., M. E. KLINGENBERG, E. QUAGLIARIELLO, and N. SILIPRANDI, eds.), p. 245. Amsterdam-London: North-Holland Publishing Co. New York: American Elsevier Publishing Co.

PANDE, S. V., and M. C. BLANCHAER, 1971: Reversible inhibition of mitochondrial adenosine diphosphate phosphorylation by long chain acyl coenzyme A esters. J. Biol. Chem. **246**, 402.

PANET, R., and Z. SELINGER, 1972: Synthesis of ATP coupled to Ca^{2+} release from sarcoplasmic reticulum vesicles. Biochim. biophys. Acta, **255**, 34.

PANINI, S. R., and C. K. RAMKRISHNA KURUP, 1974 a: Mode of inhibition of mitochondrial energy transduction by chlorophenoxyisobutyrate. Biochem. J. **142**, 253.

— — 1974 b: Cooperative interactions in mitochondrial membrane function. In: Biomembranes. Architecture, Biogenesis, Bioenergetics, and Differentiation. (PACKER, L., ed.), p. 279. New York-London: Academic Press.

PAOLETTI, C., G. RIOUS, and J. PAIRAOULT, 1972: Circular oligomers in mitochondrial DNA of human and beef non-malignant thyroid glands. Proc. nat. Acad. Sci. (U.S.) **69**, 847.

PAPA, S., and G. PARADIES, 1974: On the mechanism of translocation of pyruvate and other monocarboxylic acids in rat liver mitochondria. Eur. J. Biochem. **49**, 265.

— R. D'ALOYA, A. J. MEIJER, J. M. TAGER, and E. QUAGLIARIELLO, 1969 a: d-oxoglutarate transport in rat-liver mitochondria. In: The energy level and metabolic control in mitochondria. (PAPA, S., J. M. TAGER, E. QUAGLIARIELLO, and E. C. SLATER, eds.), p. 159. Bari: Adriatica Editrice.

— N. E. LOFRUMENTO, M. LOGLISCI, and E. QUAGLIARIELLO, 1969 b: On the transport of inorganic phosphate and malate in rat-liver mitochondria. Biochim. biophys. Acta **189**, 311.

— F. GUERRIERI, M. LORUSSO, and E. QUAGLIARIELLO, 1970: On the proton translocation system of the inner mitochondrial membrane. FEBS Lett. **10**, 295.

— A. FRANCAVILLA, G. PARADIES, and B. MEDURI, 1971: Transport of pyruvate in rat liver mitochondrial. FEBS Lett. **12**, 285.

— F. GUERRIERI, M. LORUSSO, and S. SIMONE, 1973 a: Proton translocation and energy transduction in mitochondria. Biochimie **55**, 703.

— — S. SIMONE, M. LORUSSO, and D. LAROSA, 1973 b: Mechanism of respiration-driven proton translocation in the inner mitochondrial membrane. Biochim. biophys. Acta **292**, 20.

PAPPAS, G. D., and P. W. BRANDT, 1959: Mitochondria. I. Fine structure of the complex patterns in the mitochondria of *Pelomyxa carolinensis* Wilson (Chaos chaos L.). J. Cell Biol. **6**, 85.

PARISI, B., and R. CELLA, 1971: Origin of the ribosome specific factors responsible for peptide chain elongation in yeast. FEBS Lett. **14**, 209.

PARK, R. B., and A. PFEIFHOFER, 1974: Chemical composition of fractured membrane halves. In: Membrane Proteins in Transport and Phosphorylation. (AZZONE, G. F., M. E. KLINGENBERG, E. QUAGLIARIELLO, and N. SILIPRANDI, eds.), p. 97. Amsterdam: North-Holland Publishing Co. New York: American Elsevier Publishing Co.

PARSONS, D. F., 1963: Mitochondrial structure: two types of subunits on negatively stained mitochondrial membranes. Science **140**, 985.

— and Y. YANO, 1967: The cholesterol content of the outer and inner membranes of guinea-pig liver mitochondria. Biochim. biophys. Acta **135**, 362.

— G. R. WILLIAMS, W. THOMPSON, D. WILSON, and B. CHANCE, 1967: Improvements in the procedure for purification of mitochondrial outer and inner membrane. Comparison of the outer membrane with smooth endoplasmic reticulum. In: Mitochondrial Structure and Compartmentation. (QUAGLIARIELLO, E., S. PAPA, E. C. SLATER, and J. M. TAGER, eds.), p. 29. Bari: Adriatica Editrice.

PARSONS, J. A., and R. C. RUSTAD, 1968: The distribution of DNA among dividing mitochondria of *Tetrahymena pyriformis*. J. Cell Biol. **37**, 683.

PASCAUD, M., 1964: Les phospholipides de la cellule hépatique. Interprétation functionnelle de leur renouvellement. II. Renouvellement des acides gras des phosphoglycerides. Biochim. biophys. Acta **84**, 528.

PASQUALI-RONCHETTI, I., J. W. GREENAWALT, and E. CARAFOLI, 1969: On the nature of the dense matrix granules of normal mitochondria. J. Cell Biol. **40**, 565.

PEACHEY, L. D., 1964: Electron microscopic observations on the accumulation of divalent cations in intramitochondrial granules. J. Cell Biol. **20**, 95.

PEDERSEN, P. L., H. LE VINE, III, and N. CINTRON, 1974: Activation and inhibition of mitochondrial ATPase of rat liver mitochondria. In: Membrane Proteins in Transport and Phosphorylation. (AZZONE, G. F., M. E. KLINGENBERG, E. QUAGLIARIELLO, and N. SILIPRANDI, eds.), p. 43. Amsterdam-London: North-Holland Publishing Co. New York: American Elsevier Publishing Co.

PENEFSKY, H. S., 1974: Mitochondrial and chloroplast ATPases. In: The Enzymes. (BOYER, P. D., ed.), 3rd edition, p. 375. New York-London: Academic Press.

— and R. C. WARNER, 1965: Partial resolution of the enzymes catalyzing oxidative phosphorylation. VI. Studies on the mechanism of cold inactivation of mitochondrial adenosine triphosphatase. J. biol. Chem. **240**, 4694.

— M. E. PULLMAN, A. DATTA, and E. RACKER, 1960: Partial resolution of the enzymes catalyzing oxidative phosphorylation. II. Participation of a soluble adenosine triphosphatase in oxidative phosphorylation. J. biol. Chem. **235**, 330.

PENMAN, S., H. FAN, S. PERLMAN, M. ROSBASH, R. WEINBERG, and E. ZYLBER, 1970: Distinct RNA synthesis systems of the HeLa cell. Cold Spring Harbor Symp. Quant. Biol. **35**, 561.

PENNIAL, R., 1960: The 2,4 dinitrophenol-responsive adenosine-triphosphatase of rat-liver mitochondria. Biochim. biophys. Acta **44**, 395.

PENNINGTON, J. T., R. A. HARRIS, J. ASAI, and D. E. GREEN, 1968: The conformational basis of energy transformations in membrane systems. I. Conformational changs in mitochondria. Proc. nat. Acad. Sci. (U.S.) **59**, 624.

PERKINS, M., J. M. HASLAM, and A. W. LINNANE, 1972: The effects of physiological and genetic manipulation on anion transport systems of yeast mitochondria. FEBS Lett. **25**, 271.

— — 1973: Biogenesis of mitochondria 31. The effects of physiological and genetic manipulation of *Saccharomyces cerevisiae* on the mitochondrial transport systems for tricarboxylate-cycle anions. Biochem. J. **134**, 923.

PERLMAN, P. S., and H. R. MAHLER, 1970: Formation of yeast mitochondria. III. Biochemical properties of mitochondria isolated form a cytoplasmic petite mutant. J. Bioen. **1**, 113.

— — 1974: Derepression of mitochondria and their enzymes in yeast: regulatory aspects. Arch. Biochem. Biophys. **162**, 248.

PERLMAN, S., and S. PENMAN, 1970: Mitochondrial protein synthesis: resistance to emetine and response to RNA synthesis inhibitors. Biochem. biophys. Res. Commun. **40**, 941.

— H. T. ABELSON, and S. PENMAN, 1973: Mitochondrial protein synthesis: RNA with the properties of eukaryotic messenger RNA. Proc. nat. Acad. Sci. (U.S.) **70**, 350.

PFAFF, E., and M. KLINGENBERG, 1968: Adenine nucleotide translocation of mitochondria. I. Specificity and control. Eur. J. Biochem. **6**, 66.

— H. W. HELDT, and M. KLINGENBERG, 1969: Adenine nucleotide translocation of mitochondria. Kinetics of the adenine nucleotide exchange. Eur. J. Biochem. **10**, 484.

PIHL, E., and G. F. BAHR, 1970: Matrix structure of critical point dried mitochondria. Exp. Cell Res. **63**, 391.

PINTO DA SILVA, P., and D. BRANTON, 1970: Membrane splitting in freeze-etching. J. Cell Biol. **45**, 598.

PIPERNO, G., G. FONTY, and G. BERNARDI, 1972: The mitochondrial genome in wild-type yeast cells. II. Investigation on the compositional heterogeneity of mitochondrial DNA. J. molec. Biol. **65**, 191.

PITTMAN, D., 1959: Ultraviolet induction of respiration-deficient variants of *Saccharomyces* and their stability during vegetative growth. Cytologia **24**, 315.

— J. M. WEBB, A. ROSHANMANESH, and L. E. COKER, 1960: Evidence for the genetic control of photoreactivation. Genetics. **45**, 1023.

PLATTNER, H., and G. SCHATZ, 1969: Promitochondria of anaerobically grown yeast. III. Morphology. Biochem. **8**, 339.

POLZ, G., and KREIL, 1970: Presence of N-formyl and N-acetyl-methionine in the proteins of honey bee thorax. Biochem. biophys. Res. Commun. **39**, 516.

PORTER, K., 1964: (see PEACHEY, L. D.) Electron microscope observations on the accumulation of divalent cations in intramitochondrial granules. J. Cell Biol. **20**, 95.

— 1966: Mitochondrial ion transport: Mechanism and physiological significance. (See RASMUSSEN, H.) Fed. Proc. **25**, 903.

POYTON, R. O., and G. S. GROOT, 1975: Biosynthesis of polypeptides of cytochrome c oxidase by isolated mitochondria. Proc. nat. Acad. Sci. (U.S.) **72**, 172.

— and G. SCHATZ, 1975 a: Cytochrome-c oxidase from bakers yeast. III. Physical characterization of isolated subunits and chemical evidence for two different classes of polypeptides. J. Biol. Chem. **250**, 752.

— — 1975 b: Cytochrome-c oxidase from bakers yeast. IV. Immunological evidence for participation of a mitochondrially synthesized subunit in enzymatic activity. J. Biol. Chem. **250**, 762.

PRESSMAN, B. C., 1968: An apparatus for observing multiparameter changes in cation transport system. Ann. N.Y. Acad. Sci. **148**, 285.

— 1970: Energy-linked transport in mitochondria. In: Membranes of mitochondria and chloroplasts. (RACKER, E., ed.), p. 213. New York: Van Nostrand Reinhold Co.

PRESTIPINO, G., D. CECCARELLI, F. CONTI, and E. CARAFOLI, 1974: Interactions of a mitochondrial Ca^{2+}-binding glycoprotein with lipid bilayer membranes. FEBS Lett. **45**, 99.

PRINGLE, J. R., 1970: The molecular weight of the undegraded polypeptide chain of yeast hexokinase. Biochem. biophys. Res. Commun. **39**, 46.

PROUDLOCK, J. W., J. M. HASLAM, and A. W. LINNANE, 1969: Specific effect of unsaturated fatty acid depletion on mitochondrial oxidative phosphorylation in *Saccharomyces cerevisiae*. Biochem. biophys. Res. Commun. **37**, 847.

— — — 1971: Biogenesis of mitochondria 19. The effect of unsaturated fatty acid depletion and the lipid composition and energy metabolism, of a fatty acid desaturase mutant of *Saccharomyces cerevisiae*. J. Bioenerg. **2**, 327.

PULLMAN, M. E., and G. C. MONROY, 1963: A naturally occurring inhibitor of mitochondrial adenosine triphosphatase. J. biol. Chem. **238**, 3762.

— H. S. PENEFSKY, A. DATTA, and E. RACKER, 1960: Partial resolution of enzymes catalyzing oxidative phosphorylation. I. Purification and properties of soluble, dinitrophenol-stimulated adenosine triphosphatase. J. biol. Chem. **235**, 3322.

PURVIS, J. L., and J. M. LOWENSTEIN, 1961: The relation between intra- and extra-cellular pyridine nucleotides. J. Biol. Chem. **236**, 2794.

QUAGLIARIELLO, E., and F. PALMIERI, 1968: Control of succinate oxidation by succinate-uptake by rat liver mitochondria. Eur. J. Biochem. **4**, 20.

— — G. PREZIOSO, and M. KLINGENBERG, 1969: Kinetics of succinate uptake by rat-liver mitochondria. FEBS Lett. **4**, 251.

QUAGLIARIELLO, E., G. GENCHI, and F. PALMIERI, 1971: Respiration-dependent anion uptake by rat liver mitochondria. FEBS Lett. **13**, 253.

RABINOWITZ, M., and H. SWIFT, 1970: Mitochondrial nucleic acids and their relation to the biogenesis of mitochondria. Physiol. Rev. **50**, 376.
— J. CASEY, P. GORDON, J. LOCKER, H.-J. HSU, and G. S. GETZ, 1974: Characterization of yeast *grande* and *petite* mitochondrial DNA by hybridization and physical techniques. In: The biogenesis of mitochondria. (KROON, A. M., and C. SACCONE, eds.), p. 89. New York-London: Academic Press.

RACKER, E., 1964: The reconstituted system of oxidative phosphorylation. Biochem. biophys. Res. Commun. **14**, 75.
— 1972: Reconstitution of a calcium pump with phospholipids and a purified Ca^{++}-adenosine triphosphatase from sarcoplasmic reticulum. J. biol. Chem. **247**, 8198.
— and E. EYTAN, 1973: Reconstitution of an efficient calcium pump without detergents. Biochem. biophys. Res. Commun. **55**, 174.
— and L. L. HORSTMAN, 1967: Partial resolution of the enzymes catalyzing oxidative phosphorylation. XIII. Structure and function of submitochondrial particles completely resolved with respect to coupling factor 1. J. biol. Chem. **242**, 2547.
— and A. KANDRACH, 1971: Reconstitution of the third site of oxidative phosphorylation. J. biol. Chem. **246**, 7069.
— and W. STOECKENIUS, 1974: Reconstitution of purple membrane vesicles catalyzing light-driven proton uptake and adenosine triphosphate formation. J. biol. Chem. **249**, 662.
— D. D. TYLER, R. W. ESTABROOK, T. E. CONOVER, D. F. PARSON, and B. CHANCE, 1965: Correlations between electron transport activity, ATPase and morphology of submitochondrial particles. In: Oxidases and related systems. (KING, T. E., H. S. MASON, and M. MORRISON, eds.), p. 1077. New York: Wiley.
— C. BRUNENSTEIN, A. LOYTER, and R. O. CHRISTIANSEN, 1970: The sidedness of the inner mitochondrial membrane. In: Electron transport and energy conservation. (TAGER, T. H., S. PAPA, E. QUAGLIARIELLO, and E. C. SLATER, eds.), p. 235. Bari: Adriatica Editrice.
— A. LOYTER, and R. O. CHRISTIANSEN, 1971: In: Probes of Structure and Function of Macromolecules and Membranes. (CHANCE, B., C. P. LEE, and J. K. BLAISE, eds.), Vol. 1, p. 407. New York: Academic Press.

RADSAK, K., K. KATO, N. SATO, and H. KOPROWSKI, 1971: Effect of ethidium bromide on mitochondrial DNA and cytochrome synthesis in HeLa cells. Exp. Cell Res. **66**, 410.

RAISON, J. K., 1973: The influence of temperature-induced phase changes in the kinetics of respiratory and other membrane-associated enzyme systems. J. Bioenerg. **4**, 285.

RAPATZ, G. L., L. J. MENZ, and B. J. LUYET, 1966: Anatomy of the freezing process in biological materials. In: Cryobiology. (MERYMAN, H. T., ed.), p. 138. New York-London: Academic Press.

RASMUSSEN, H., J. FISCHER, and C. ARNAND, 1965: Parathyroid hormone. Ion exchange and mitochondrial swelling. Proc. nat. Acad. Sci. (U.S.) **52**, 1198.

RAUT, C., 1953: A cytochrome deficient mutant of *Saccharomyces cerevisiae*. Exp. Cell Res. **4**, 295.

REDMAN, C. M., 1967: Studies on the transfer of incomplete polypeptide chains across rat liver microsomal membranes *in vitro*. J. biol. Chem. **242**, 761.

REICH, S. E., and D. J. L. LUCK, 1966: Replication and inheritance of mitochondrial DNA. Proc. nat. Acad. Sci. (U.S.) **55**, 1600.

REIJNDERS, L., and P. BORST, 1972: The number of 4 S RNA genes on yeast mitochondrial DNA. Biochem. biophys. Res. Commun. **47**, 126.
— C. M. KLEISEN, L. A. GRIVELL, and P. BORST, 1972: Hybridization studies with yeast mitochondrial RNAs. Biochim. biophys. Acta **272**, 396.

REILLY, C., and F. SHERMAN, 1965: Glucose repression of cytochrome *a* synthesis in cytochrome-deficient mutants of yeast. Biochim. biophys. Acta **95**, 640.

RENDI, R., 1959: The effect of chloramphenicol on the incorporation of labelled amino acids into proteins by isolated subcellular fractions from rat liver. Exp. Cell Res. **18**, 187.

RENTHAL, R., and J. K. LANYI, 1975: Light-dependent changes in electrical potential of cell envelope vesicles from *Halobacterium halobium* measured with a cyanine dye. Biophys. J. **15**, 68 a (Abstract).

RESNICK, M. A., and R. K. MORTIMER, 1966: Unsaturated fatty acid mutant of *Saccharomyces cerevisiae*. J. Bact. **92**, 597.

REVEL, J. P., D. W. FAWCETT, and C. W. PHILPOTT, 1963: Observations on mitochondrial structure. Angular configuration of the cristae. J. Cell Biol. **16**, 187.

REYNAFARJE, B., and A. L. LEHNINGER, 1969: High affinity and low affinity binding of Ca^{++} by rat liver mitochondria. J. biol. Chem. **244**, 584.

RICHTER, D., and F. LIPMANN, 1970: Separation of mitochondrial and cytoplasmic peptide chain elongation factors from yeast. Biochem. **9**, 5065.

RICHTER, E., 1971: Production of mitochondrial peptide-chain elongation factors in yeast deficient in deoxyribonucleic acid. Biochem. **10**, 4422.

RIESKE, J. S., 1971: Changes in oxidation-reduction potential of cytochrome *b* observed in the presence of antimycin A. Arch. Biochem. Biophys. **145**, 179.

— R. E. HANSEN, and W. S. ZAUGG, 1964 a: Studies on the electron transfer system. LVIII. Properties of a new oxidation-reduction component of the respiratory chain as studied by electron paramagnetic resonance spectroscopy. J. biol. Chem. **239**, 3017.

— W. S. ZAUGG, and R. E. HANSEN, 1964 b: Studies on the electron transfer system. LIX. Distribution of iron and of the component giving an electron paramagnetic resonance signal as g = 1.90 in subfractions of complex III. J. biol. Chem. **239**, 3023.

RIFKIN, M. R., D. D. WOOD, and D. J. L. LUCK, 1967: Ribosomal RNA and ribosomes from mitochondria of *Neurospora crassa*. Proc. nat. Acad. Sci. (U.S.) **58**, 1024.

ROBBERSON, D. L., Y. ALONI, and G. ATTARDI, 1971: Expression of the mitochondrial genome in HeLa cells. VI. Size determination of mitochondrial ribosomal RNA by electron microscopy. J. molec. Biol. **60**, 473.

— H. KASAMATSU, and J. VINOGRAD, 1972: Replication of mitochondrial DNA. Circular replicative intermediates in mouse L cells. Proc. nat. Acad. Sci. (U.S.) **69**, 737.

ROBERTON, A. M., C. T. HOLLOWAY, I. G. KNIGHT, and R. B. BEECHEY, 1968: A comparison of the effects of NN′-dicyclohexylcarbodi-imide, oligomycin A and aurovertin on energy-linked reactions in mitochondria and submitochondrial particles. Biochem. J. **108**, 445.

ROBINSON, B. H., 1971: Transport of phosphoenolpyruvate by tricarboxylate transport systems in mammalian mitochondria. FEBS Lett. **14**, 309.

— and J. B. CHAPPELL, 1967: The inhibition of malate tricarboxylate and oxoglutarate entry in to mitochondria by 2-n-butyl-malonate. Biochem. biophys. Res. Commun. **28**, 249.

ROODYN, D. B., 1962: Protein synthesis in mitochondria. 3. The controlled disruption and subfractionation of mitochondria labelled *in vitro* with radioactive valine. Biochem. J. **85**, 177.

— P. J. REIS, and T. S. WORK, 1961: Protein synthesis in mitochondria. Requirements for the incorporation of radioactive amino acids into mitochondrial protein. Biochem. J. **80**, 9.

ROSING, J., and E. C. SLATER, 1972: The value of ΔG° for the hydrolysis of ATP. Biochim. biophys. Acta **267**, 275.

ROSS, E., E. EBNER R. O. POYTON, T. L. MASON, B. ONO, and G. SCHATZ, 1974: The biosynthesis of mitochondrial cytochromes. In: The biogenesis of mitochondria. (KROON, A. M., and C. SACCONE, eds.), p. 477. New York-London: Academic Press.

ROSSI, C., A. AZZI, and G. F. AZZONE, 1967 a: Ion transport in liver mitochondria. I. Metabolism-independent Ca^{++} binding and H^+ release. J. biol. Chem. **242**, 951.

— G. F. AZZONE, and A. AZZI, 1967 b: Ionic transport in rat liver mitochondria. 3. Stoicheometry of proton release during aerobic calcium ion translocation. Eur. J. Biochem. **1**, 141.

ROSSI, C. S., and A. L. LEHNINGER, 1964: Stoichiometry of respiratory stimulation, accumulation of Ca^{++} and phosphate and oxidative phosphorylation in rat liver mitochondria. J. biol. Chem. **239**, 3971.

ROSSI, E., and G. F. AZZONE, 1969: Ion transport in liver mitochondria, energy barrier and stoicheometry of aerobic K+ translocation. Eur. J. Biochem. **7**, 418.

ROSSI, E., and G. F. AZZONE, 1970: The mechanism of ion translocation in mitochondria. 3. Coupling of K+ efflux and ATP synthesis. Eur. J. Biochem. **12**, 319.

ROTTENBERG, H., 1970: ATP synthesis and electrical membrane potential in mitochondria. Eur. J. Biochem. **15**, 22.

— 1973: The mechanism of energy-dependent ion transport in mitochondria. J. Memb. Biol. **11**, 117.

— and A. SCARPA, 1974: Calcium uptake and membrane potential in mitochondria. Biochem. **13**, 4811.

— and A. K. SOLOMON, 1969: The osmotic nature of the ion induced swelling of rat liver mitochondria. Biochim. biophys. Acta **193**, 48.

ROUILLER, CH., and A. M. JÉZÉQUEL, 1963: Electron microscopy of the liver. In: The liver, VI. (ROUILLER, CH., ed.), p. 195. New York-London: Academic Press.

ROUSER, G., G. J. NELSON, S. FLEISCHER, and G. SIMON, 1968: Lipid composition of animal cell membranes, organelles and organs. In: Biological Membranes, Physical Fact and Function. (CHAPMAN, D., ed.), p. 5. New York-London: Academic Press.

ROWE, M. J., R. A. LANSMAN, and D. O. WOODWARD, 1974: A comparison of mito-chondrially synthesized protein from whole mitochondria and cytochrome oxidase in *Neurospora*. Eur. J. Biochem. **41**, 25.

RUBIN, M. S., and A. TZAGOLOFF, 1973 a: Assembly of the mitochondrial membrane system. IX. Purification, characterization, and subunit structure of yeast and beef cytochrome oxidase. J. biol. Chem. **248**, 4269.

— — 1973 b: Assembly of the mitochondrial membrane system. X. Mitochondrial synthesis of three of the subunit proteins of yeast cytochrome oxidase. J. biol. Chem. **248**, 4275.

RUPEC, M., 1969: Mitochondriale Innenmembranpartikeln im Schnittpräparat. Cytobiol. **1**, 184.

RUSKA, C., and H. RUSKA, 1969: Compartments and membrane structure in freeze-etched heart muscle mitochondria. Z. Zellforsch. **97**, 298.

SABADIE-PIALOUX, N., and D. GAUTHERON, 1971: Free-SH variations during ATP synthesis by oxidative phosphorylation in heart muscle mitochondria. Biochim. biophys. Acta **234**, 9.

SACCONE, C., M. N. GADALETA, and E. QUAGLIARIELLO, 1967: Effect of atractyloside on nucleoside triphosphate incorporation into RNA of rat-liver mitochondria. Biochim. biophys. Acta **138**, 474.

— — and R. GALLERANI, 1969: RNA synthesis in isolated mitochondria. Eur. J. Biochem. **10**, 61.

— C. DE GIORGI, P. CANTATORE, and R. GALLERANI, 1974: Ribonucleotide polymerizing activities in rat liver mitochondria. In: Biomembranes, Architecture, Biogenesis, Bio-energetics, and Differentiation, p. 87. (PACKER, L., ed.), New York-London: Academic Press.

SAGER, R., 1972: Cytoplasmic genes and organelles. New York-London: Academic Press.

SAITO, A., and S. FLEISCHER, 1971: Intramitochondrial tubules in adrenal glands of rat. J. Ultrastruct. Res. **35**, 642.

— M. SMIGEL, and S. FLEISCHER, 1974: Membrane junctions in the intermembrane space of mitochondria from mammalian tissues. J. Cell Biol. **60**, 653.

SAKAI, A., 1971: Some factors contributing to survival of rapidly cooled plant cells. Cryobiol. **8**, 225.

SALA, F., and H. KÜNTZEL, 1970: Peptide chain intiation in homologous and heterologous systems from mitochondria and bacteria. Eur. J. Biochem. **15**, 280.

SANDERS, J. P. M., R. A. FLAVELL, P. BORST, and J. N. M. MOL, 1973: Nature of the base sequence conserved in the mitochondrial DNA of a low-density *petite*. Biochim. biophys. Acta **312**, 441.

SANDS, R. H., and H. BEINERT, 1959: On the function of copper in cytochrome oxidase. Biochem. biophys. Res. Commun. **1**, 175.

SANI, B. P., K. M. LAM, and D. R. SANADI, 1970: A complex of mitochondrial factor A and a new factor involved in oxidative phosphorylation. Biochem. biophys. Res. Commun. **39**, 444.

SATO, N., D. F. WILSON, and B. CHANCE, 1971 a: Two b cytochromes in pigeon heart mitochondria. FEBS Lett. **15**, 209.

SATO, N., D. F. WILSON, and B. CHANCE, 1971 b: The spectral properties of the b cytochrome in intact mitochondria. Biochim. biophys. Acta **253**, 88.

— and K. KUROSOMI, 1965: Gunma Symp. Endocrinol. (Maebashi) **2**, 61.

SCARPA, A., and G. F. AZZONE, 1970: The mechanism of ion translocation in mitochondria. 4. Coupling of K^+ efflux and Ca^{2+} uptake. Eur. J. Biochem. **12**, 328.

— and P. GRAZIOTTI, 1973: Mechanisms for the intracellular calcium regulation in heart. I. Stopped flow measurements of Ca^{++} uptake by cardiac mitochondria. J. gen. Physiol. **62**, 756.

SCHÄFER, K. P., and H. KÜNTZEL, 1972: Mitochondrial genes in *Neurospora:* a single cistron for ribosomal RNA. Biochem. biophys. Res. Commun. **46**, 1312.

— G. BUGGE, M. GRANDI, and H. KÜNTZEL, 1971: Transcription of mitochondrial DNA *in vitro* from *Neurospora crassa.* Eur. J. Biochem. **21**, 478.

SCHATZ, G., 1968: Impaired binding of mitochondrial adenosine triphosphate in the cytoplasmic petite mutant of *Saccharomyces cerevisiae.* J. biol. Chem. **243**, 2192.

— 1970: Biogenesis of mitochondria. In: Membranes of mitochondria and chloroplasts. (RACKER, E., ed.), p. 251. New York: Van Nostrand Reinhold Co.

— and T. L. MASON, 1974: The biosynthesis of mitochondrial proteins. Ann. Rev. Biochem. **43**, 51.

— and J. SALTZGABER, 1969: Protein synthesis by yeast promitochondria *in vivo.* Biochem. biophys. Res. Commun. **37**, 996.

— H. S. PENEFSKY, and E. RACKER, 1967: Partial resolution of the enzymes catalyzing oxidative phosphorylation. XIV. Interaction of purified mitochondrial adenosine triphosphatase from baker's yeast with submitochondrial particles from beef liver. J. biol. Chem. **242**, 2552.

— G. S. P. GROOT, T. MASON, W. ROUSLIN, D. C. WHARTON, and J. SALTZGABER, 1972: Biogenesis of mitochondrial inner membranes in baker's yeast. Fed. Proc. **31**, 21.

SCHMITT, H., 1970: Characterization of a 72 S mitochondrial ribosome from *Saccharomyces cerevisiae.* Eur. J. Biochem. **17**, 278.

SCHNEDL, W., 1974: Veränderung des Mitochondrienbestandes während des Zellzyklus. Cytobiologie **8**, 403.

SCHNEIDER, D. L., and E. RACKER, 1971: Cytochrome c_1 and cytochrome oxidase localization in the inner mitochondrial membrane. Fed. Proc. **30**, 1190 Abstr.

— Y. KAGAWA, and E. RACKER, 1972: Chemical modification of the inner mitochondrial membrane. J. biol. Chem. **247**, 4074.

SCHOLTE, H. R., 1973: The separation and enzymatic characterization of inner and outer membranes of rat-heart mitochondria. Biochim. biophys. Acta **330**, 283.

SCHUSTER, F. L., 1965: A deoxyribose nucleic acid component in mitochondria of *Didymium nigipes,* a slime mold. Exp. Cell Res. **39**, 329.

SCHWAB, A. J., 1974: Precursor proteins of cytochrome *c* oxidase in cytochrome *c* deficient copper-depleted *Neurospora.* In: The biogenesis of mitochondria. (KROON, A. M., and C. SACCONE, eds.), p. 501. New York-London: Academic Press.

SCHWEYEN, R., and F. KAUDEWITZ, 1970: Protein synthesis by yeast mitochondria *in vivo.* Quantitative estimate of mitochondrially governed synthesis of mitochondrial proteins. Biochem. biophys. Res. Commun. **38**, 728.

SCOTT, K. M., V. A. KNIGHT, C. T. SETTLEMIRE, and G. P. BRIERLEY, 1970: Differential effects of mercurial reagents on membrane thiols and the permeability of the heart mitochondrion. Biochem. **9**, 714.

— K. M. HWANG, M. JURKOWITZ, and G. P. BRIERLEY, 1971: Ion transport by heart mitochondria. XXIII. The effects of lead on mitochondrial reactions. Arch. Biochem. Biophys. **147**, 557.

SCRAGG, A. H., 1971: Chain elongation factors of yeast mitochondria. FEBS Lett. **17**, 111.

— H. MORIMOTO, V. VILLA, J. NEKHOROCHEFF, and H. O. HALVORSON, 1971: Cell-free protein synthesizing system from yeast mitochondria. Science, **171**, 908.

SEBALD, W., H. WEISS, and G. JACKL, 1972: Inhibition of the assembly of cytochrome oxidase in *Neurospora crassa* by chloramphenicol. Eur. J. Biochem. **30**, 413.

SEBALD, W., W. MACHLEIDT, and J. OTTO, 1973: Products of mitochondrial protein synthesis in *Neurospora crassa*. Determination of equimolar amounts of three products in cytochrome oxidase on the basis of amino-acid analysis. Eur. J. Biochem. **38**, 311.

— — — 1974: Cooperation of mitochondrial and cytoplasmic protein synthesis in the formation of cytochrome *c* oxidase. In: The biogenesis of mitochondria. (KROON, A. M., and C. SACCONE, eds.), p. 453. New York-London: Academic Press.

SEIDLER, R. J., and M. MANDEL, 1971: Quantitative aspects of deoxyribonucleic acid renaturation: base composition state of chromosome replication and polynucleotide homologies. J. Bact. **106**, 608.

SELINGER, A., M. KLEIN, and A. AMSTERDAM, 1969: Properties of particles prepared from sarcoplasmic reticulum by deoxycholate. Biochim. biophys. Acta **183**, 19.

SELWYN, M. J., 1967: Preparation and general properties of soluble adenosine triphosphatase from mitochondria. Biochem. J. **105**, 279.

— A. P. DAWSON, M. STOCKDALE, and N. GAINS, 1970: Chloridehydroxide exchange across mitochondrial erythrocyte and artifical lipid membranes mediated by trialkyl and triphenyltin compounds. Eur. J. Biochem. **14**, 120.

SENA, E. E., 1971: Mitochondrial DNA replication in yeast. Ph.D. dissertation, University of Wisconsin, Madison.

SENIOR, A. E., 1973 a: The structure of mitochondrial ATPase. Biochim. biophys. Acta **301**, 249.

— 1973 b: Relationship of cysteine and tyrosine residues to adenosinetriphosphate hydrolysis by mitochondrial adenosine triphosphatase. Biochem. **12**, 3622.

— 1975: Mitochondrial adenosine triphosphatase. Location of sulfhydril groups and disulfide bonds in the soluble enzyme from beef heart. Biochem. **14**, 660.

— and J. C. BROOKE, 1970: Studies on the mitochondrial oligomycin insensitive ATPase. L. An improved method of purification and the behavior of the enzyme in solutions of various depolymerizing agents. Arch. Biochem. Biophys. **140**, 257.

SETTLEMIRE, C. T., G. R. HUNTER, and G. P. BRIERLEY, 1968: Ion transport in heart mitochondria. XIII. The effect of ethylenediaminetetra-acetate on monovalent ion uptake. Biochim. biophys. Acta **162**, 487.

SHAKESPEARE, P. G., and H. R. MAHLER, 1971: Purification and some properties of cytochrome *c* oxidase from the yeast *Saccharomyces cerevisiae*. J. biol. Chem. **246**, 7649.

SHANNON, C., R. ENNS, L. WHEELIS, K. BURCHIEL, and R. S. CRIDDLE, 1973: Alternation of mitochondrial triphosphatase activity resulting from mutation of mitochondrial deoxyribonucleic acid. J. biol. Chem. **248**, 3004.

SHAPIRO, A. L., and J. V. MAIZEL, JR., 1969: Molecular weight estimation of polypeptides by SDS-polyacrylamide gel electrophoresis: further data concerning resolving power and general considerations. Annal. Biochem. **29**, 505.

— E. VIÑUELA, and J. V. MAIZEL, 1967: Molecular weight estimation of polypeptide chains by electrophoresis in SDS-polyacrylamide gels. Biochem. biophys. Res. Commun. **28**, 815.

SHERIDAN, M. N., and W. D. BELT, 1964: Fine structure of guinea pig adrenal cortex. Anat. Rec. **149**, 73.

— and R. J. REITER, 1970: Observations on the pineal system in the hamster. II. Fine structure of the deep pineal. J. Morph. **131**, 163.

SHERMAN, F., 1964: Mutants of yeast deficient in cytochrome *c*. Genetics (Princeton) **49**, 39.

— and P. P. SLONIMSKI, 1964: Respiration-deficient mutants of yeast. II. Biochemistry. Biochim. biophys. Acta **90**, 1.

— H. TABER, and W. CAMPBELL, 1965: Genetic determination of iso-cytochromes *c* in yeast. J. molec. Biol. **13**, 21.

— J. W. STEWART, E. MARGOLIASH, J. PARKER, and W. CAMPBELL, 1966: The structural gene for yeast cytochrome *c*. Proc. nat. Acad. Sci. (U.S.) **55**, 1498.

— — J. H. PARKER, G. J. PUTTERMAN, B. B. L. AGRAWAL, and E. MARGOLIASH, 1970: The relationship of gene structure and protein structure of iso-I-cytochrome *c* from yeast. In: Control of organelle development. (MILLER, P., ed.), p. 85. Cambridge: Cambridge Univ. Press/Academic Press.

SHERMAN, J. K., 1972: Comparison of *in vitro* and *in situ* ultrastructural cryoinjury and cryoprotection of mitochondria. Cryobiology **9**, 112.

SHERMAN, J. K., and K. S. KIM, 1964: Correlation of cellular ultrastructure before freezing, while frozen and after thawing in assessing freeze-thaw-induced injury. Cryobiology **4**, 61.

— and K. C. LIU, 1973: Ultrastructural cryoinjury and cryoprotection of rough endoplasmic reticulum. Cryobiology **10**, 104.

SHERTZER, H. G., and E. RACKER, 1974: Adenine nucleotide transport in submitochondrial particles and reconstituted vesicles derived from bovine heart mitochondria. J. biol. Chem. **249**, 1320.

SHIMADA, K., and E. ASAHINA, 1972: Types of cell freezing and post-thawing survival of individual HeLa cells. Cryobiology **9**, 51.

SHUG, A. L., and E. SHRAGO, 1973: Inhibition of phosphenolpyruvate transport via tricarboxylate and adenine-nucleotide carrier systems of rat-liver mitochondria. Biochem. biophys. Res. Commun. **53**, 659.

SIMPSON, M. V., 1962: Protein biosynthesis. Ann. Rev. Biochem. **31**, 333.

SIMS, P. Y., A. S WAGGONER, C.-H. WANG, and J. F. HOFFMAN, 1974: Studies on the mechanism by which cyanine dyes measure membrane potential in red blood cells and phosphatidyl choline vesicles. Biochem. **13**, 3315.

SINCLAIR, J. H., and D. D. BROWN, 1971: Retention and common nucleotide sequences in the ribosomal deoxyribonucleic acid of eukaryotes and some of their physical characteristics. Biochem. **10**, 2761.

— and B. J. STEVENS, 1966: Circular DNA filaments from mouse mitochondria. Proc. nat. Acad. Sci. U.S.) **56**, 508.

SINGH, V. N., E. RAGHUPATHY, and I. L. CHAIRKOFF, 1964: Incorporation of amino acid carbon into proteins by sheep thyroid gland mitochondria. Biochem. biophys. Res. Commun. **16**, 12.

SISLER, H. D., and M. R. SIEGEL, 1967: In: Antibiotic mechanism of action. (GOTTLIEB, D., and P. D. SHAW, eds.). Berlin-Heidelberg-New York: Springer-Verlag.

SJÖSTRAND, F. S., 1953: Ultra-structure of rod-shaped mitochondria. Nature **171**, 30.

— and L. BARAJAS, 1968: Effect of modifications in conformation of protein molecules on structure of mitochondrial membranes. J. Ultrastruct. Res. **25**, 121.

— — 1970: A new model for mitochondrial membranes based on structural and biochemical information. J. Ultrastruct. Res. **32**, 293.

SKINNER, D. M., and M. S. KERR, 1971: Characterization of mitochondrial and nuclear satellite deoxyribonucleic acids of five species of *Crustacea*. Biochem. **10**, 1864.

SKULACHEV, V. P., A. A. SHARAF, and E. A. LIBERMAN, 1967: Proton conductors in the respiratory chain and artificial membranes. Nature **216**, 718.

— — L. S. YAGUZINSKY, A. A. JASAITIS, E. A. LIBERMAN, and V. P. TOPALI, 1968: The effect of uncouplers on mitochondria, respiratory enzyme complexes and artificial phospholipid membranes. Curr. Mod. Biol. **2**, 98.

SLATER, E. C., 1971: The coupling between energy-yielding and energy-ultilizing reactions in mitochondria. Quart. Rev. Biophys. **4**, 35.

— 1973: Mitochondrial cytochromes *b* and their possible role in energy conservation. In: Mechanism in bioenergetics. (AZZONE, G. F., L. ERNSTER, S. PAPA, E. QUAGLIARIELLO, and N. SILIPRANDI, eds.), p. 405. New York-London: Academic Press.

— 1974: Electron transfer and energy conservation. In: Dynamics of Energy Transducing Membranes. (ERNSTER, L., R. W. ESTABROOK, and E. C. SLATER, eds.), p. 1. Amsterdam: Elsevier Scientific Publishing Co.

— and H. F. TER WELLE, 1969: Applications of oligomycin and related inhibitors in bioenergetics. In: Inhibitors, Tools in Cell Research. (BÜCHER, TH., and H. SIES, eds.), p. 258. Berlin-Heidelberg-New York: Springer-Verlag.

— B. F. VAN GELDER, and K. MINNAERT, 1965: Cytochrome *c* oxidase. In: Oxidase and related redox systems. (KING, T. E., H. S. MASON, and M. MORRISON, eds.), Vol. 2, p. 617. New York: John Wiley.

— C. P. LEE, J. A. BERDEN, and H. J. WEGDAM, 1970 a: High energy forms of cytochrome *b*. Nature **226**, 1248.

— — — — 1970 b: High energy forms of cytochrome *b*. I. Effect of ATP and antimycin on cytochrome *b* in phosphorylation of submitochondrial particles. Biochim. biophys. Acta **223**, 356.

SLATER, E. C., J. A. ROSING, D. A. HARRIS, R. J. VAN DE STADT, and A. KEMP, JR., 1974: The identification of functional ATPase in energy transducing membranes. In: Membrane proteins in transport and phosphorylation. (AZZONE, G. F., M. E. KLINGENBERG, E. QUAGLIARIELLO, and N. SILIPRANDI, eds.), p. 137. Amsterdam: North-Holland Publishing Co.

SLAYMAN, C. L., W. S. LONG, and C. Y.-H. LU, 1973: The relationship between ATP and an electrogenic pump in the plasma membrane of Neurospora crassa. J. Membr. Biol. 14, 305.

SLAYMAN, C. W., D. C. REES, P. P. ORCHARD, and C. L. SLAYMAN, 1975: Generation of adenosine triphosphate in cytochrome-deficient mutants of Neurospora. J. Biol. Chem. 250, 396.

SLUSE, F. E., M. RANSOM, and C. LIÉBECQ, 1972: Mechanism of exchanges catalyzed by the oxoglutarate translocator of rat-heart mitochondria. Kinetics of the exchange reactions between 2-oxoglutarate, malate and malonate. Eur. J. Biochem. 25, 207.

— G. GOTTART, and C. LIÉBECQ, 1973: Mechanism of the exchanges catalyzed by the oxoglutarate translocator of rat heart mitochondria. Kinetics of the external product inhibition. Eur. J. Biochem. 32, 283.

SMITH, A. E., and K. A. MARCKER, 1968: N-formylmethionyl transfer RNA in mitochondria from yeast and rat liver. J. molec. Biol. 38, 241.

SO, A. G., and E. W. DAVIE, 1968: The incorporation of amino acids into protein in a cell-free system from yeast. Biochem. 2, 132.

SONE, N., E. FURUYA, and B. HAGIHARA, 1969: Purification and properties of mitochondria adenosine triphosphatase from yeast, Endomyces magnusii. J. Biochem. (Tokyo) 65, 935.

SORDAHL, L. A., Z. R. BLAILOCK, G. H. KRAFT, and A. SCHWARTZ, 1969: The possible relationship between ultrastructure and biochemical state of heart mitochondria. Arch. Biochem. Biophys. 132, 404.

SOTTOCASA, G. M., G. SANDRI, E. PANFILI, B. DE BERNARD, P. GAZZOTTI, F. D. VASINGTON, and E. CARAFOLI, 1972: Isolation of a soluble Ca^{2+} binding glycoprotein from ox liver mitochondria. Biochem. biophys. Res. Commun. 47, 808.

SOUTH, D. J., and H. R. MAHLER, 1968: RNA synthesis in yeast mitochondria, a derepressible activity. Nature 218, 1226.

SOUTHARD, J. H., and D. E. GREEN, 1974 a: High affinity binding of Ca^{++} in mitochondria: a reappraisal. Biochem. biophys. Res. Commun. 59, 30.

— — 1974 b: Control of the energy coupling modes in mitochondria by mercurials. Biochem. biophys. Res. Commun. 61, 1310.

— J. T. PENNINSTON, and D. E. GREEN, 1973: Induction of transmembrane proton transfer by mercurials in mitochondria. I. Ion movement accompanying transmembrane proton transfer. J. biol. Chem. 248, 3546.

— G. A. BLONDIN, and D. E. GREEN, 1974: Induction of transmembrane proton transfer by mercurials in mitochondria. II. Release of a Na^+/K^+ ionophore. J. biol. Chem. 249, 678.

SOUVERIJN, J. H. M., L. A. HUISMAN, J. ROSING, and A. KEMP, JR., 1973: Comparison of ADP and ATP as substrates for the adenine nucleotide translocator in rat liver mitochondria. Biochim. biophys. Acta 305, 183.

SOUZU, H., 1973: The phospholipid degradation and cellular death caused by freeze-thawing or freeze-drying of yeast. Cryobiology 10, 427.

STEINERT, M., 1969: The ultrastructure of mitochondria. Proc. roy. Soc. (London), Ser. B 173, 63.

STEVENS, B. J., J. J. CURGY, H. G. LEDOIGT, and J. ANDRÉ, 1974: Analysis of mitoribosomes from Tetrahymena by polyacrylamide gel electrophoresis and electron microscopy. In: The Biogenesis of Mitochondria. (KROON, A. M., and C. SACCONE, eds.), p. 327. New York-London: Academic Press.

STILES, J. W., J. T. WILSON, and F. L. CRANE, 1968: Membrane fibrils in cristae and grana. Biochim. biophys. Acta 162, 631.

STOFFEL, W., and H.-G. SCHIEFER, 1968: Biosynthesis and composition of phosphatides in outer and inner mitochondrial membranes. Hoppe-Seyler's Z. Physiol. Chem. 349, 1017.

STONER, C. D., and H. D. SIRAK, 1969: Passive induction of the "energized-twisted" conformational state in bovine heart mitochondria. Biochem. biophys. Res. Commun. 35, 59.

ŠUBÍK, J., Š. KUŽELA, J. KOLAROV, L. KOVÁČ, and T. M. LACHOWICZ, 1970: Oxidative phosphorylation in yeast. VI. ATPase activity and protein synthesis in mitochondria isolated from nuclear mutants deficient in cytochromes. Biochim. biophys. Acta 205, 513.

SUTTIE, J. W., 1962: The existence of two routes from incorporation of amino acids into protein of isolated rat-liver mitochondria. Biochem. J. 84, 382.

SUYAMA, Y., 1967: The origins of mitochondrial ribonucleic acids in Tetrahymena pyriformis. Biochem. 6, 2829.

— and J. EYER, 1968: Ribonucleic acid synthesis in isolated mitochondria from Tetrahymena. J. biol. Chem. 243, 320.

— and K. MIURA, 1968: Size and structural variation of mitochondrial DNA. Proc. nat. Acad. Sci. (U.S.) 60, 235.

SUZUKI, T., and F. K. MOSTOFI, 1967: Intramitochondrial filamentous bodies in the thick limb of Henle of the rat kidney. J. Cell Biol. 33, 605.

SVOBODA, D. J., and J. HIGGINSON, 1964: Ultrastructural changes produced by protein and related deficiencies in the rat liver. Amer. J. Pathol. 45, 353.

— and R. T. MANNING, 1964: Chronic alcoholism with fatty metamorphosis of the liver. Mitochondrial alterations in hepatic cells. Amer. J. Pathol. 44, 645.

TABAK, H. F., 1972: Ph. D. Thesis, Amsterdam.

TAKEHARA, I., and A. W. ROWE, 1971: Increase in ATPase activity in red cell membranes as a function of freezing regimen. Cryobiol. 8, 559.

TALEN, J. L., J. P. M. SANDERS, and R. A. FLAVELL, 1974: Genetic complexity of mitochondrial DNA from Euglena gracilis. Biochim. Biophys. Acta 374, 129.

TANDLER, B., and F. H. SHIPKEY, 1964: Ultrastructure of Warthin's Tumor. I. Mitochondria. J. Ultrastruct. Res. 11, 292.

TANI, E., T. AMETANI, N. HIGASHI, and E. FUJIHARA, 1971: Atypical cristae in mitochondria of human glioblastoma multiforme cells. J. Ultrastruct. Res. 36, 211.

TANIGUCHI, K., and R. L. POST, 1974: ATP synthesis and P_i-ATP exchange in guinea pig kidney, Na^+, K^+-ATPase. Fed. Proc. 33, 1289 Abstract.

TAYLOR, C. B., E. BAILEY, and W. BARTLEY, 1967: Studies on the biosynthesis of protein and lipid components of rat liver mitochondria. Biochem. J. 105, 605.

TEDESCHI, H., 1959: The structure of the mitochondrial membrane: inferences from permeability properties. J. Cell Biol. 6, 241.

— 1961: Osmotic reversal of mitochondrial swelling. Biochim. biophys. Acta 46, 159.

— 1965: Some observations on the permeability of mitochondria to sucrose. J Cell Biol. 25, 229.

— 1971 a: Are there electrochemical or mechanochemical coupling mechanisms in mitochondria? In: Energy transduction in respiration and photosynthesis. (QUAGLIARIELLO, E., S. PAPA, and C. S. ROSSI, eds.), p. 767. Bari: Adriatica Editrice.

— 1971 b: Mitochondrial compartments; a comparison of two models. Curr. Top. Membr. Transp. 2, 207.

— 1974: Mitochondrial membrane potential: evidence from studies with a fluorescent probe. Proc. nat. Acad. Sci. (U.S.) 71, 583.

— and D. L. HARRIS, 1955: The osmotic behavior and permeability to non-electrolytes of mitochondria. Arch. Biochem. Biophys. 58, 52.

— — 1958: Some observations on the photometric estimation of mitochondrial volume. Biochim. biophys. Acta 28, 392.

— and H. J. HEGARTY, 1965: Osmotic reversal of Ca^{2+}-induced mitochondrial swelling. Biochem. biophys. Res. Commun. 19, 558.

— — 1966: Some observations on the apparent shrinkage induced by Ca^{2+} on mitochondrial suspensions. Life Sci. 5, 1949.

— — and J. M. JAMES, 1965: Osmotic reversal of phosphate-induced mitochondrial swelling. Biochim. biophys. Acta 104, 612.

TELFER, A., and J. BARBER, 1974: Twofold effect of valinomycin on isolated spinach chloroplasts: uncoupling and inhibition of electron transport. Biochim. biophys. Acta **333**, 343.

TELFORD, J. N., and E. RACKER, 1973: A method of increasing contrast of mitochondrial inner membrane spheres in thin section of epon-araldite embedded tissues. J. Cell Biol. **57**, 580.

TEORELL, T., 1953: Transport processes and electrical phenomena in ionic membranes. Progr. in Biophys. molec. Biol. **3**, 305.

TER SCHEGGET, J., and P. BORST, 1971 a: DNA synthesis by isolated mitochondria. I. Effect of inhibitors and characterization of the product. Biochim. biophys. Acta **246**, 239.

— — 1971 b: DNA synthesis by isolated mitochondria. II. Detection of product DNA hydrogen-bonded to closed duplex circles. Biochim. biophys. Acta **246**, 249.

— H. VAN DEN BOSCH, M. A. VAN BAAK, K. Y. HOSTETLER, and P. BORST, 1971 a: The synthesis and utilization of dCDP-diglyceride by a mitochondrial fraction from rat liver. Biochim. biophys. Acta **239**, 234.

— R. A. FLAVELL, and P. BORST, 1971 b: DNA synthesis by isolated mitochondria. III. Characterization of d-loop DNA, a novel intermediate in mtDNA synthesis. Biochim. biophys. Acta **254**, 1.

TEWARI, J. P., S. K. MALHOTRA, and J. C. TU, 1971: A study of the structure of mitochondrial membranes by freeze-etch and freeze-fracture techniques. Cytobios **4**, 97.

— J. C. TU, and S. K. MALHOTRA, 1972: Structure of the mitochondria of *Neurospora crassa* as revealed by thin sectioning and freeze-etch techniques. Cytobios **5**, 261.

— J. JAYARAMAN, and H. R. MAHLER, 1965: Separation and characterization of mitochondrial DNA from yeast. Biochem. biophys. Res. Commun. **21**, 141.

THAYER, W. S., and P. C. HINKLE, 1973: Stoichiometry of adenosine triphosphate-driven proton translocation in bovine heart submitochondrial particles. J. biol. Chem. **248**, 5395.

THE, R., and W. HASSELBACH, 1972: The modification of the reconstituted sarcoplasmic ATPase by monovalent cations. Eur. J. Biochem. **30**, 318.

THOMAS, D. Y., and D. WILKIE, 1968: Inhibition of mitochondrial synthesis in yeast by erythromycin: cytoplasmic and nuclear factors controlling resistance. Gen. Res. **11**, 33.

— and D. H. WILLIAMSON, 1971: Products of mitochondrial protein synthesis in yeast. Nature N.B. **233**, 196.

THOMAS, R. S., and J. W. GREENAWALT, 1968: Microincineration, electron microscopy, and electron diffraction of calcium phosphate-loaded mitochondria. J. Cell Biol. **39**, 55.

THOMPSON, J. E., R. COLEMAN, and J. B. FINEAN, 1968: Comparative X-ray diffraction and electron microscope studies of isolated mitochondrial membranes. Biochem. biophys. Acta **150**, 405.

THOMPSON, T. E., and B. D. MCLEES, 1961: An electrophoretic study of suspensions of intact mitochondria and fragments of mitochondrial membranes. Biochim. biophys. Acta **50**, 213.

TILLACK, T. W., and V. T. MARCHESI, 1970: Demonstration of the outer surface of freeze-etched red blood cell membranes. J. Cell Biol. **45**, 649.

TINBERG, H. M., R. L. MELNICK, J. MAGUIRE, and L. PACKER, 1974: Studies on mitochondrial proteins. II. Localization of components of the inner mitochondrial membrane: labeling with diazobenzene-sulfonate, a non-penetrating probe. Biochim. biophys. Acta **345**, 118.

TRUMAN, D. E. S., and A. KORNER, 1962: Incorporation of amino acids into the protein of isolated mitochondria. A search for optimum conditions and a relationship to oxidative phosphorylation. Biochem. J. **83**, 588.

TSUDZUKI, T., and D. F. WILSON, 1971: The oxidation-reduction potential of the hemes and copper of cytochrome oxidase from beef heart. Arch. Biochem. Biophys. **145**, 149.

TUPPER, J. T., and H. TEDESCHI, 1967: Observations on low amplitude Ca^{2+} induced swelling in mitochondria. Life Sci. **6**, 2021.

— — 1969 a: Microelectrode studies of the membrane properties of isolated mitochondria. Proc. nat. Acad. Sci. (U.S.) **63**, 370.

— — 1969 b: Microelectrode studies on the membrane properties of isolated mitochondria. II. Absence of a metabolic dependence. Proc. nat. Acad. Sci. (U.S.) **63**, 713.

TUPPER, J. T., and H. TEDESCHI, 1969 c: Mitochondrial potentials measured with micro-electrodes: probable ionic basis. Science **166**, 1539.

TYLER, D. D., 1968: The inhibition of phosphate entry in rat liver mitochondria by organic mercurials and by formaldehyde. Biochem. J. **107**, 121.

TZAGOLOFF, A., 1969: Assembly of the mitochondrial membrane system. II. Synthesis of the mitochondrial adenosine triphosphatase, F_1. J. biol. Chem. **244**, 5027.

— 1970: Assembly of mitochondrial membrane system. III. Function and synthesis of oligomycin sensitivity-conferring protein of yeast mitochondria. J. biol. Chem. **245** 1545.

— 1971 a: Structure and biosynthesis of the membrane adenosine triphosphatase of mito-chondria. Curr. Top. Membr. Transp. **2**, 157.

— 1971 b: Assembly of the mitochondrial membrane system. IV. Role of mitochondrial and cytoplasmic protein synthesis in the biosynthesis of the rutamycin-sensitive adenosine triphosphatase. J. biol. Chem. **246**, 3050.

— 1972: A model of membrane biogenesis. J. Bioenerg. **3**, 39.

— 1974: Assembly of inner membrane complexes. Ann. N.Y. Acad. Sci. **227**, 521.

— and A. AKAI, 1972: Assembly of the mitochondrial membrane system. VIII. Properties of the products of mitochondrial protein synthesis in yeast. J. biol. Chem. **247**, 6517.

— and P. MEAGHER, 1971: Assembly of mitochondrial membrane system. V. Properties of a dispersed preparation of the rutamycin-sensitive adenosine triphosphatase of yeast mitochondria. J. biol. Chem. **246**, 7328.

— — 1972: Assembly of mitochondrial membrane system. VI. Mitochondrial synthesis of subunit proteins of the rutamycin-sensitive adenosine triphosphate. J. biol. Chem. **247**, 594.

— K. H. BYINGTON, and D. H. MacLENNAN, 1968 a: Studies on mitochondrial adenosine triphosphatase system. II. The isolation of an oligomycin-sensitive adenosine triphos-phatase from bovine heart mitochondria. J. biol. Chem. **243**, 2405.

— D. H. MacLENNAN, and K. H. BYINGTON, 1968 b: Studies on the mitochondrial adenosine triphosphatase system. III. Isolation from the oligomycin-sensitive adenosine triphosphatase complex of the factors which bind F_1 and determine oligomycin sen-sitivity of bound F_1. Biochem. **7**, 1596.

— A. AKAI, and M. F. SIERRA, 1972: Assembly of the mitochondrial membrane system: VII. Synthesis and integration of F_1 subunits into the rutamycin-sensitive adenosine triphosphate. J. biol. Chem. **247**, 6511.

— M. S. RUBIN, and M. F. SIERRA, 1973: Biosynthesis of mitochondrial enzymes. Biochim. biophys. Acta **301**, 71.

— A. AKAI, and M. S. RUBIN, 1974: Mitochondrial products of yeast ATPase and cyto-chrome oxidase. In: The biogenesis of mitochondria. (KROON, A. M., and C. SACCONE, eds.), p. 405. New York-London: Academic Press.

ULRICH, F., 1959: Ion transport by heart and skeletal muscle mitochondria. Amer. J. Physiol. **197**, 997.

UPHOLT, W. B., and P. BORST, 1974: Accumulation of replicative intermediates of mito-chondrial DNA in *Tetrahymena pyriformis* grown in ethidium bromide. J. Cell Biol. **61**, 383.

URBAN, P. F., and M. KLINGENBERG, 1969: On the redox potentials of ubiquinone and cytochrome *b* in the respiratory chain. Eur. J. Biochem. **9**, 519.

URRY, D. W., 1972: Conformation of protein in biological membranes and a model trans-membrane channel. Ann. N.Y. Acad. Sci. **195**, 108.

UTUSUMI, K., and L. PACKER, 1967: Oscillatory states of mitochondria. II. Factors con-trolling period and amplitude. Arch. Biochem. Biophys. **120**, 404.

VAARTJES, W. J., A. KEMP, JR., J. H. M. SOUVERIJN, and S. G. VAN DEN BERGH, 1972: Inhibition by fatty acyl esters of adenine nucleotide translocation in rat liver mitochondria. FEBS Lett. **23**, 303.

VAIL, W. J., and R. K. RILEY, 1971: Ultrastructure of isolated heavy beef heart mito-chondria revealed by the freeze-etching technique. Nature **231**, 525.

— — and C. H. WILLIAMS, 1972: The morphology and configurational states of isolated heavy beef heart mitochondria by the freeze fracture technique. J. Bioenerg. **3**, 467.

VAIL, W. J., D. PAPAHADJOPOULOS, and M. A. MOSCARELLO, 1974: Interaction of a hydrophobic protein with liposomes: evidence for particles seen in freeze fracture as being proteins. Biochim. biophys. Acta **345**, 463.

VALENTINE, R. C., and R. W. HORNE, 1962: An assessment of negative staining techniques for revealing ultrastructure. In: Interpretation of ultrastructure. (HARRIS, R. J. C., ed.), p. 263. New York-London: Academic Press.

VAN BRUGGEN, E. F. G., P. BORST, G. J. C. M. RUTTENBERG, M. GRUBER, and A. M. KROON, 1966: Circular mitochondrial DNA. Biochim. biophys. Acta **119**, 437.

VAN BUUREN, K. J. H., and G. J. A. SCHILDER, 1973: Inhibition of cytochrome c oxidase by cyanide. Ninth International Congress of Biochemistry, Abstracts, p. 216.

VAN DE STADT, R. J., B. L. DE BOER, and K. VAN DAM, 1973: The interaction between the mitochondrial ATPase (F_1) and the ATPase inhibitor. Biochim. biophys. Acta **292**, 338.

VAN GELDER, B. F., and H. BEINERT, 1969: Studies on the heme components of cytochrome c oxidase by e.p.r. spectroscopy. Biochim. biophys. Acta **189**, 1.

— and R. H. TIESJEMA, 1973: Reductive titrations of cytochrome c oxidase followed by CD measurements. Ninth International Congress of Biochemistry, Abstracts, p. 216.

VAN ZUTPHEN, H., A. J. MEROLA, G. P. BRIERLEY, and D. G. CORNWELL, 1972: The interaction of non-ionic detergents with lipid bilayer membranes. Arch. Biochem. Biophys. **152**, 755.

VANNESTE, W. H., 1966: Molecular proportion of the fixed cytochromes of the respiratory chain components of Keilin-Hartree particles and beef heart mitochondria. Biochim. biophys. Acta **113**, 175.

VASINGTON, F. D., and J. W. GREENAWALT, 1968: Osmotically lysed rat liver mitochondria. Biochemical and ultrastructural properties in relation to massive ion accumulation. J. Cell Biol. **39**, 661.

— and J. V. MURPHY, 1962: Ca^{2+} uptake by rat liver mitochondria and its dependence on respiration and phosphorylation. J. biol. Chem. **237**, 2670.

— P. GAZZOTTI, R. TIOZZO, and E. CARAFOLI, 1972: The effect of ruthenium red on Ca^{2+} transport and respiration in rat liver mitochondria. Biochim. biophys. Acta **256**, 43.

VELDSEMA-CURRIE, R. D., and E. C. SLATER, 1970: The kinetics of changes in redox states of ubiquinone on the transition from state 4 to state 3 in rat-liver mitochondria. Biochim. biophys. Acta **197**, 113.

VERDOUX, H., and R. M. BERTINA, 1974: Affinities of ATP for the dinitrophenol induced ATPase. Biochim. biophys. Acta **325**, 385.

VERMA, I. M., M. EDELMAN, M. HERZBER, and U. Z. LITTAUER, 1970: Size determination of mitochondrial ribosomal RNA from *Aspergillus nidulans* by electron microscopy. J. molec. Biol. **52**, 137.

— — and U. Z. LITTAUER, 1971: A comparison of nucleotide sequences from mitochondrial and cytoplasmic ribosomal RNA of *Aspergillus nidulans*. Eur. J. Biochem. **19**, 124.

VIGNAIS, P. M., and P. V. VIGNAIS, 1973: Fuscin, in inhibitor of mitochondrial SH-dependent transport-linked functions. Biochim. biophys. Acta **325**, 357.

VIGNAIS, P. V., and P. M. VIGNAIS, 1972: Effect of SH reagents on atractyloside binding to mitochondria and ADP translocation Potentiation by ADP and its prevention by the uncoupler FCCP. FEBS Lett. **26**, 27.

— — C. S. ROSSI, and A. L. LEHNINGER, 1963: Restoration of ATP-induced contraction of pretreated mitochondria by "contractile protein". Biochem. biophys. Res. Commun. **11**, 307.

— — and G. DEFAYE, 1971: Gummiferin, an inhibitor of the adenine-nucleotide translocator. Studies of its binding properties to mitochondria. FEBS Lett. **17**, 281.

— B. J. STEVENS, J. HUET, and J. ANDRÉ, 1972: Mitoribosomes from *Candida utilis*. Morphological, physical, and chemical characterization of the monomer form and of its subunits. J. Cell Biol. **54**, 468.

— P. M. VIGNAIS, G. LAUQUIN, and F. MOREL, 1973: Binding of adenosine-diphosphate and of antagonist ligands to mitochondrial ADP carrier. Biochim. **55**, 763.

— — and G. DEFAYE, 1973: Adenosine diphosphate translocation in mitochondria. Nature of the receptor site for carboxyatractyloside (gummiferin). Biochem. **12**, 1508.

VINOGRADOV, A., and A. SCARPA, 1973: The initial velocities of calcium uptake by rat liver mitochondria. J. Biol. Chem. **248**, 5527.

VOGELL, W., 1963: Struktur und funktionelle Biochemie der Mitochondrien. I. Die Morphologie der Mitochondrien. In: Funktionelle und morphologische Organisation der Zelle. (KARLSON, P., ed.), p. 55—67. Berlin-Göttingen-Heidelberg: Springer-Verlag.

VON HUNGEN, K., H. R. MAHLER, and W. J. MOORE, 1968: Protein and RNA turnover in synaptic subcellular fractions from rat brain. J. biol. Chem. **243**, 1415.

VON JAGOW, G., and M. KLINGENBERG, 1970: Pathways of hydrogen in mitochondria of *Saccharomyces carlbergensis*. Eur. J. Biochem. **12**, 583.

— 1972: Close correlation between antimycin titer and cytochrome b_{T} content in mitochondria of chloramphenicol treated *Neurospora crassa*. FEBS Lett. **24**, 278.

— H. WEISS, and M. KLINGENBERG, 1973: Comparison of respiratory chain of *Neurospora crassa* wild-type and mimutants MI-1 and MI-3. Eur. J. Biochem. **33**, 140.

WAGNER, R. P., and H. K. MITCHELL, 1955: Genetics and metabolism. New York: Wiley and Sons.

WARD, R. T., 1962: The origin of protein and fatty yolk in *Rana pipiens*. J. Cell Biol. **14**, 309.

WARTIOVAARA, J., and D. BRANTON, 1970: Visualization of ribosomes by freeze-etching. Exp. Cell Res. **61**, 403.

WARREN, G. B., P. A. TOON, N. J. M. BIRDSALL, A. G. LEE, and J. C. METCALFE, 1974: Reconstitution of a calcium pump using defined membrane components. Proc. nat. Acad. Sci. (U.S.) **71**, 622.

WATSON, K., 1972: The organization of ribosomal granules within mitochondrial structures of aerobic and anaerobic cells of *Saccharomyces cerevisiae*. J. Cell Biol. **55**, 721.

WEBER, A. F., E. A. USENIK, and S. C. WHIPP, 1962: Experimental production of electron dense intramatrical bodies in calves' adrenal zona glomerulosa cells. 5th Congress of Electron Microscopy **2**, YY7.

WEBER, K., and M. OSBORN, 1969: The reliability of molecular weight determinations by dodecyl sulfate polyacrylamide gel electrophoresis. J. biol. Chem. **244**, 4406.

WEBER, N. E., and P. V. BLAIR, 1969: Ultrastructural studies of beef heart mitochondria. I. Effects of adenosine diphosphate in mitochondrial morphology. Biochem. biophys. Res. Commun. **36**, 987.

WEGDAM, H. J., J. A. BERDEN, and E. C. SLATER, 1970: High-energy forms of cytochrome *b*. II. The effect of ATP and antimycin on cytochrome *b* in intact mitochondria. Biochim. biophys. Acta **223**, 365.

WEIDMANN, M. J., H. ERDELT, and M. KLINGENBERG, 1969: Elucidation of a carrier site for adenine nucleotide translocation in mitochondria with the help of attractyloside. In: Inhibitors, tools in cell research. (BUCHER, T. H., and H. SIES, eds.), p. 324. New York-Heidelberg-Berlin: Springer-Verlag.

WEINBACH, E. C., and J. GARBUS, 1965: The interaction of uncoupling phenols with mitochondria and with mitochondrial protein. J. biol. Chem. **240**, 1811.

— — and H. G. SHEFFIELD, 1967: Morphology of mitochondria in the coupled, uncoupled and recoupled state. Exp. Cell Res. **46**, 129.

WEISLOGEL, P. O., and R. A. BUTOW, 1971: The fate of mitochondrial membrane proteins and mitochondrial deoxyribonucleic acid during petite induction. J. biol. Chem. **246**, 5113.

WEISS, H., 1972: Cytochrome *b* in *Neurospora crassa* mitochondria. A membrane protein containing subunits of cytoplasmic and mitochondrial origin. Eur. J. Biochem. **30**, 469.

— and TH. BÜCHER, 1970: Chromatographic separation of membrane proteins on lipophilic ion exchange resins. The influence of various resin-linked aliphatic chains. Eur. J. Biochem. **17**, 561.

— and B. ZIGANKE, 1974 a: Cytochrome *b* in *Neurospora crassa* mitochondria-site of translation of the heme protein. Eur. J. Biochem. **41**, 63.

— — 1974 b: Biogenesis of cytochrome *b* in *Neurospora crassa*. In: The biogenesis of mitochondria. (KROON, A. M., and C. SACCONE, eds.), p. 491. New York-London: Academic Press.

WEISS, H., W. SEBALD, and T. BÜCHER, 1971: Cycloheximide resistant incorporation of amino acids into a polypeptide of the cytochrome oxidase of *Neurospora crassa*. Eur. J. Biochem. **22**, 19.

— B. LORENZ, and W. KLINOW, 1972: Contribution of mitochondrial protein synthesis to the formation of cytochrome oxidase in *Locusta migratoria*. FEBS Lett. **25**, 49.

WERKHEISER, W. C., and W. BARTLEY, 1957: The study of steady-state concentration of internal solutes of mitochondria by rapid centrifugal transfer to a fixation medium. Biochem. J. **66**, 79.

WERNER, S., 1974 a: Isolation and characterization of a mitochondrially synthesized precursor protein of cytochrome oxidase. Eur. J. Biochem. **43**, 39.

— 1974 b: Antibodies to subunits of cytochrome *c* oxidase and their relation to precursor proteins of the enzyme. In: The biogenesis of mitochondria. (KROON, A. M., and C. SACCONE, eds.), p. 505. New York-London: Academic Press.

WEST, D. W., J. F. A. CHASE, and P. K. TUBBS, 1972: The separation and properties of two forms of carnitine palmitoyltransferase from ox liver mitochondria. Biochem. biophys. Res. Commun. **42**, 912.

WESTERGAARD, O., and B. LINDBERG, 1972: An induced mitochondrial DNA polymerase from *Tetrahymena*. Eur. J. Biochem. **28**, 422.

— K. A. MARCKER, and J. KELDING, 1970: Induction of a mitochondrial DNA polymerase in *Tetrahymena*. Nature **227**, 708.

WHEELDON, L. W., and A. L. LEHNINGER, 1966: Energy-linked synthesis and decay of membrane protein in isolated rat liver mitochondria. Biochem. **5**, 3533.

— A.-C. DIANOUX, M. BOF, and P. V. VIGNAIS, 1974: Stable and labile products of mitochondrial protein synthesis *in vitro*. Eur. J. Biochem. **46**, 189.

WIKSTRÖM, M. K. F., 1971 a: Inhibition of oxidative phosphorylation by hydroxylamine in sonicated particles from beef-heart mitochondria. Biochim. biophys. Acta **234**, 16.

— 1971 b: Properties of three cytochrome *b*-like species in mitochondria and submitochondrial particles. Biochim. biophys. Acta **253**, 332.

— 1971 c: Effect of ^2H_2O on energy dependent oxidoreduction of cytochrome *b*. Biochim. biophys. Acta **245**, 512.

— 1973: The different cytochrome *b* compenents in the respiratory chain of animal mitochondria and their role in electron transport and energy conservation. Biochim. biophys. Acta **301**, 155.

— and J. A. BERDEN, 1973: On the behavior of cytochrome *b* in the energized mitochondrial membrane. In: Mechanisms in bioenergetics. (AZZONE, G. F., L. ERNSTER, S. PAPA, E. QUAGLIARIELLO, and N. SILIPRANDI, eds.), p. 545. New York-London: Academic Press.

— and N. E. L. SARIS, 1970: The reversal of electron transfer across the terminal energy-conservation site. In: Electron transport and energy conservation. (TAGER, J. M., S. PAPA, E. QUAGLIARIELLO, and E. C. SLATER, eds.), p. 77. Bari: Adriatica Editrice.

WILKIE, D., G. SAUNDERS, and A. W. LINNANE, 1967: Inhibition of respiratory enzyme synthesis in yeast by chloramphenicol: Relationship between chloramphenicol tolerance and resistance to other anti-bacterial antibiotics. Gen. Res. **10**, 199.

WILLIAMS, M. A., 1967: More intramitochondrial bodies. J. Cell Biol. **35**, 730.

WILLIAMS, R. J. P., 1961: Possible functions of chains of catalysts. J. theor. Biol. **1**, 1.

— 1969: Electron transfer and energy conservation. Curr. Top in Bioenerg. **3**, 80.

— 1972: An analytical appraisal of energy transduction mechanisms. J. Bioenerg. **3**, 81.

— 1974: The separation of electrons and protons during electron transfer: the distinction between membrane potentials and transmembrane gradients. Ann. N.Y. Acad. Sci. **227**, 98.

WILLS, E. J., 1965: Crystalline structures in mitochondria of normal human liver parenchymal cells. J. Cell Biol. **24**, 511.

WILSON, D. F., and P. L. DUTTON, 1970 a: The oxidation-reduction potentials of cytochromes *a* and a_3 in intact rat liver mitochondria. Arch. Biochem. Biophys. **136**, 583.

— — 1970 b: Energy dependent changes in the oxidation-reduction potential of cytochrome *b*. Biochem. biophys. Res. Commun. **39**, 59.

WILSON, D. F., M. KOPPELMAN, M. ERECIŃSKA, and P. L. DUTTON, 1971 a: Energy conservation in detergent-treated mitochondria and purified succinate-cytochrome c reductase. Biochem. biophys. Res. Commun. **44**, 759.

— H. P. TING, and M. S. KOPPELMAN, 1971 b: Mechanism of action of uncouplers of oxidative phosphorylation. Biochem. **10**, 2897.

— M. ERECIŃSKA, J. S. LEIGH, JR., and M. KOPPELMAN, 1972 a: The properties of the mitochondrial succinate-cytochrome c reductase. Arch. Biochem. Biophys. **151**, 112.

— — and P. NICHOLLS, 1972 b: An energy-dependent transformation of a ferrocytochrome of the mitochondrial respiratory chain. FEBS Lett. **20**, 61.

— P. L. DUTTON, M. ERECIŃSKA, J. G. LINDSAY, and N. SATO, 1972 c: Mitochondrial electron transport and energy conservation. Accounts Chem. Res. **5**, 234.

— J. G. LINDSAY, and E. S. BROCKLEHURST, 1972 d: Heme-heme interaction in cytochrome oxidase. Biochim. biophys. Acta **256**, 277.

— P. L. DUTTON, and M. WAGNER, 1973: Energy transducing components of mitochondria respiration. Curr. Top. in Bioenerg. **5**, 233.

WINTERSBERGER, E., 1964: DNA-abhängige RNA-Synthese in Rattenlebermitochondrien. Hoppe Seyler's Z. physiol. Chem. **336**, 285.

— 1965: Proteinsynthese in isolierten Hefemitochondrien. Biochem. Z. **341**, 409.

— 1966: Synthesis and function of mitochondrial ribonucleic acid. In: Regulation of metabolic processes in mitochondria. (TAGER, J. M., S. PAPA, E. QUAGLIARIELLO, and E. C. SLATER, eds.), p. 439. Amsterdam-London-New York: Elsevier Publishing Co.

— 1967: A distinct class of ribosomal RNA components in yeast mitochondria as revealed by gradient centrifugation and by DNA-RNA-hybridization. Hoppe Seyler's Z. physiol. Chem. **348**, 1701.

— 1972: Synthesis of mitochondrial RNA. Fed. Eur. Biochem. Soc., Eighth Meeting, Amsterdam, p. 21. Amsterdam-London: North-Holland/American Elsevier.

— und H. TUPPY, 1965: DNA-abhängige RNA-Synthese in isolierten Hefemitochondrien. Biochem. Z. **341**, 399.

— and G. VIEHHAUSER, 1968: Function of mitochondrial DNA in yeast. Nature **220**, 699.

WIRTZ, K. W. A., and D. B. ZILVERSMIT, 1968: Exchange of phospholipids between liver mitochondria and microsomes in vitro. J. Biol. Chem. **243**, 3596.

— — 1970: Partial purification of phospholipid exchange protein from beef heart. FEBS Lett. **7**, 44.

— H. H. KAMP, and L. L. VAN DEENEN, 1972: Isolation of a protein from beef liver which specifically stimulates the exchange of phosphatidylcholine. Biochim. biophys. Acta **274**, 606.

WITT, H. T., 1971: Coupling of quanta, electrons, fields, ions, and phosphorylation in the functional membrane of photosynthesis. Results by pulse spectroscopic methods. Quart. Rev. Biophys. **4**, 365.

— and A. ZICKLER, 1973: Electrical evidence for the field indicating absorption change in bioenergetics of membranes. FEBS Lett. **37**, 307.

— — 1974: Vectorial electron flow across the thylakoid membrane. Further evidence by kinetic measurements with an electrochromic and electrical method. FEBS Lett. **39**, 205.

WOLSTENHOLME, D. R., K. KOIKE, and P. COCHRAN-FOUTS, 1973 a: Single strand containing replicating molecules of circular mitochondrial DNA. J. Cell Biol. **56**, 230.

— — — 1973 b: Replication of mitochondrial DNA: Replicative forms of molecules from rat tissues and evidence for discontinuous replication. Cold Spring Harbor Symp. on Quant. Biol. **38**, 267.

WOOD, D. D., and D. J. L. LUCK, 1969: Hybridization of mitochondrial ribosomal RNA. J. molec. Biol. **41**, 211.

WOZNIAK, M., D. CIESIELSKI, J. BOPINIGIS, and M. ŻYDOWO, 1973: Biocarbonate transport through mitochondrial membrane. Phys. Chem. **5**, 237.

WRIGGLESWORTH, J. M., L. PACKER, and D. BRANTON, 1970: Organization of mitochondrial structure as revealed by freeze-etching. Biochim. biophys. Acta **205**, 125.

WU, M., N. DAVIDSON, G. ATTARDI, and Y. ALONI, 1972: Expression of the mitochondrial genome in HeLa cells. XIV. The relative positions of the 4 S RNA genes and of the ribosomal RNA genes in mitochondrial DNA. J. molec. Biol. **71**, 81.

YAMADA, E., 1965: Gunma Symp. Endocrinol. (Maebashi) **2**, 1.

YAMADA, S., and Y. TONOMURA, 1972: Phosphorylation of the Ca^{2+}-Mg^{2+}-dependent ATPase of the sarcoplasmic reticulum coupled with cation translocation. J. Biochem. **71**, 1101.

— M. SUMIDA, and Y. TONOMURA, 1972: Reaction mechanism of the Ca^{2+}-dependent ATPase of sarcoplasmic reticulum from skeletal muscle. VIII. Molecular mechanism of the conversion of osmotic energy to chemical energy in the sarcoplasmic reticulum. J. Biochem. **72**, 1537.

YAMASHINA, I., K. IZUMI, H. OKAWA, and E. FURUYA, 1965: Hexosamine and sialic acid in mitochondria and microsomes from rabbit liver. J. Biochem. **58**, 538.

YEATES, R. A., 1974: Interaction of beef-heart mitochondrial ATPase, coupling factor F_1 with aurovertin. Biochim. biophys. Acta **333**, 173.

YOUNG, J. H., G. A. BLONDIN, and D. E. GREEN, 1971: Conformational model of active transport, role of protons. Proc. nat. Acad. Sci. (U.S.) **68**, 1364.

YU, C. A., L. YU, and T. E. KING, 1972: Spectral evidence of multiple cytochrome *b* present in succinate-cytochrome *c* reductase. Biochim. biophys. Acta **267**, 300.

ZAAR, K., 1974: Mitochondrial inner membrane particles seen in sections of *in situ* large amplitude swollen mitochondria in rhizodermal cells of cress (*Lepidium sativum* L.). J. Bioenerg. **6**, 57.

ZIEGLER, D. M., and K. A. DOEG, 1962: Studies on the electron transport system. XLIII. The isolation of succinic-coenzyme Q reductase from beef heart mitochondria. Arch. Biochem. Biophys. **97**, 41.

ZUCKERMAN, B. M., M. KISIEL, and S. HIMMELHOCH, 1973: Unusual mitochondrial cristae in the vinegar eelworm. J. Cell Biol. **58**, 476.

ZUDUNAISKY, J. A., J. F. GENNARO, JR., N. BAHIRELAHI, and M. HILTON, 1968: Intracellular redistribution of sodium and calcium during stimulation of sodium transport in epithelial cells. J. Gen. Phys. **51**, 290s.

ZYLBER, E. A., S. PERLMAN, and S. PENMAN, 1971: Mitochondrial RNA turnover in the presence of cordycepin. Biochim. biophys. Acta **240**, 588.

Subject Index